THE CRISIS OF US HOSPICE CARE

THE CRISIS OF US HOSPICE CARE

Family and Freedom at the End of Life

HAROLD BRASWELL

JOHNS HOPKINS UNIVERSITY PRESS, BALTIMORE

Johns Hopkins University Press
2715 North Charles Street
Baltimore, Maryland 21218-4363
www.press.jhu.edu

Library of Congress Cataloging-in-Publication Data

Names: Braswell, Harold, 1981– author.
Title: The Crisis of US Hospice Care : Family and Freedom at the End
    of Life / Harold Braswell.
Description: Baltimore : Johns Hopkins University Press, 2019. |
    Includes bibliographical references and index.
Identifiers: LCCN 2018048619 | ISBN 9781421429823 (hardcover : alk.
    paper) | ISBN 9781421429830 (electronic) | ISBN 1421429829 (hard-
    cover : alk. paper) | ISBN 1421429837 (electronic)
Subjects: | MESH: Hospice Care—ethics | Hospice Care—history |
    Right to Die | History, 20th Century
Classification: LCC R726 | NLM WB 310 | DDC 179.7—dc23
LC record available at https://lccn.loc.gov/2018048619

A catalog record for this book is available from the British Library.

*Special discounts are available for bulk purchases of this book. For more
information, please contact Special Sales at 410-516-6936 or specialsales
@press.jhu.edu.*

Johns Hopkins University Press uses environmentally friendly book
materials, including recycled text paper that is composed of at least 30
percent post-consumer waste, whenever possible.

To Nikki, Stella, and Augie

CONTENTS

ACKNOWLEDGMENTS

I could not have written this book without the support of two institutions that value interdisciplinary scholarship. The first is Emory University's Graduate Institute for the Liberal Arts (ILA), where I obtained my PhD. The second is Saint Louis University's Albert Gnaegi Center for Health Care Ethics, where I currently work.

At Emory, I benefited most from the guidance of my dissertation committee: Gary Belkin, who generously offered to serve as an external reader; Chikako Ozawa-de Silva, who taught me medical anthropology—and also taught me to love it; Rosemarie Garland-Thomson, who has been a mentor, supporter, and friend since before I arrived at Emory; and my advisor, Howard I. Kushner, who taught me how to be a teacher, a scholar, and a dissertation advisor.

There were many other faculty members who helped me at Emory: Angelika Bammer, Kevin Corrigan, Kirk Elifson, Martha Fineman, Sander Gilman, Elizabeth Goodstein, Anna Grimshaw, Lynne Huffer, Ivan Karp, Corrie Kratz, Michael Moon, Robert Paul, Mark Risjord, Deboleena Roy, Ani Satz, Michael Sullivan, Colin Talley, Peter Wakefield, and Kimberly Wallace-Sanders. My fellow graduate students at the ILA provided a rich network of intellectual and emotional support. I am particularly grateful to the students who were colleagues of mine in studying the applied history of medicine: Claire Clark, Melissa Creary, Mary Horton, Leslie Leighton, and Jennifer Sarrett.

Long before I came to Saint Louis University, I benefited from the generosity of Jeffrey Bishop. And since my arrival at SLU, Jeff has been an incredible mentor and a great friend. I am similarly indebted to my colleagues at the Gnaegi Center: Jill Burkemper, Stephanie Solomon Cargill, Kelly Dineen, Jason Eberl, Jason Keune, Kimbell Kornu, Elizabeth Quiros, Erica Salter, Griffin Trotter, and Tobias Winwright. Adrienne McCarthy has been tremendously helpful. I have also benefited from the generosity of colleagues throughout the university. Of particular note are the members of the Ethnographic Workshop: Elizabeth Chiarello, Amy Cooper, Terra Edwards, Monica Eppinger, Bruce O'Neill, and Christopher Prener. I would also highlight the members of the Center for Health Law Studies, particularly Robert Gatter, Jesse Goldner, Sandra Johnson, Elizabeth Pendo,

Amy Sanders, Sidney Watson, and Ruqaiijah Yearby. Darcy Scharff at the College for Public Health and Social Justice has also been very generous in supporting my work.

I thank my students at Emory and SLU, who have helped me to develop my ideas at every stage of this project. In particular I thank my TAs, who saved me a lot of time: Kathrine Bendsten, Brandy Fox, Catherine Gale, Melissa Porterhouse, Clare (Mauri) Puttmann, and Karen Rieffel. Most deserving of thanks is Jaime Konerman-Sease, who was my research assistant throughout much of this work.

I have participated in five academic organizations over the past decade: the American Society for Bioethics and Humanities, the American Association for the History of Medicine, the Society for Disability Studies, the Conference on Medicine and Religion, and the International Academy for Bioethical Inquiry. I thank the administrators of these groups for their work in creating such stimulating environments for intellectual exchange.

Among the academic colleagues whom I have met through these organizations, I am particularly grateful to two fellow historians of American end-of-life care: Emily Abel and Carla Keirns. I also thank other colleagues whose insight and support have been of great benefit: Rachel Adams, Alex Alexander, Rachelle Barina, Gil Ben-Herut, Liat Ben-Moshe, Gaymon Bennett, Pat Blanchfield, Teresa Blankmeyer Burke, Cindy Cain, Steve Campbell, Allison Carey, Mel Chen, Merlin Chowkwanyun, James Crowe, Brooke Dodson-Lavelle, Jim DuBois, Jacalyn Duffin, April Dworetz, Elaine Eisenbaum, Celia Feinstein, Jim Ferris, Kate Fialkowski, Michele Friedner, Kelly Fritsch, Phil Fung, Joe Gabriel, Rebecca Garden, Daniel Goldberg, Jeremy Greene, Lauren Guilmette, Kristina Gupta, Jasmine Harris, Cassandra Hartblay, Haim Hazan, Alvan Ikoku, Adria Imada, Douglas Kidd, Eunjung Kim, Priya Lalvani, Erin Lamb, Shai Lavi, Armando Mastrogiovanni, Simon May, Adam Newman, Kim Nielsen, Abraham Nussbaum, William Peace, Govind Persad, Margaret Price, Nic John Ramos, James Redfield, Alison Reiheld, Benjamin Reiss, Lizzie Reiss, Mike Rembis, Tarris Rosell, Paul Scherz, Jennifer Scuro, David Serlin, Lisa Sonnenborn, Devan Stahl, Joseph Stramondo, Sandra Sufian, Sunaura Taylor, Sara van den Berg, Amy Vidali, Jillian Weise, Jacqueline Wolf, Michelle Wolf, Megan Wright, Jarret Zigon, and Laurie Zoloth. I apologize to anyone whom I have inadvertently left off this list.

Several institutions invited me to present on the research that makes up this book. I thank Bentley University, the Gateway End-of-Life Coalition, Johns Hopkins University, the University of Kansas Medical Center, and the long-term care ombudsman organization VOYCE. I am very grateful to the individuals who organized these events: Joan Bretthauer, Cynthia Clark, Christopher Crenner, Mary

Lynn Faunda Donovan, Ryan Fagan, Chien Hung, Jeffrey Kahn, Carla Keirns, Kavitha Lakshmanan, Lindy Landzaat, Allison Netson, Kristen Nill, Sharon Orlet, Karin Porter-Williamson, Lisa Smith, Tracie Ugamoto, and Cara Wallace.

This book has been immeasurably aided by my engagement with psychoanalysis. I will always be grateful to Sander Gilman who, in his capacity as the head of Emory's Psychoanalytic Studies Program, provided funding for me and other doctoral students to complete coursework at Emory's Psychoanalytic Institute. I am grateful to my professors at the institute and to the other students in my cohort. The Saint Louis Psychoanalytic Institute has been a second home since my arrival in this city. I am particularly grateful to Cathy Krane for her hospitality.

The American Psychoanalytic Association's fellowship program has been tremendously helpful . I am grateful to the fellowship committee for selecting me and to Fran Arnold, Melinda Gellman, and Lynne Zeavin in particular. I also thank Keri Brenner and Al Marguiles for commenting on my work; Stephanie Brody and David Buxton for encouraging me in studying the end of life; and Moisy Shopper for being a generous and insightful mentor. I am most grateful to the other fellows who celebrated with me the news of this manuscript's acceptance. Finally, I thank the two analysts whom I saw during the process of writing this book. Without their patience, generosity, and insight, this work would not exist.

Many friends listened to me talk through the ideas in this book. I thank in particular Ari Friedlander, Leigh Goldstein, Adam Kushner, Michael Otterman, Joe Rater, and Kira Walsh. I also thank the entire Otterman family, especially Bernard Otterman, who was the first person who taught me what it means to be an intellectual.

Johns Hopkins University Press has been extremely supportive throughout the writing and editing process. Jackie Wehmueller reached out to me about this project when I was a graduate student. I thought a lot about our conversations as I wrote this book. Matt McAdam has been very sensitive in moving this project through the publication process, as has Will Krause. I will always be grateful to Merryl Sloane for her care in copyediting the manuscript and to Juliana McCarthy for guiding me through production. I also thank Farr Curlin for reviewing the proposal, as well as the two anonymous reviewers, both of whom gave me extremely thoughtful feedback.

A section of chapter 4 was previously published as part of the article "Putting the 'Right to Die' in Its Place: Disability Rights and Physician-Assisted Suicide in the Context of US End-of-Life Care." I am grateful to the journal *Studies in Law, Politics and Society*, edited by Austin Sarat, and to Emerald Group Publishing for allowing me to reprint it here.

The research for chapter 2 relies on the Florence and Henry Wald Papers, which are housed at Yale University's Sterling Memorial Library. I thank the staff of the Manuscripts and Archives room for their help.

I also thank the staff of the facility I refer to here as Amberview Hospice. I wish I could directly acknowledge the people who work there. I admire both them and the facility very much, and I will always be grateful for their openness to my research.

I will similarly always be grateful to the Dominican Sisters of Hawthorne, who are some of the most amazing people I have ever met. I particularly thank Sister Edwin, who gave me unyielding support and who was a constant and creative dialogue partner. I also thank Sister de Paul for helping me do research in the papers of Rose Hawthorne Lathrop, and I thank the entire staff at Our Lady of Perpetual Help Home. I wish I could be hanging out with them right now.

I thank all the patients and families whom I interviewed and whose care I observed. I hope that this research honors them.

My own family has given me everything. I first thank the parents who raised me: Estelle Sechster and Bud Stirber—my heroes for life. I also thank my biological parents: Andrea Braswell, whose courage, strength, and beauty becomes more evident to me with each passing day, and Douglas Braswell, whom I have enjoyed getting to know better. The entire Stirber family has always been extremely welcoming to me. I thank Bob, Donna, Hedy, Joyce, Lee, Michele, Ron, and Yossi. I also thank Ann and Harry Harris and the Rosenwachs.

I am also very grateful to the Braswell family for being so wonderful to me over the years, even though I appeared in their lives a bit later than might have been expected. I am especially thankful to Jane and Fran and Rob and Sharon. Getting to know my cousin Taylor Braswell has been a highlight of recent years. I've learned a lot from our conversations.

The Karalekas/Buckley family have been so warm in their embrace of me, especially considering the shambles that my life was in when I walked through their door. I thank Cindy, Homer, Sophia, Steve, Cathy, Walter, Thomas, Nick, Andrew, and Bella.

My children, Stella and Augie, are the best things to ever happen to me. I never would have written this without you two. I love you both so much.

Most of all, I thank my wife, Nikki Karalekas. She gave me the first line of this book. And basically everything else. The process of writing was difficult for me—but much worse for her because she had to deal with me throughout it. (I whine.) She's a genius, the best editor I know. Also, the best friend. Only she knows what she's been through with me. She taught me to love.

THE CRISIS OF US HOSPICE CARE

Introduction

Death is personal. It happens to a person, someone who is not like any other person in the world. When their life ends, it cannot and will not be replaced. The projects that they were in the middle of, the relationships they had, their hopes and dreams for the future—everything dies. In a sense perhaps they live on, in the memories of those around them, in memorials and scraps of paper, in items that once were theirs. But not really. As the singer-songwriter Phil Elverum puts it: "Someone's there, and then they're not."[1]

This personal context is also evident in the period immediately before death, a time I refer to as the "end of life." This period is often characterized by the diagnosis of a terminal disease: a medical condition that, a doctor predicts, will end the person's life in six months or less.[2] These predictions are often wrong: some people live much longer, some much shorter.[3] But even if they were always right, they would be limited. A prognosis is just a number. Its meaning resides in the person who has just been told that this number applies to *them*. Any assessment of the end of life must be based on the lives of the dying.

It should also include the people who live with the dying, who care about them, and for whom their deaths matter. Following physician Ira Byock, I refer to these people as "family."[4] This definition of family is not based on biology or law. It is based on the extent to which a person cares for the dying. I mean "care" in a sense that is itself personal: care as love. The family members of the dying are losing a person who is important to them, someone whom they love. In this sense, the end of life is not just personal. It is *inter*personal, in that it affects the relationships between people. Since these relationships shape the identities of their participants, the end of life is even *intra*personal. It impacts both the dying person and their family *from within*. When a family member loses a loved one, they lose a way of being themselves.

Caring at the end of life frequently involves more than love. It also involves work. Dying people are still people. But they are not as they were before. They need love. But they also need help with things that previously they might have considered to be second nature. Family members of the dying often provide such help. They assist dying people with basic tasks: feeding and clothing, bathing and grooming, and even general safety in a world suddenly laced with menace. Caring, in this sense, is not just a question of our love for the dying. It is also a matter of our ability to put in the work.

These are two different ways of thinking about familial care at the end of life: as love and as labor. These ways are both essential to appropriate care. But they are quite different in what they ask of the caregiver. To love a dying person does not require expert knowledge, physical strength, or geographic proximity. I can love a dying person when I am far away, whether or not I know how to prevent bedsores, or even if I am debilitated or dying myself. But such love, however important, is not labor. Labor requires the ability and willingness to carry out tasks that are physically, mentally, and emotionally demanding, time consuming, and sometimes highly technical.

Love and labor can be complementary. A daughter, for example, helps her dying father get dressed because she loves him. This love is why she undertakes the labor. It may also be part of the reason why she does it well: with a degree of sensitivity that may in fact be higher than if she were working for monetary remuneration. Love, in this case, does not just support labor. It elevates it, making it into a manifestation of love itself.

Things do not always match up that clearly, however. A family member can love the dying person, but they may not be able to do the work. There can be a number of reasons for this inability: perhaps they are disabled; perhaps they have to work a job; perhaps they have emotional ambivalence about caregiving; perhaps they lack the money to buy the dying person the necessary food; perhaps they live in a neighborhood so unsafe that they cannot go out at all. For any of these reasons, labor can fail. The person dying, in such cases, will receive caregiving that is "inadequate," meaning insufficient to their needs.

To label someone an "inadequate familial caregiver" might seem to be judgmental, even cruel. Perhaps it is impossible to avoid this implication, but it is not my intent. I consider "inadequate familial caregiver" to be a neutral descriptor. It is not a judgment of a caregiver's love for the dying person or their character as a human being. It is rather an assessment that they lack three related qualities: skill at tasks that are highly technical, for which they were likely never trained; certain physical, mental, and emotional abilities; and resources that they likely were never told they needed and probably would not have been able to amass even if they had been told years in advance. Referring to someone as an inadequate familial caregiver in the context of the end of life, therefore, is much like referring to them as an inadequate neurosurgeon if they spent their entire life training to be a carpenter; as an inadequate professional basketball player if they lack the ability to jump; or as an inadequate purchaser of private airplanes if they cannot afford to take a bus. To be an inadequate familial caregiver is to lack skills, abilities, and resources. It is not to lack love.

In this book, I discuss the causes and impacts of inadequate familial caregiving at the end of life. As part of the research I conducted, I observed familial caregivers for the dying. I saw the ways in which they gave their loved ones much-needed assistance and also the ways in which they failed at this task. I saw many cases of inadequate familial caregiving, but I did not see any in which the caregiver, even at their most inadequate, was lacking in love. Anyone who puts themselves in the position of caring for a dying family member has already committed themselves to love. But part of making that commitment requires exposing ourselves to the possibility of our failure: the despairing reality that love, sometimes, is not enough.

Take the example of a woman I will refer to only as Maya.[5] Maya was the familial caregiver for her husband, Frank. Frank had been diagnosed with lung cancer around a year before I met them. He had recently stopped chemotherapy, and his doctor had told him that he had only a few more months to live. Maya wanted to care for him while he was dying. There was just one problem. She had recently been diagnosed with breast cancer. It was not terminal, but she needed to begin treatment immediately. To receive this treatment, she had to travel, leaving her husband alone for hours at a time. And once she returned home, she was often too debilitated to assist him. Indeed, she was frequently in need of assistance herself. Maya loved her husband, but due to her condition, she was not able to be an adequate familial caregiver.

To be diagnosed with cancer while your family member is dying is an extreme situation. But there are many other medical conditions that, though less debilitating, can significantly hinder our ability to provide adequate care. When such conditions are not present, other factors can impinge: financial, geographic, emotional, psychological, technological, and more. Taken in isolation, any one factor can be enough to make a familial caregiver inadequate. But they rarely occur in isolation. Maya, for example, did not "just" have breast cancer. She also had a job, the income from which she and her husband depended on, particularly as her husband could no longer work. Even without breast cancer, adequate familial caregiving might not have been possible for her. Maya's failure to be an adequate caregiver, however, is not an indictment of her love.

I know about this from personal experience. I was a familial caregiver for a dying person: my mother. And, like Maya, I was inadequate. I know now that there were things that I could have done differently. I wish I had known then. But I didn't, and it was hard. I was twenty-seven years old when she got sick. And I was a very green twenty-seven, quite the mama's boy. I depended on her for a lot, and when I lost that ability—the ability to depend—I lost much of who I was. I tried to paper over this loss and to do things for her. But my general lack of competence undermined me. I knew nothing of medicine, had no hands-on knowledge of caring for the sick. I am neurotic and a mild hypochondriac. I lived hundreds of miles away and was in the midst of a PhD program that neither she nor I wanted me to leave. There were also issues among the members of our family—people that I should have stood up to but didn't because they were older than me, because I wrongly thought that they "knew." All these things colluded against me. All these things thwarted my ability to express my love through adequate care. My love was real. But as much as I loved my mother, my love was not enough.

This is a book about when love fails. It is a book about familial caregivers like me: inadequate ones. I do not deny the personal nature of this caregiving. Nor do I deny the highly personal feelings of disappointment when it fails. But I do seek to place both of them in their proper context. This context is not personal. It is political.

Inadequate familial caregiving at the end of life is not primarily a personal failure. It is, rather, a failure of the political structure of the country in which this book's action is set: the United States of America. Within our political structure, the problem of inadequate familial caregiving for dying people originates in a place that seems unlikely, first, because we do not generally think of it as political, and second, because it is generally not considered to be a cause of inadequate familial caregiving, but a resource that caregivers can turn to when they are most in need.[6]

That place is hospice, which is the dominant form of end-of-life care in the United States. Though privately managed—largely through for-profit corporations—hospice is in general financed by the US government.[7] The largest payer of US hospice care is Medicare, the federal health insurance program for the elderly.[8] The high percentage of services paid for by Medicare makes individual hospices dependent on Medicare certification. To achieve this certification, they must structure their caregiving in a way that complies with Medicare guidelines. Medicare thus determines the ability of US hospices to function and determines the kinds of caregiving that they can—and cannot—afford to provide.

The result of the dependence of US hospices on Medicare is that they have a highly centralized structure. It is tempting to think of US hospices as individual entities, as Kindred Hospice, Vitas Hospice, or HCR Manor. To be sure, individual differences matter. But an individualistic approach misses that the differences among hospices occur within a structure that makes them all generally the same. I refer to this structure as the "US hospice system," a term by which I emphasize the federally centralized, standardized nature of hospice in this country.[9] Though there are hospices that operate outside of this system—for example, hospices that are primarily funded by charity or private payments—they are exceptions and do not disprove the norm of the system itself.[10]

The US hospice system provides many forms of assistance that are beneficial to dying people and their families: medicine, nursing, social work, chaplaincy. It does not, however, include what is referred to as "long-term care." Such care is designed to help individuals with the "activities of daily living" (ADLs), such as feeding, bathing, general safety, and routine hygienic maintenance.[11] Dying people need this care. But as a result of the reliance on Medicare financing, it is not included in hospice.

Such care is instead frequently carried out by an informal network of unpaid caregivers: the family.[12] Long-term care makes up the bulk of the care that the dying person receives. In this sense, although hospice is the country's primary form of end-of-life care, hospice providers are not the country's primary caregivers. The primary caregivers in the United States at the end of life are the family members of dying people.[13] Sometimes they provide this care directly by clipping toenails and washing limbs. Other times, they might hire an aide, if they can afford one (most cannot), or arrange for their loved one to be sent to a nursing home or other long-term care facility.[14] Even if they are not performing every act of long-term care, family members of the dying carry an enormous amount of responsibility for coordinating it, financing it, and generally making it work.

Family members sometimes provide such care out of personal choice. But often they have little choice in the matter. Their loved ones need long-term care, and someone has to provide it. That someone, by default, is them. The conflation of love and labor is essential to the working of US hospice care. The US hospice system thus creates the problem of inadequate familial caregiving. The love of family members will, in general, not be enough. But our hospice system is designed as if it will be.

When love is not enough—when familial caregiving fails—hospice fails too. Dying people are not the only ones who depend on their family members. Hospice providers also depend on the family members of dying people to provide adequate care. This care is the essential context in which hospice services can be delivered. As a result, inadequate familial caregiving is not only harmful to dying people in itself. It is also harmful because it keeps dying people from effectively receiving hospice services. Without suitable familial caregiving, it may be impossible to deliver these services; even if delivered, they may be so attenuated by the caregiving environment that they are unable to ameliorate the dying person's suffering. Hospice services, as a result, become inadequate. In such instances, the US hospice system's dependence on familial caregiving seems to sabotage itself. When self-sabotage of this sort is endemic—when hospice becomes dependent on a level of care that most American families cannot provide—then the hospice system can fairly be described as in crisis.

In the United States, we are experiencing just such a crisis of hospice care. Our hospice system requires a level of familial caregiving that is beyond the abilities of most families in the country. The result is the systemic undermining of hospice delivery. This crisis does not impact all people equally. It is mediated by various factors: race, class, gender, sexual orientation, geography, religion, disability, and more. Depending on these factors—as well as on personal issues that are idiosyncratic but potentially significant—this crisis can have a greater effect on some and a lesser one on others. But it stretches across what might seem to be otherwise intractable demographic divides.

The crisis of US hospice care, then, is not simply a black crisis or a white one; not one of the poor, the middle class, or even, in some cases, the rich; not one of Christians, Jews, Muslims, or all the believers and nonbelievers in between. It is an *American* crisis, and it impacts an astoundingly broad cross-section of the people who call this nation their home.

It is also an American crisis in another sense. It is caused, in part, by the way that we, as Americans, see our own identity. More specifically, it is caused by how we understand our signature political value: freedom. I argue that there is no place for dying either in our national imaginary or in our shared political vocabulary. Though this rejection of the end of life might seem merely rhetorical, it is central to the material problems that have created a crisis for dying people, for hospice providers, and for family members who care.

Rectifying the current state of US hospice care does not, then, just require crafting newer and better hospice policy, though certainly that is essential. It requires, I believe, rewriting the very meaning of "America." We must make our country into one that can still call itself the "home of the free," while understanding that, for that to be true, we must also be the "home of the dying." We must transform this nation into one that dying people can call their home.

To do so, we can turn to a resource that, given what I have just written, might seem unlikely: hospice itself. This book is not just a critique of US hospice care. It is also an appreciation of the work of hospice professionals and the American hospice tradition. This tradition, though flawed, contains within it the resources to provide not just a better way of doing hospice, but also a better way of being American. Hospice is in crisis, in part, because of a failure in our larger national project. But through hospice, we may find the resources to ameliorate both the particular crisis of US hospice care and the broader crisis of American identity.

The goal of this book is to provoke just such a resolution. But I must first consider a key obstacle to its realization: the American family itself. As I've already mentioned, the crisis of US hospice care is primarily political. But it is not a top-down imposition on US families. In part, this crisis is a product of the way we in America think about the family. More specifically, it comes from how American familial caregivers—people like me—think about ourselves.

Bioethicist Bruce Jennings has argued that a major impediment to the improvement of US end-of-life care is that Americans see it as an issue that is solely personal.[15] This lack of a political understanding of end-of-life care leads, in turn, to a lack of political action on behalf of dying people. Thus, we have an end-of-life care system that is grossly underfunded, bereft of the resources necessary to support dying people in their most basic needs.[16]

Jennings's argument is both confirmed and deepened by the work of sociologist Sandra Levitsky, who argues the lack of adequate long-term care in the United States is a product of the reluctance of familial caregivers to see their work as political.[17] They view caregiving as the family's responsibility. This makes them reticent to rally for more resources from the state. They view such requests as an abdication of their responsibility and ultimately of their role as family members. The resulting lack of political will is, for Levitsky, a major source of responsibility for the lack in America of a feasible system of long-term care.

Levitsky's research provides empirical evidence of the psychological and social dynamics underlying Jennings's argument about US end-of-life care. But it is also relevant because the crisis of US hospice care is not *just* a crisis of US hospice care. It is caused, in part, by the lack of a functioning long-term care system.[18] The crisis of US hospice care is thus a specific instance of what Levitsky describes as a more general "caregiving crisis."[19] This crisis has been caused by many factors. One of them is the way that familial caregivers think about the work that they do. American families want, desperately, to care for their loved ones when they are sick or dying. But this very desire precludes them from asking for resources from the state. The result is a lack of the care that dying people need. In a gutting paradox, our national crisis of caregiving is a product of the zeal with which American families care.

Rectifying the problems of US hospice care thus requires challenging a definition of familial caregiving that is commonly held. This definition equates familial caregiving with carrying out long-term, end-of-life care for dying people. In this book, I redefine such caregiving to mean not primarily *providing* such care, but rather recognizing that it is likely to be beyond our current and future abilities to do so without significant governmental support. This inability is not a failure of the caregiver. It is a failure of the current hospice system. Familial caregiving thus requires changing this system. Such change *is* political. But it is *also* personal. Political activism on behalf of the dying is, I believe, a necessary component of familial care.

In this book I ask readers to reimagine what it means to be caregivers for dying people. In the process, I ask us to expand our definition of what "family" means. If we are to ameliorate the crisis of US hospice care, we must see the family as political, and politics as familial. Such a politicization of the family does not diminish the personal nature of familial connections. It deepens these connections and creates a more fertile ground for them to flourish.

In no sense am I arguing against familial caregiving at the end of life. I support familial caregiving for dying people and would like to see the United States become a country that is more hospitable to it. But there is a diametrical opposition between a hospice system that *supports* familial caregiving and one that *depends* on it. A hospice system that supports familial caregiving provides families with the resources they need to provide care. One that depends on it denies them these resources. When caregiving fails—predictably, systematically—the current system implicitly rationalizes this failure as a personal shortcoming. A hospice system that seems to blame US familial caregivers for its own failures of design cannot be described as one that supports them.

Nor does this system support the hospice professionals who labor in its grip. In researching this book, I was greatly moved by the technical skill of American hospice professionals, as well as their abundance of love for the patients and families under their care. This book does not indict their competence, and I appreciate the frequently heroic extent to which they care. What I do indict is a system that, in many cases, keeps them from doing the work to which they—often at great personal sacrifice—have dedicated their lives. If we are to take their work seriously, then we must consider fundamental change.

Before we can enact such change, we must examine how we got here: how hospice in America came to take the form that it has today.

The Hospice Family Romance

In *The Family Romance of the French Revolution*, historian Lynn Hunt argues that revolutionary movements are based on collective images of the family. She calls such images "family romances."[20] This phrase comes from the founder of psy-choanalysis, Sigmund Freud, who used it to discuss an individual's fantasy of replacing their current family members with others who are "as a rule" of higher social status.[21] Hunt's rethinking of the family romance refers not to individuals in families, but rather to revolutionary political movements. Such movements are, she argues, driven by desires—often unconscious—to transition from one model of the family to another, superior alternative.[22] Revolutionary attempts to reimagine the political world are thus ways of reimagining the family.

Hospice is not generally thought of as a revolutionary movement. This is understandable. At present, hospice—in America at least—is not revolutionary. And it is difficult to imagine it ever having been. Hospice care in the United States seems as representative of the "establishment" as any multibillion-dollar industry whose largest members have been accused of defrauding the federal government.[23] But even if hospice were not a multibillion-dollar industry, any radical origins would still seem odd. Hospice is a form of health care generally referred to in terms that seem suited for familial intimacy, not revolutionary pol-itics: care, not conflict; hospitality, not creative destruction; mourning, not zeal. Yet this placid image papers over what was initially and, in some ways remains, hospice's radical edge.

The US hospice industry of today began in the early 1970s and was called by its leaders the "hospice movement."[24] The term "movement" referred to what had been the great social undertakings of the previous decade: feminism and civil rights.[25] Hospice leaders in the United States thought of these movements as models for the revolution that they wanted to provoke on behalf of a pop-ulation that had, to that point, flown under the radar of those seeking radical change: dying people. Hospice was from the beginning a form of health care and, yes, a business—albeit one not always oriented toward profit. But it was also much more than either of those things. It was a spark that would ignite a change in the way that Americans thought of the dying, cared for them, and, at a fundamental level, *were* dying themselves.

This revolution, like the French Revolution at the center of Hunt's study, was based on a certain family romance, which went as follows: The family was once the natural caregiver for dying people, and caring for dying people was the natu-ral role of the family. This state of nature was upset by the rise of the field of med-icine, specifically hospitals. Hospitals removed dying people from their families. The care they provided was often futile, even harmful. The result was terrible for everyone. Hospice would remedy this situation by returning dying people to their natural state under the family's care.[26]

This family romance differentiated the modern hospice movement from the radical movements it had taken as a model. Both the civil rights and the women's liberation movements had their own family romances.[27] They generally did not imagine the ideal family to exist in the past, however, but in the future: they were trying to create a new kind of family. Hospice, in contrast, imagined the ideal family to be a kind of return to the way things were prior to the field of medicine's rise. It was not seeking just the family that *should be* but also the family that *had been* and was no longer. The result made hospice a hybrid movement that wedded a desire for progressive social change to a conservative reverence for times gone by.[28]

This hybrid vision was partially correct. Hospice leaders in the United States were right that the rise of medicine had not been a positive development for dying people, but they were wrong in their belief that dying had necessarily been better before.[29] People dying in the nineteenth century had significant medical needs. But those needs seemed lesser in large part because, since modern pain medicine did not yet exist, there was no expectation of a painless death.[30] In that context of diminished expectations, it may have been easier to be a familial caregiver. But it was not easier to be the person dying.

Indeed, dying in the early years of America was in many ways much worse for those groups that would benefit from the great liberation movements of the nineteenth and twentieth centuries: women and African Americans. For women, who had effectively no choice but to care for the dying, familial caregiving was not a simple expression of love. And dying could not be described as an idyllic experience for African Americans in bondage, whose families were often broken up, not by medicine, but to serve the slaver's gain.

This misunderstanding of history shaped the way that hospice leaders confronted the present. Because of their focus on medicine, they did not consider that the decline in familial caregiving might also be due to changes in US families themselves. Hospice leaders also neglected to consider the implications of their model for women and nonwhite communities. They gave little thought, for example, to how housing discrimination might hinder the ability of black families to participate in a form of end-of-life care based in the home. Nor did they adequately consider the degree to which familial caregiving was a burden that many American women were trying to escape.

The result was an overestimation of the ability and willingness of American families to provide end-of-life care. Dying Americans did need to be taken out of hospitals and given appropriate hospice care. And in some cases they did prefer to be cared for by their families. But their families needed a much higher level of social support than US hospice leaders had anticipated. Such a need for social support was at odds with the idealized family of the hospice family romance. For this reason, the family romance contributed—and continues to contribute—to a gap between the abilities of familial caregivers and the needs of dying patients. This gap is at the root of the crisis in US hospice care.

When Romance Leads to Crisis

The biggest contribution of the hospice family romance to this crisis was not its overestimation of the abilities of US families, however. It was the influence this romance exerted on the hospice movement's orientation toward the state.

The revolutionary movements of the 1960s promoted a vision of the state that was expansive. They wanted government to intervene in the private sphere, whether through the provision of resources or the elimination of barriers to access.[31] The US hospice movement, at least initially, held a similar view. Its leaders did want to return care to the family, but they also understood that families required significant support. They thus requested, like other social movements, that the government take a more expansive role—in this case, by subsidizing hospice care.

The US government has generally not been supportive of such requests for public support.[32] A key reason is the central concept of American political philosophy: freedom. The United States was founded "in liberty," and "freedom" has remained what political theorist Corey Robin refers to as the "keyword" of American politics.[33] But as historian Gary Gerstle has noted, this keyword has typically been equated with the freedom of individuals *from* government intervention. This understanding of freedom as limited government has been a barrier to the expansion of social benefits to American citizens. Such benefits generally require a larger governmental role. They have therefore been maligned as attacks on freedom and, by extension, on America itself.[34]

This antithetical relationship between freedom and social benefits shifted during the period from 1940 to 1970. This time saw the emergence of a new understanding of American freedom, one that equated freedom with the obligation of the federal government to provide more substantial benefits to individuals in the private sphere.[35] In this view, freedom is not just freedom from government intervention. It is also the freedom to do certain basic things: to eat, to work, to have a home, to be protected from discrimination, to receive a basic level of health care. This redefinition of American freedom began with Franklin Roosevelt's New Deal and stretched throughout the civil rights movement, the women's rights movement, and Lyndon Johnson's War on Poverty.[36]

Hospice leaders were fully supportive of this redefinition of American freedom. It was central to the movements that they took as their model. There was
just one problem. Though hospice leaders were supportive of the extension of
social benefits, the federal government no longer was. The modern US hospice
movement did not begin between 1940 and 1970. It began, rather, in 1971. And by
then, another shift in the meaning of American freedom had already taken place.
The name given to this shift by both its opponents and many of its proponents
is neoliberalism. Nowadays, the term "neoliberalism" is often used recklessly,
at times more to police the boundaries of online disputes than to impart actual
insight into reality. But the term does have value for our understanding of the
current state of US hospice care and the predicament of our country as a whole.

The US economy during the 1970s was characterized by a combination of
stagnation and inflation.[37] This "stagflation" produced an employment crisis.
Prominent economists attributed this crisis to the excessive size of the US state.
The solution, they argued, was to remove the government from the private
sphere. This would allow private interactions to take the form of a market: efficient and characterized by voluntary contractual acts between individuals. Its
proponents saw this as promoting economic growth.

But it also promoted something that was much more important than money:
freedom. Neoliberals argued that their vision of economic growth was not just
economic; it was also a return to the bedrock of American political philosophy.
In this view, the individual, choosing among existing options in the market, became the essence of freedom, and *homo economicus* became the model American
citizen.[38] This redefinition of freedom as private economic activity is what I mean
when I talk about neoliberalism.[39]

Sociologist Melinda Cooper has shown that this neoliberal view of freedom as
private economic activity depends on a strong conception of the family.[40] Neoliberals understand that there will be times when individuals are unable to participate in the market due to illness, disability, age, or proximity to death. In such
times, individuals need to depend on others. But rather than depending on the
state, neoliberals argue that, ideally, they should depend on their family. Such familial dependence does not, in theory, increase the size of government. Thus, it
is not anathema to freedom. On the contrary, the ability of individuals to exercise
their freedom in the market depends on the caregiving provided by the family.
Neoliberals thus understand familial caregiving to be essential to freedom.

They also believe that good familial caregiving depends on the *absence* of state
support. For neoliberals, state involvement in the private sphere replaces the family's proper function: caregiving. Such caregiving solidifies the family, establishing

the intimate affective bonds that are essential for families to remain together. Thus, more social support does not in fact support the family. It rips the family apart. Rolling back social benefits thus facilitates familial caregiving, even as such caregiving is essential to the new definition of freedom as the ability to participate in the market.[41]

The leaders of the modern US hospice movement were not neoliberals. They believed that familial caregiving at the end of life requires significant state support. But their valorization of family caregiving gave them and neoliberals a significant common ground. This common ground expanded when hospice leaders began in the early 1970s to argue that familial caregiving was economically efficient—significantly lowering governmental expenditures at the end of life (see chapter 2). This led the hospice family romance to become increasingly aligned with the neoliberal conception of the family.[42]

This coherence of views was abetted by the hospice movement's lack of interest in politics. The US hospice movement wanted to revolutionize medicine and society. But hospice leaders did not rethink the relationship between dying people and the state. Indeed, freedom was, to them, a completely foreign word. For this reason, neoliberal policy makers did not understand the US hospice movement to be a challenge to their vision of either the US government or American freedom. Neither did hospice leaders themselves.

This compatibility with neoliberalism led the US hospice movement to its greatest success: the 1982 incorporation of hospice into Medicare through the Medicare Hospice Benefit (MHB). But this success came at a price. The MHB did provide dying people and their families with government-funded care, but it also attempted to save the government money by shifting long-term care onto the family. Even at the time, US hospice leaders worried that this shift was too radical, that the MHB was placing a greater burden on American families than they would be able to bear.

The result was a mismatch between the amount of familial caregiving required to sustain US hospice care and the abilities of American families. Over the almost forty years since the benefit's passage, this initial mismatch has grown even wider, in part due to the effects that neoliberal reforms have had both in hospice and in US society as a whole. This has led to the crisis that we have today: the abilities of familial caregivers in the US hospice system are generally insufficient for the needs of the people under their care.

This crisis is, in a terrible irony, incredibly costly. The excessive burden of care on American families leads to people dying in hospitals and nursing homes. Such deaths are extremely cost inefficient; indeed, such cost inefficiencies are in part what hospice was designed to avoid. But by trying to support dying people and their families on the cheap, the designers of the US hospice system inadvertently prolonged and exacerbated the problem of overly expensive end-of-life care.

This crisis has negative impacts on hospice professionals, family members, and the US health system and economy. But here I focus on its primary victims: dying people themselves.

The Nature of the Crisis

What happens to dying people who are left in the gap between the requirements of hospice and the abilities of the family members responsible for their care? They find themselves without access to essential medical care and social services and in environments that restrict every aspect of their lives. The resulting impact could be described in many ways. But I think that the best way to describe it is in terms of freedom. The crisis of US hospice care limits and in some cases destroys the freedom of dying people, their individual liberty to govern their own lives.[43] Dying Americans caught in the mismatch between US hospice requirements and familial capacity are deprived of the ability to make choices for themselves.[44] In part, this deprivation is due to their terminal medical conditions. But only in part. It is also a result of our hospice system. Without a dramatic change to this system, their freedom will continue to be denied. Until this crisis is resolved, dying Americans should not be considered free.

This is not to say that the lack of freedom is the only way to describe this crisis. It is also a crisis of health care, of human rights, of justice, of systemic neglect. The deprivations that dying Americans suffer are numerous and can be described in numerous ways. But even if freedom were not the most philosophically accurate term to describe this crisis, I would still use it. That is because my goal in this book is not merely philosophical accuracy. It is political change. And in the United States, no term has been as effective in provoking change as "freedom." It has provided impetus to social movements dating back to the American Revolution.[45] This is true across the political spectrum, with the term being used by both liberals and conservatives alike.[46]

My goal in this book is not just to describe the crisis of US hospice care, but also to begin to establish the political base necessary to ameliorate it. Even if this crisis were not one of freedom—and it is—freedom would be the best concept to accomplish this goal. In the US context, it may well be the only appropriate one.

There are arguments against the use of the term "freedom" to describe this crisis, and the strongest comes from political philosopher Isaiah Berlin. Berlin argued that freedom should be understood only as the freedom from obstruction by other people, which he called "negative liberty."[47] Berlin opposed arguments that state-funded resources were necessary for freedom. Such arguments lead to a philosophical misunderstanding. An individual living in poverty might be very limited. But if these limitations do not come from the actions of other people, they are not limitations on the individual's freedom.[48]

This misunderstanding can be dangerous. It gives the state the power to determine what freedom is to individuals, even if they might themselves disagree. For Berlin, this danger was not speculative. He found evidence for it throughout history, including most notably in the Soviet Union, perhaps the dominant world power at the time of his writing in the late 1950s. Berlin was in favor of more robust social benefits. But calling such benefits "freedom" would cause unnecessary categorical confusion and likely political despair.[49]

The United States was not the focus of Berlin's work, and he wrote nothing about the state of terminally ill Americans. But his argument about freedom has implications for this book. From his perspective, terminally ill people caught in the crisis of US hospice care might well be suffering, and perhaps should be provided with public support. But the degree to which they lack control over their lives would seem to be inherent to their terminal disease. Their constraints would therefore be medical, not political. For this reason, the crisis of US hospice care might, for Berlin, be described as one of insufficient care, but it should not be considered one of freedom.

Berlin's critique rests on an underlying belief: that it is possible, even easy, to separate a medical impediment from a political one.[50] A political impediment created by human action would, for Berlin, be an impediment to freedom. A medical one, in contrast, would be a quirk of biology, not a human-caused limitation. This separation of medicine and politics would seem to negate the idea that the crisis of US hospice care is one of freedom. But this very separation has over the past forty years come under attack by the leaders of a movement that marks an important chapter in the story of freedom in America: the movement for disability rights.

In the Tradition of Disability Rights

The disability rights movement emerged at roughly the same time as the US hospice movement: the early 1970s.[51] In many ways, the two movements were similar. They both advocated on behalf of individuals whose medical conditions were incurable and who, because of this incurability, suffered in the US medical establishment. Both were critical of hospitals, which tried to cure the incurable, as well as nursing homes, which kept people in conditions that were inadequate and hidden from public view (see chapter 2). Further, both categorized their target populations in terms that were not primarily medical. The US hospice movement did this by arguing for care that treated the dying as "whole persons."[52] The disability rights movement took a different route.

Disability rights advocates argued that Americans with disabilities were oppressed.[53] They lived in institutions that were segregated from society and had significantly limited opportunities for employment and for enjoying the shared social goods necessary for a basic quality of life. This oppression was a product of the organization of US society. But most Americans did not realize the political nature of this oppression—or that disabled people were even oppressed at all—because of the actions of medical providers. Medical providers created the mistaken impression that being disadvantaged was inherent to the biology of disability: it was "natural" for disabled people to be segregated and unemployed. The disability rights movement resisted this view, which required redefining disability as a condition that was not primarily medical, but political.[54]

This political redefinition of disability involved rethinking the relationship between disabled people and the state. Disability rights advocates argued that disabled people in the United States were not, at present, free. To achieve their freedom, there was a need for political change. In part, this change involved eliminating discriminatory barriers that prohibited people with disabilities from participating as equal members of US society. In addition, the state needed to provide disabled individuals with the resources necessary to access society. Disability rights required not just the negative freedom from interference—the kind of freedom that Isaiah Berlin supported—but also the positive freedom to realize their desires through the receiving of social support.[55] Indeed, the lack of such support was itself an interference with their freedom.

The culmination of this movement was the 1990 passage of the Americans with Disabilities Act. The ADA does not merely mandate that the federal government provide disabled people with resources. It considers such resources as necessary to their very freedom. The act created a federal obligation to provide disabled people with social support.[56] Such support is not external to their freedom. It is freedom itself.

In its redefinition of freedom, the ADA was different from the US hospice movement. The hospice movement did not link the provision of social benefits to the freedom of dying people. For this reason, it based its call for support on the idea that these resources would, in reality, shrink the size of the state. The result has been the dependence of both the hospice system and dying people on familial caregiving. The ADA, in contrast, linked state benefits to the freedom of people with disabilities. By doing so it established a stronger obligation on the part of the state to provide disabled people with much-needed resources—and created a greater ability for people with disabilities to choose to live on their own.[57]

This movement—away from the family and toward the state—is the direction in which I seek to take end-of-life care. Just as the ADA defined disability as a political category, I highlight the political nature of terminal illness and the political character of the oppression that dying people face. This is not an argument against familial caregiving. But such caregiving, to be effective, must be accompanied by a stronger state obligation to provide resources to people who are dying.

The ADA defines disability as a protected class subject to discrimination, similar to race and gender.[58] I support the adoption of such an approach to dying. I have argued elsewhere that dying people can be subject to discrimination.[59] And I believe that they should be protected by the ADA. To the degree that the ADA does not apply to dying people, they should be the beneficiaries of a separate set of civil rights legislation for the terminally ill—a modern-day "rights of the dying."[60] But though I support such rights, this book is not an argument on their behalf.

The ADA has significantly improved the lives of disabled Americans. But disability rights scholars have recognized its limitations.[61] Employment rates for people with disabilities have not significantly risen as a result of the ADA, and the legislation does not include the long-term care services that are, from a disability rights perspective, essential to freedom. Though it is a watershed in the history of America's treatment of disabled people, the ADA has in many ways had an effect that is highly limited. There are a number of reasons for this, including hostile interpretations of the act from US courts.[62] But as legal scholar Samuel Bagenstos has argued, these limitations are inherent to antidiscrimination law. Antidiscrimination law is limited because it operates on a case-by-case basis and in contexts in which it is very difficult to prove intent.[63] This is not an argument against the necessity of antidiscrimination laws. Rather, it is an argument that such laws must be accompanied by other approaches to the freedom of people with disabilities. Bagenstos in particular argues that more robust social benefits should be considered complementary to an antidiscrimination approach.

While I support antidiscrimination laws for dying people, they will be of significantly less utility than they are for people with disabilities. Terminally ill people are generally too physically weak to work and may be uninterested in doing so. This eliminates a major area in which antidiscrimination statutes might be relevant. The antidiscrimination approach can be more relevant in other areas: for example, involuntary institutionalization. I do not believe, however, that it is the most effective way to support the freedom of dying people.[64] In this book, my approach is not litigious.

I am recommending the reformulation of the Medicare Hospice Benefit. I argue that the MHB was not designed with the freedom of dying people in mind. This has made hospice into a caregiving modality that inadvertently thwarts their freedom. An antidiscrimination approach will have limited utility if the US hospice system retains its current form. For this reason, my goal is to redesign the hospice system from the perspective of freedom at the end of life.

Health policy is not external to freedom. Some healthcare benefits can subvert it. For example, political scientist Jamila Michener has argued that Medicaid maintains its socioeconomically impoverished beneficiaries in a state of stigmatized dependency that discourages their political participation.[65] From this perspective Medicare, which does not implicitly stigmatize its recipients as the "undeserving poor," is more liberating.[66] Though I agree with this generally, I argue that the liberating quality of Medicare is severely curtailed in the case of dying Americans. By reimagining the MHB, I hope to correct this flaw.

And yet, it is not enough to conceptually redesign Medicare. We must also garner the political will to make that design a reality. The disability rights movement is of limited utility in this regard. Unlike, for example, the civil rights movement, it did not change policy by amassing a substantial popular base.[67] Instead, the movement largely worked behind the scenes in Washington, DC. Though this strategy was successful, the absence of broad popular support for— or even understanding of—disability rights has limited the degree to which the ADA has been enforced. A movement for the freedom of dying people must, to avoid such pitfalls, have a broader popular base. To achieve this, the movement must be carried out by an actor that is unique in American politics.

The Dying Family

Familial advocacy has always played a significant role in the disability rights movement.[68] But in disability rights, it has generally been assumed that the major agents of political change should be disabled people themselves. This view —captured in the slogan "nothing about us without us"—is more difficult to implement with dying people.[69] The severity of terminal illness is such that the dying are generally precluded from participating in any political activity on their own behalf. It is also the case that under current hospice guidelines most dying people do not even gain consciousness of their own dying until they are effectively incapacitated—if they gain consciousness of it at all.[70] Though there will occasionally be terminally ill people who can mobilize politically, their numbers will never be sufficient to enact political change.

As a result, any movement for the freedom of dying people must, in general, be led by people other than those who are dying. These are members of the "dying family," which is not a biological category but rather a relationship that is claimed through acts of caring for dying people. Often such care is provided only privately. This is appropriate and largely unavoidable. While their relative is dying, it is unrealistic to expect family members to mobilize politically on their behalf. They may advocate in their immediate environment with doctors and nursing home administrators, with noisy neighbors and unhelpful kin. Given the demanding nature of familial caregiving, such advocacy will almost certainly be all-consuming. It is entirely correct, then, that while individuals are dying, familial caregiving will just be focused on them.

The politicized familial advocacy of the dying family must thus occur when we are not in the context of the end of life. This advocacy can only occur after our loved one has died. Because such advocacy comes too late to help our own deceased family member, it will naturally be suffused with mourning. This mourning often is not only for the dead, but also for the way that they died: in a situation of political oppression that destroyed their freedom. Grief thus will generally coexist with anger, anger that should be directed, at least in part, at a system, a society, and a country that can no longer harm the dead but is harming the dying.

Political advocacy on behalf of those who have died requires us to make connections with those who have not yet died but are dying and even with those who are not yet actively dying at all. It requires looking outside of our private family and seeing our own particular loved one as a member of a class of people: the dying. Mourning is perhaps an ideal emotional process for such advocacy. As the philosopher Judith Butler has argued, to be in mourning requires a generative loss of self.[71] The person in mourning has lost someone to whom they were attached—a person who made them who they are. But this loss is generative because, now broken open, the person in mourning can form new connections with others, can expand their circle of kinship and become part of a family that is larger than the one to which they had previously belonged.

In this sense, mourning, far from an apolitical, private process, can form the basis for a new form of politics. It can create what the philosopher Peter Singer has called the "expanding circle," an ever-increasing community of kinship in which we look beyond our tribal affiliations to claim relationship with others.[72] But while the dying family enacts Singer's vision of an expanding circle, it does not do so by moving *beyond* our familial affiliations. In the dying family, care for the others who are here now is a way of continuing to care for those who have passed. The new recipients of care become intermingled in the mind of the care-giver with those who are no longer here. The result is a continuation of the obli-gations of kinship even after a person has died. Joining in the dying family and forming kinship with strangers are ways of simultaneously caring for others and for our own dead.

But the orientation of the dying family is not solely toward the past. Whether or not we have been caregivers for our dying family members in the past, it is extremely likely that we will be caregivers for them in the future. We owe it to our family members to provide them with the best care possible when they do begin to die. Such care, however, will be beyond our control as individuals. With-out drastic changes, the political arrangement of the US hospice system will be a serious impediment to our ability to provide adequate care. Thus, unless we advocate now on behalf of our family members who will, in the future, be dying, we condemn them to die without freedom. It is never too early, from this per-spective, to begin to care.

This work on behalf of others is also a form of advocacy for ourselves. This book is not just an appeal to former, current, and future caregivers for dying people. It is also an appeal to anyone—regardless of their interest or experience in caregiving—to think of their own life from the perspective of its end. The end of life is not just death. It is also the days, weeks, and months before death, the moments when we are not yet dead but dying. Given the current arrangement of US hospice care, it is extremely likely that any given American person will die without freedom. This is concerning in a general sense. But it is also concerning in a particular sense: as it pertains to me and to you. If we do not want to be stripped of freedom when we are at our most vulnerable, we should begin now by advocating for the transformation of US end-of-life care.

Such self-advocacy is not just self-oriented. Surveys indicate that Americans are afraid of being a burden on their family members at the end of life.[73] Whether we identify with this fear or not—and I do—it comes from a relatively selfless, even admirable place. But the degree to which we will burden our loved ones is not solely determined by the medical aspects of dying. It is also a product of how we have designed our country's system of end-of-life care. This design currently maximizes the extent to which we will be a burden.

Indeed, it is extremely likely that the days, weeks, and months before our deaths will place our family members in situations that are more than they can handle. They will experience extremely negative effects during these situations and even after them: physical and mental exhaustion, trauma, financial expenses that drive many Americans to bankruptcy, irregular mourning that will haunt them for long after we die.[74] Therefore, claiming membership in the dying family should be of interest to those understandably concerned about burdening their loved ones at the end of life. In the context of the current arrangement of US hospice care, this concern is entirely rational.

At present, discussions of end-of-life planning are almost entirely oriented around individual decision making: specifically, decisions regarding how we want our surrogates to act in the event that we lose consciousness at the end of life.[75] Such end-of-life planning is an admirable expression of individual freedom and of concern for our kin. But without a larger, political process of end-of-life planning, it will not be enough.

The goal of this book is to help readers to understand why such a process is necessary and why they should take part in it. My project here is to try to create the ideological and political basis for a movement on behalf of the freedom of dying people. I have structured the following chapters with this goal in mind.

What's to Come

In this volume, each chapter can be read in isolation, as a stand-alone entity, but they also function as a whole. The book's argument takes the reader from a consideration of existing debates about freedom at the end of life to an understanding of the meaning of freedom in US politics.

I understand hospice as a site that because of its focus on the end of life, places a particular strain on the way we understand freedom. This strain has created problems—indeed, a crisis—but also opens up possibilities that can impact us as both individuals and members of a larger political community. By bringing together the personal and political aspects of freedom at the end of life, I hope to convince you to join the dying family that I have described above.

Chapter 1 examines current debates in US bioethics about the so-called right to die. Such debates conflate the practice of physician-assisted suicide with the broader topic of freedom at the end of life. This conflation is a misunderstanding. Freedom at the end of life is the ability not just to choose to die, but also to exercise control over one's life while dying. To determine whether such freedom is available to dying Americans, it is necessary to move beyond the right to die and to consider the design of US hospice care itself.

Chapter 2 studies how the relationship of hospice to familial caregiving developed through an examination of the first US hospice: Hospice Inc. Hospice Inc.'s leaders depended on familial caregiving for two functions: to provide better clinical care and to cut costs. But by the end of the 1970s, they were concerned that these two functions had come into conflict. This conflict was, I argue, inherent to the US hospice movement's dependence on the family. This dependence enabled hospice to spread but limited its effectiveness.

In chapter 3, I examine the culmination of this process: the passage of the Medicare Hospice Benefit. The MHB based hospice on the work of familial caregivers. But, as US hospice leaders recognized, the degree to which it did so was already excessive in 1982. Over the almost forty years since the benefit's passage, this initial mismatch between hospice requirements and familial capability has dramatically expanded. The result is the crisis in US hospice care that we face today.

Chapter 4 considers how this crisis impacts dying people. Based on an ethnographic study of hospice care in the Atlanta area, I argue that in our healthcare system, people dying with inadequate familial support generally face two options: remain in a home environment that is neglectful or be sent to a nursing home. Both options cause the destruction of their freedom.

In chapter 5, I examine an end-of-life care facility called Our Lady of Perpetual Help Home. The home provides integrated long-term and end-of-life care to patients whose families cannot sustain the work required by hospice. By doing so, it promotes the freedom of dying people. This care is grounded in the facility's Catholic theology. But this theology, though generative, limits the ability of Our Lady to serve as a model for the resolution of the crisis of US hospice care. What the home represents, however, is the possibility of a political movement for dying people that cuts across the culture wars that have divided our country for the past half century.

Chapter 6 posits some of the basic goals of the movement to change the structure of US hospice care. But I also look beyond hospice at a range of problems that, though not principally pertaining to the end of life, strongly influence hospice delivery. Ultimately, we must be cognizant of how the end of life is influenced by events throughout the lifespan. Only by recognizing that the end of life does not begin at the end of life can we solve the crisis of freedom in US hospice care.

I conclude the book by arguing that dying must become foundational to our conception of the American family. Adopting this perspective will create a new basis for how we understand freedom, our collective mythology, and our national identity. That basis is hospice. By making hospice the foundation of our identity, we can become a nation that is more hospitable to dying people—and to all. This

requires linking the personal and the political: reimagining the relationship between our country and ourselves.

In the afterword, I recount the story of my mother's death. This story is, for
me, quite personal. But it was shaped by the political structure of US hospice
care and of America itself. By telling it, I hope to give you tools to perceive such
connections in your own experiences with death and to inspire you to join the
dying family whose contours I here describe. It is only through such a coming
together that we can make it possible for dying Americans to be free.

CHAPTER ONE

Beyond the Right to Die

Ann Neumann's father was dying. He had been dying for quite some time. After ten years with non-Hodgkin's lymphoma, his body was debilitated. And the cancer's effects had spread to his brain. For the previous three months, Neumann had cared for him. She gave him his morphine, helped him to the bathroom, fed him, clothed him, and tried to comfort him as he faced the end of his existence, as his mind and body were withering away.[1]

Toward the end of his illness, Neumann's father began to kick and punch at her and her sister. He did not seem to recognize who they were. He wanted to go home. But he *was* home. There was nothing they could do to make him see that, nothing they could do to keep him calm. So they called the hospice nurse. She said that he would have to be sent to the hospice inpatient unit, that the drugs that could pacify him were too strong to be delivered at home. Neumann and her sister wanted to give their father the home death he wished for. But that was no longer an option.

And that's how Ann Neumann's father died, against his wishes, thirty minutes from his house.

Even after her father died, Neumann kept caring. One product of this care is her book *The Good Death*, the subtitle of which is "An Exploration of Dying in America." And it is that. But it is also a thorough discussion of the right to die, which I, unlike Neumann, define as "the ability of dying people to end their lives with medical assistance." Neumann believes that if her father had been able to pursue what she calls "aid in dying," he might have been spared his painful death. Later, in *The Good Death*, when Neumann discusses the passage of Death with Dignity laws across the country, she writes: "While my father might never have pursued aid in dying had it been legal in Pennsylvania, he was in pain. He did not die a peaceful death. Some of that suffering could have been according to his wish, but I had to wonder how much of it could we have done away with if hospice had a more inclusive understanding of end-of-life options. . . . Sometimes hospice is not enough."[2] Neumann is not alone in becoming a right-to-die advocate in response to a family member's death.[3] But her argument also includes an acknowledgment that there are many more ways—beyond the right to die—in which hospice in the United States is not enough.

Forty-five pages before the paragraph quoted above, Neumann makes an observation about the state of US hospice care. While hospice does provide some assistance, "the burden of daily care . . . falls to the families of those still at home." These burdens are significant for family members: "cooking, cleaning, bathroom assistance, bathing, sorting medications, bills." But there are also patients who fall into a "gap." They do not have a caregiver at home, and they lack the funds to pay for one. Such patients may receive four hours of daily care from hospice, but they will be "isolated and alone for the other twenty."[4]

Neumann is aware of the dependence of the US hospice system on familial caregiving, and she is aware that there is a gap between the level of familial caregiving required by hospice and that which many dying people receive. To note that this gap is also part of Neumann's own story is not to indict her own efforts as a caregiver. It is to point out, rather, that there was much that hospice could have—and should have—done for her father so that he might have realized his final wish. Indeed, this is true not just for Ann Neumann's father but also for all patients in our hospice system.

Hospice could offer patients stronger drugs so that they could stay at home longer. It could offer them round-the-clock assistance on a far more regular basis. And it could offer a much better understanding of what the dying process looks like. Hospice could also provide caregivers with not just pointers but comfort: the sense that they are not in this situation by themselves.

Finally, if all these things still fail the families who are focused on keeping their loved ones at home, hospice could move them to a facility that feels *like home*. It could transfer patients to that facility earlier, so that they would have time to adjust. A reformed hospice could provide caregivers who, though professional, are known by both the patient and the family—caregivers who, perhaps, with time, even come to feel like family themselves.

But this is often not what happens. The result is that families can feel that they are abandoned by the hospice that has taken them under its ostensible care. This abandonment makes the caregiving that families provide inadequate, but this inadequacy is not their fault. On the contrary, Neumann's story does not just illustrate the gap between hospice requirements and familial capability. It illustrates how unreasonable these requirements are in the first place.

Ann Neumann was, by any measure, an extremely sensitive and dedicated caregiver for her dying father. When she could not obtain leave from work, she quit her job. She moved back to her childhood home and dedicated herself to her father's needs full time. She did everything possible to make him feel comfortable in his transition to death. She had help from her sister and the hospice team. Neumann provided her father with the best familial caregiving possible. But in our hospice system, even the best familial caregiving is not enough.

There are many ways in which the US hospice system can go wrong as a result of its dependence on familial caregiving. This is because even in the best possible circumstances, providing care at the end of life is extremely hard. This raises the question of how we might improve the hospice system for caregivers and dying people. The right to die is important. But it does not prevent patients and their families from falling into the gap between hospice requirements and familial capability. Its relevance is at best secondary, perhaps even nil. Yet, too often, it turns our collective attention away from the broader problems with hospice in America. This skewed focus has unfortunately been encouraged by an academic field that has exercised a significant influence over how Americans think about the end of life: bioethics.

Bioethics emerged largely in the United States in the late 1960s and early 1970s in response to the development of new medical and scientific technologies. Such technologies raised a series of ethical questions that concerned doctors yet were beyond their professional abilities to answer. There was a need for a new group of professionals to address them, professionals trained in ethics, yet not as an abstract subspecialty of philosophy. Rather, ethics, for them, would be applied to the medical setting. This required broadening the term's definition and including in it a range of academic disciplines other than philosophy, including biology, theology, and law. This group of professionals called themselves "bioethicists."[5] I count myself among them. Yet, though I work as a bioethicist, there are many things about my field that I find concerning. These concerns are perhaps best epitomized by the manner in which bioethicists think about dying—and the effect of their thought on the actual experience of dying in America.

Bioethicists have, in theory, been discussing dying since our field's origin. In practice, however, the topic has rarely come up. What we bioethicists call "dying" is largely just the right to die.[6] Our discussions of this "right" have been constant— and constantly repetitive. Debates continue—and in some ways improve—but almost no one ever changes their mind. The result is less an exchange of ideas than a poignant illustration of what Friedrich Nietzsche called "the eternal recurrence of the same."[7]

Amid this library of motionless debate, there is not one article about Medicare.[8] This might seem shocking. Medicare is, after all, the principal funder of US end-of-life care. It thus exerts an enormous impact on the way Americans die. This impact would seem to be relevant to the decisions dying Americans make about whether to end their lives. Surely, a field dedicated to assessing those decisions would have *something* to say about this matter.

Alas, no. The impact of our country's primary funder of end-of-life care on dying people has somehow eluded the notice of those of us preoccupied with decision making at the end of life. It is not the only thing that isn't being discussed. There are no bioethical disquisitions on the brutalization wreaked on dying people by inadequate fall prevention. Nor on the distressing fact that Americans are increasingly spending their final days in facilities that are not designed for dying at all.[9] There is also nothing on how the end of life is impacted by the collapse of the housing market, the mass incarceration of black men, or the widening chasm between the haves and the have-nots.

All of this—and much more—lies outside of our bioethical gaze. Were this just a problem of an academic field, it would be significant. But the situation is much worse.

Bioethicists are *public* scholars. We exercise our authority in a range of venues outside the university's walls: through the Presidential Commission for the Study of Bioethical Issues; through the Department of Bioethics at the National Institutes of Health; through appearances on MSNBC, Fox News, and NPR; and through the research underpinning books and movies whose viewers number in the millions and that go on to win prestigious awards.

People talking about dying in hospitals and barbershops, in locker rooms and mosques may not have read a bioethical article or know what "bioethics" is. But their conversations have been shaped by the work that we do. The limits of our conversations as bioethicists are inseparable from the limits of our conversations as a country. They perhaps even mark the limits of *your* conversations: the intimate discussions that you have with the people you love.

The harshness of these limits has become increasingly evident. As hospice physician Ira Byock has noted, "the question of whether or not to legalize physician-assisted suicide has become a proxy for how we die." This question has come to "conscript all the legislative energy and editorial page attention . . . that might actually resolve the sorry state of dying in America."[10] For Byock, our national focus on the right to die is therefore not just analytically limiting. It is actively harmful. Byock has long been, in his words, a "combatant" in this debate. But recognizing its harmful effects and political futility, he is choosing to abstain now, instead focusing on "constructive policies" that cut across the right-to-die divide.[11]

Byock is right. But before we can set the right-to-die debate aside, we must first examine why it has so monopolized our attention. I argue that this monopoly is due to our conflation of "assisted suicide" with the most enduring ideal of American national identity: freedom. This conflation saps much of our political energy and obscures the broad range of factors relevant to the freedom of dying people. One such factor is the gap between hospice requirements and the capacities of US families. But we cannot consider this gap to be relevant to freedom until we rethink freedom at the end of life.

The problem is not that the right to die represents a freedom that is too radical. On the contrary, the freedom of physician-assisted suicide is nowhere near radical enough.

Here, I attempt to radicalize the US debate about freedom at the end of life. But by "radicalize," I do not mean just dramatically change. I also use the term in its original meaning: to return to the root. By looking beyond the right to die, we can gain a better understanding of and have a deeper commitment to what we in the United States mean when we talk about freedom at the end of life, freedom in general, and indeed America itself. I begin with the issue that, more than any other, frames our right-to-die discussion: physician-assisted suicide.

What Is Physician-Assisted Suicide?

Physician-assisted suicide (PAS) is a form of voluntarily ending one's life with medical assistance. A medical doctor provides a prescription for a fatal drug to a patient who has requested it. The doctor does not administer this drug. Instead, the patient takes it—or elects not to take it at all. Any lethal action comes from the patient directly and from the physician only indirectly.[12]

This is not how doctors generally treat requests by their patients for help in ending their lives. Generally, doctors are legally and professionally obligated to prevent suicide. Any doctor who "assisted" a suicide would normally face professional condemnation and legal sanction. But in PAS, this is not the case. It is seen differently because of what is believed to be the cause of the patient's wish to die.

Patients who petition for PAS have a medical condition. Normally, the goal of a physician would be to ameliorate this condition, but in this case, the condition is incurable. This incurable medical condition, in theory, causes suffering. Because this suffering originates in an incurable medical condition, it too is surmised to be incurable. This incurable medical suffering is presumably the cause of the individual's desire to end their life through PAS.[13]

This cause changes the nature of suicidal ideation. Such ideation is no longer seen as pathological. Rather, it may be seen as rational, because it is rational to choose the absence of suffering—even via death—over its ineradicable presence. As a result, incurably ill individuals who petition for assisted suicide are not considered mentally ill. They are considered sane. Because they are sane, they are competent to make their own medical decisions, including the decision to die. Consequently, physicians can assist in realizing this decision without professional compromise. Incurable medical suffering thus provides a rationale for physicians to help suicidal patients to end their lives.[14]

This legitimization of suicidal ideation has reached such an extent that in the United States, supporters of PAS no longer refer to it as "suicide."[15] Instead, they prefer the terms "aid in dying" or "assisted death." The reasons for this language are in part for political expediency. Polls show that PAS garners more public support when it is not referred to as "suicide."[16] But there are also ideologically coherent reasons that American supporters of physician-assisted suicide reject the term.

Advocates reject the idea that those who seek PAS are *choosing* to die. In the United States, PAS is only legal for people who are dying already.[17] These people do not choose death. This "choice" is being forced on them by their fatal medical condition. Would that they could choose otherwise! To call such people suicidal is, at a basic level, incorrect. But really, it is cruel to smear as death-seeking someone who would likely give almost anything to live.

Death in terminal cases is outside of human control. It cannot be stopped by anyone, but it can be facilitated. And that is what those who seek aid in dying want. They do not *want* to die, but they are going to. They want aid in dying *faster*. This aid is not the cause of death. The cause of death, rather, remains the individual's terminal disease. Deaths that follow aid in dying are thus as "natural" as any other.[18] Their cause is not suicide, but nature itself.

I sympathize with these arguments against the word "suicide." But in this book, I use the term "physician-assisted suicide." This term should in no way diminish the ability of someone to support this practice. On the contrary, the vast majority of arguments for PAS explicitly refer to it as "suicide."[19] At the same time, utilizing the term "aid in dying" undermines the arguments of opponents of PAS, who begin with the premise that the practice is a form of suicide.[20] It is perhaps impossible to make an argument against aid in dying if one supports the use of that term; by accepting the legitimacy of the term "aid in dying," one concedes the very point of debate. "Physician-assisted suicide," in contrast, is a term that has consistently been used by both supporters and opponents of the practice. It is thus more ideologically neutral. Since my intention is not to take sides in this debate—but to move beyond it—a more neutral term is appropriate.

The practice of PAS exists in relationship to two other medical interventions: voluntary active euthanasia (VAE) and the withdrawal of life-sustaining treatment (WLST). In VAE, the medical professional kills an incurably ill individual who has given consent.[21] In WLST, the medical professional removes the patient from the medical technology that was keeping them alive.[22] Together, VAE, PAS, and WLST form a spectrum of options for individuals who wish to end their lives in response to an incurable illness.

What defines this spectrum is the degree to which medical providers cause death. Voluntary active euthanasia is on the radical end because such providers are death's *direct cause*.[23] Withdrawal of life-sustaining treatment is on the conservative end of the spectrum because the cause of death is not considered to be the medical provider, but rather the underlying disease entity. Physician-assisted suicide occupies a midway point between these options: the medical provider causes death only indirectly; its direct cause is the patient.

This midway point has been the focus of our country's deliberation of the right to die. There are no substantial debates in the United States about the legalization of VAE; indeed, prominent PAS organizations emphasize that this is not their goal.[24] And there are no moves to ban WLST—even by those who argue that the practice is routinely abused.[25] Our debates, rather, are about PAS.

These debates persist in part because they have legal consequences. The US Supreme Court has elected neither to ban PAS nor to legalize it throughout the country.[26] Instead it has left the decision up to individual states. This has converted each state into a battleground in which PAS advocates and opponents discuss the merits and demerits of the practice. Such debates frequently focus on freedom.[27] This might be surprising since what I have described thus far is a medical procedure—one that holds no intrinsic relationship to that term. I now explain why its proponents consider this procedure to be a representative of "freedom" both in America and in general.

Freedom—to Its Ultimate Extent

Physician-assisted suicide "is a simple expression of respect for human freedom," claims theologian Ronald Green.[28] A "terminally ill person has a fundamental liberty to choose to die with the assistance of a physician," writes political scientist Howard Ball.[29] "Denying mentally capable individuals the right to end their lives in a peaceful manner is a denial of their individual rights to self-determination and freedom of choice," argues journalist Rafia Zakaria.[30] Such claims have been echoed by others, ranging from professional PAS activists to prominent legal and political philosophers.[31]

The argument for PAS as an expression of human freedom depends on the following claim: the fundamental nature of freedom is *personal autonomy*, or the ability of the individual to control their own life.[32] What this means in practice is that the state cannot prohibit individuals from taking certain actions unless those actions will harm *others*.[33] Individuals are free to harm themselves. Smoking a cigarette may be harmful to me, but so long as I am not hurting others—for example, through secondhand smoke—I am free to puff.[34]

In the United States, however, there are certain limitations placed on this freedom. Some substances—such as heroin—are considered to be so harmful that they are considered fair justifications for limiting personal autonomy. But even such restrictions are considered limitations *on freedom*.[35] As such, they reinforce an understanding of freedom *as* personal autonomy. This conception of freedom is widely held in modern liberal democracies, which generally give individuals in the private sphere significant latitude to make their own decisions regarding such matters as family, career, leisure, and, yes, medicine. It has a particularly high value in the United States.[36]

Such freedom has generally *not* been extended, however, to the right of an individual to take their own life. Suicide has typically been prohibited or, at the very least, discouraged, whether by medical, legal, or cultural means—or some combination of all three.[37] The suicidal individual has been seen as the ward of the state, a medical doctor, or their local community. But they typically have not been given governance over themselves—until now. That is the claim of PAS advocates. Their argument is that PAS represents a radical realization of the individual's self-governance.[38] An individual can do whatever they want with their own life—including even ending it—and can do so without the impediment of others. In this sense, PAS represents a kind of culmination of democracy. It gives the individual citizen the most radical form of power in a political order: the power to inflict death. But by limiting this power to the individual's own body, PAS ensures that it will in no way impinge on the freedom of anyone else. Physician-assisted suicide, from this perspective, is a simple win-win.

But for its supporters, PAS does not just extend the incurably ill individual's freedom of choice. It liberates them from a situation that PAS advocates consider to be lacking in freedom.

Escape from Hell

The Spanish author Ramón Sampedro was a quadriplegic. He was also an advocate for what he called "euthanasia" but which coheres with the definition that I have given here of physician-assisted suicide. He published a best-selling book making his argument for this practice, and his life story was made into the Oscar-winning movie *The Sea Inside* (Mar Adentro).[39]

Like most PAS advocates, Sampedro made his claim based on a language of "freedom." In part, this freedom was based in his ability to make decisions about his own life, but in part it was a response to his condition. Sampedro referred to his paralyzed body as "hell." As an inhabitant of hell, he had no freedom—no ability to move on his own, to follow his own desires—just a life of seemingly incurable dependence. Assisted suicide was his freedom, in part, because it was an escape from this unfree state. "Whoever commits suicide," he wrote, "does so because they desire to free themselves from hell."[40]

Sampedro's interpretation of his predicament is not uncommon. In fact, 92.4 percent of terminally ill individuals in the state of Oregon—where PAS has been legal since 1997—petition for PAS because they fear the loss of their "autonomy."[41] They believe that their biological condition takes away their control over their body and their lives. They do not just want freedom *from* dying. Dying itself has rendered them unfree.

The idea that illness and disability are constraining is arguably the premise of medicine. People show up at the doctor's office because their body is behaving in a way that they do not want. Their suffering and pain are indications of this loss of control and also its result. By alleviating it, medicine allows them to regain governance over their bodies. Medicine therefore can be said to promote freedom, if one accepts the definition of freedom that has been used in the PAS debate: control over our body.

This understanding goes against the way that medicine and freedom are typically understood in scholarly discussions of their relationship. In such discussions, freedom is considered to be the ability to make our own decisions about medicine.[42] The medical treatment itself does not, in this view, increase or decrease our liberty. Academic discussions thus understand medicine and freedom to be separate entities without any inherent relationship.

But this scholarly framing of the relationship between medicine and freedom, whatever its merits, is removed from the justifications provided by advocates for the right to die. Such advocates do not consider autonomy as just the ability to make medical decisions. They consider it as the ability to control their bodies in a more general sense. From such a perspective, illness is inherently opposed to freedom, and medicine, by removing it, is a vehicle of freedom. Medicine in this view is inherently and primarily free*ing.* The ability to make decisions about medical treatment is secondary, an extension of the fundamental freedom given by medicine itself.

The problem, it would seem, is that medicine cannot free everyone. Many disabilities and illnesses cannot be cured. People with them are trapped in a state that appears to be—and is often experienced by them as—one of diminished liberty. And there seems no way for them to be freer—except for PAS. Physician-assisted suicide is thus, for its supporters, less a free choice than a choice that frees. This choice, in turn, transforms death from freedom's antithesis into its peak. This is a powerful argument. But it is also one that has been subjected to substantial critique. Often, critics concede that PAS increases human freedom, but they argue that this freedom should be limited.[43] I do not address such arguments here. Instead, I focus on a group of scholars who argue that PAS is not freedom at all—in fact, it is the opposite. These scholars belong to a field called disability studies.

No Freedom amid Discriminatory Double Standards

Not everyone can petition for physician-assisted suicide. It is not available for people who are sad following the breakup of a romantic relationship. Nor can a person receive aid in dying if they find themselves unemployed or broke, not even if they do not have any real prospects of a sustainable financial future. There are many reasons that one might want to die, but PAS supporters do not imply that giving *anyone* the right to die for *any* reason would be freeing. Instead, the "freedom" of PAS is constrained: in general, it is limited to just those who are incurably ill; in the United States, it is limited specifically to those who are dying. This constraint has been cheered by proponents of PAS as proof that they are not encouraging suicidal ideation or provoking a move down a "slippery slope."[44] But this very limitation of PAS creates another problem, one that calls into question whether it is really freedom at all.

I call this argument the "discriminatory double standard": the application of a distinct—and generally inferior—standard to the members of one particular population group is, in essence, discriminatory.[45] Such double standards are in no sense freeing. Rather, they indicate that the people subjected to them are less free: their actions are limited in a way that does not apply to other population groups. They do not have free choice. They are rather *denied* the same treatment that is given to everyone else.

This is not a difficult concept for most Americans to understand. Indeed, it is the bedrock of our legal concept of discrimination, as well as popular understandings of it. When we create distinct water fountains for black people and white people, distinct expectations of job performance for women and men, or distinct access to marriage for heterosexuals and homosexuals—these are discriminatory double standards. They limit the freedom of the targeted group.

This argument is also easy to understand when applied to suicide. We generally consider suicide a bad thing. It is so bad that we almost always seek to prevent it. If we did not offer such basic suicide prevention to any one group, we would be discriminating against them. For example, if doctors did not treat suicidal ideation in African Americans, even as they did everything to prevent it in whites, it would seem to most people in this country to be a horrible form of bigotry. Even if we subsequently celebrated this bigotry as "freedom," it would still, in reality, be a horrific limitation of the freedom of the black people whom it impacted.

This commonsensical understanding of discrimination can be applied to the right to die. By limiting PAS to chronically disabled people and terminally ill individuals, right-to-die supporters advocate a double standard. They justify this double standard with the idea that disability and terminal illness make an individual's life less worthy of protecting. Were this belief held of practically any other population in the United States—women, Jews, blonds, homosexuals—most of us would recognize it as discriminatory. That we do not see this discrimination with regard to incurably sick and disabled people does not prove that it is reasonable. Discrimination may well seem commonsensical in societies that are deeply bigoted. That it seems so does not mean that these societies are *less* bigoted. It is, rather, proof of just how bigoted they are. From this perspective the relative acceptance of "debating" the double standard in the treatment of suicidal ideation for incurably sick people and those with disabilities is an objective indicator of their disenfranchisement. Were it any other group, such a double standard would—rightly—be outside of debate.

Some proponents of this double standard argue that there is a fundamental difference between incurable illness and the other categories: incurable illness is a medical diagnosis, unlike race, religion, or gender. Those are social categories and thus subject to discrimination. Medicine, in contrast, is objective and therefore cannot be considered discriminatory. This argument has been countered by scholars in the field of disability studies, who have most forcefully advocated seeing PAS as a discriminatory double standard. Disability studies scholars argue that medicine is not just a neutral, objective science. Rather, it both reflects and contains societal norms and value judgments. The medical classification of people into categories, such as "sick" and "disabled," is an inherently social endeavor.

This categorization does not necessarily carry the implication that the individuals who fall into these groups are less valuable, nor that they are less worthy of the protections against suicide given to everyone else. That it seemingly does so today indicates that it is in no sense objective. It is, rather, deeply social—and therefore discriminatory. That such discrimination seems natural to us does not mean that it is right. Indeed, race, gender, and religion have been—in different times and places—considered medical categories.[46] In those eras, medicine came to be used as a vehicle for and a justification of discrimination against various groups. And that, disability studies scholars argue, is what is happening to sick people and those with disabilities today.

With regard to chronically disabled people, this argument has been made most forcefully by disability studies scholars Carol Gill and Paul Longmore.[47] The philosopher Felica Ackerman has extended it to the terminally ill.[48] From this perspective, any double standard in the treatment of suicidal ideation is inherently discriminatory and should be rejected. This discrimination changes the very character of the decision to die made by the incurably ill person because it transforms the issue of *who* is making the decision to begin with.

These scholars argue that the discriminatory double standard inherently compromises the decisions made by incurably ill individuals to end their lives. Proponents of PAS argue that these decisions are the epitome of individual freedom. But the disability studies scholars say that such decisions are not individual at all. The double standard in the treatment of suicidal ideation is a social one. Making the choice to die available only to incurably ill individuals is a social decision to discriminate. Incurably ill individuals might endorse this discrimination—which is not surprising, given how pervasive and uncritically accepted it is. But this endorsement does not come from them. It comes, rather, from the society they are part of. To offer the choice to them—and only them—is to manipulate them.[49]

As a result, decisions made by individuals in this situation are not free. They are responses to discrimination that negates their freedom, discrimination inherent in the very "choice" made available, which is predicated on the denial of basic suicide prevention. Thus, from the perspective of disability studies scholars, PAS is not an extension of human freedom. On the contrary, it is an objective indicator of the extent to which the incurably ill—both terminal and chronic— are oppressed.

This critique rejects the premise of right-to-die proponents: that extending the decision to die to a targeted group of individuals is itself freeing. But disability studies scholars also criticize the other way of understanding freedom advanced by proponents of the right to die: that incurable illness or disability is a condition that is inherently unfree. Ultimately, it is their understanding of the relationship between the discriminatory double standard and the question of the freedom of incurably sick people and those with disabilities that makes their argument considerably more radical.

A "Choice" That Prolongs Unfreedom

Like PAS advocates, disability studies scholars agree that "freedom" is the ability to control our life. In part, this ability requires that individuals be able to make their own decisions, including, specifically, decisions about medicine. But freedom is also a state: the state of being unconstrained. Both PAS advocates and disability studies scholars agree that many disabled people do not live in this state. And they agree that they must be freed. But they disagree on *why* they lack freedom. Advocates of PAS argue that this lack is inherent to the medical conditions of people with disabilities. Disability studies scholars say that it is a product of US society. They argue that US society discriminates against disabled people, barring them equal access to employment, housing, basic necessities, and shared social goods.[50] This discrimination strips people with disabilities of control over their lives. Instead, they are controlled by the world in which they live.

The epitome of this control is the nursing home.[51] Nursing homes are institutions that house and care for disabled people. In them, people with disabilities are made to live according to a routine that is designed in the interests of the home's management. They are bathed, fed, and clothed according to a schedule that is not theirs. The care they receive is frequently mediocre and sometimes abusive. They cannot, in general, leave. This makes it impossible for them to work, to obtain goods and services, and to interact with nondisabled people. They are effectively segregated. In this environment, people with disabilities have no control over their lives. Their institutionalization destroys their freedom.[52]

This destruction of freedom has been movingly depicted by surgeon Atul Gawande. In *Being Mortal*, Gawande describes the life of a nursing home resident as follows: "All privacy and control were gone. She was put in hospital clothes most of the time. She woke when they told her, bathed and dressed when they told her, ate when they told her. She lived with whomever they said she had to. There was a succession of roommates, never chosen with her input and all with cognitive impairments. Some were quiet. One kept her up at night. She felt incarcerated, like she was in prison for being old."[53] Gawande goes on to refer to nursing homes as "total institutions." This term was used by the sociologist Erving Goffman to describe a broad range of institutions that destroy the freedom of their inhabitants, including insane asylums and prisons. Goffman also considered nursing homes to be among their number—and Gawande agrees.[54]

The disability rights activist Harriet McBryde Johnson considered nursing homes to be a part of what she called "America's disability gulag."[55] The language that Gawande uses is more measured, but his conclusion is the same. For Gawande, nursing homes represent our collective acquiescence "to a belief that, once you lose your physical independence, a life of worth and freedom is simply not possible."[56]

Gawande is not affiliated with disability studies. But his work is very valuable to the field. It shows that one does not have to be a disability studies scholar or some radical activist in order to accept the arguments that these scholars and advocates make. All we need to do is enter the facilities where we keep disabled people—to look around and breathe.[57]

Freedom can be a scarce commodity even for those disabled people who live outside of the nursing home's walls. Disabled people routinely encounter barriers that prevent them from accessing shared social goods. These barriers can be physical: the lack of accessible sidewalks, buildings, public transportation, and schools. They can also be interpersonal: negative attitudes about people with disabilities that manifest in hate speech, dirty looks, employment rejections, and even violence. Frequently, they are both. The result can be just as limiting to the freedom of disabled people as the institutional segregation of the nursing home.[58]

To live in a highly constraining society impacts one's tendency toward suicide. Specifically, it *increases* it, making such individuals more likely to take their lives. The lack of freedom that they experience in daily life leads them to want to die soon. This is true of a variety of populations, including soldiers, women, immigrants, and racial minorities.[59] And it is true of disabled people as well.[60] Some disabled people want to end their lives because, given the lack of freedom they experience in US society, they feel that they have no better options. A decision to die, in this context, is not free. It is, in the words of psychologist Carol Gill, a "forced choice."[61] Further, for researchers like Gill, PAS is not *just* a choice without freedom. It is a choice that obscures the very reason that disabled people are not free. A premise of the right to die is that people seek it because of their incurable medical conditions. But, according to disability studies scholars, this is not true. Disabled people are deprived of freedom, but the source of this deprivation is not their medical condition. It is the society in which they—and we—live. Rather than change that society, however, the right to die destroys people with disabilities, and it does so in the name of freedom.

The claim that PAS extends freedom is a lie. But people believe it. Because they believe it, they also believe that disabled people are unfree *inherently*. This belief, in turn, leads them to ignore the society that destroys the freedom of people with disabilities. This avoidance allows the destruction to go on. The freedom to die thus contributes to—and arguably epitomizes—the lack of freedom among people with disabilities. It is not only an unfree choice. It is a choice that itself prolongs unfreedom.

In this sense, it is not sufficient to point out that PAS is based on a discriminatory double standard. Physician-assisted suicide does not just apply a distinct—and lesser—standard of suicide prevention to one population. That in itself would negate their freedom, but the reality, from a disability studies perspective, is much worse. From that perspective, PAS applies a lesser standard of suicide prevention to a population that is unusually already at risk for suicide *because they lack freedom*. But rather than recognize and ameliorate this lack of freedom, PAS seeks to eliminate disabled people and to call this elimination the summit of "freedom."

PAS as a Disability Right

Contrary to what I have just presented, there is no uniform disability studies perspective on PAS. In general, the field has been highly skeptical of it. Yet, since the 1990s there have been disability studies scholars who have argued that PAS is not itself threatening to people with disabilities. Indeed, it might be a fundamental disability right. These scholars—such as Lennard Davis and Andrew Batavia—have sought to distinguish between PAS for disabled people and for terminally ill people. They argue that terminal illness generally involves much more significant physical symptoms than chronic disability: for example, extreme physical pain coupled with a rapid escalation of debilitating medical conditions.[62] This makes terminal illness qualitatively different from—and more severe than—chronic disability.

These pro-PAS disability studies scholars do not deny that terminal illness provokes both disability as well as fears of disability. But they argue that the shortened lifespan of dying people leaves them with insufficient time to change their negative views about disability. To ban PAS in such cases is to condemn these individuals to suffering that, though social in part, is functionally incurable. To ignore such distinctions is to fail to acknowledge the specific needs of dying people. It is also a failure to acknowledge the safeguards against disability discrimination that have been included in US right-to-die legislation. The distinction between chronic disability and terminal illness is one such safeguard. There is no evidence, since the passage of the Oregon Death with Dignity Act, of PAS being extended to chronically disabled people.[63]

For terminally ill people who are eligible for PAS, there are procedures to ensure that the individual is of sound mind and is not making a decision in response to familial manipulation. Finally, because the terminally ill patient must take the fatal substance themself, PAS protects individuals from being put to death against their will. Such safeguards are, for disability studies supporters of PAS, sufficient to ensure that the practice is not a manifestation of disability discrimination.[64]

Because of the existence of the safeguards, disability studies scholars who support PAS argue that the act is a genuine reflection of freedom. The decisions made by terminally ill people to end their lives may take place in a context of disability discrimination, but this discrimination is not sufficient, given the safeguards in place, to nullify their freedom to choose to die. Thus, disability studies opponents of PAS are going against a central tenet of the disability rights movement: disabled people should have control over their own medical decisions.[65]

Restricting terminally ill people's control over their own medical decisions is bad in itself. But it also risks provoking another kind of slippery slope. Taking away the freedom to make medical decisions from dying people establishes a precedent, which justifies limiting the power that people have over their medical treatment. This precedent might, with time, be extended to people with chronic disabilities—curtailing their own freedom to decide. This would be, from any disability studies perspective, catastrophic. Protecting disability rights thus requires affirming the legitimacy of PAS.[66]

For the most part, disability studies scholars who advocate for PAS have stopped at this point: supporting the practice for the dying, but opposing it for disabled people. But there are some who have argued that this is not enough. To be truly consistent with disability rights, they claim, the right to die must be extended to disabled people themselves.[67]

Such advocates do not deny the prevalence of disability discrimination in US society as a whole and with regard to the right to die. But this discrimination is not sufficient to—and perhaps *cannot* be sufficient to—overrule individual freedom. Freedom is such a core value of disability rights that it is effectively inalienable. This means supporting PAS even when disabled people seek it, even when their doing so is, in some way, a response to disability discrimination. It means, at a basic level, supporting the choices of disabled people to do what they want with their lives, even if their choices are products of a society that devalues them in numerous ways. This is what freedom for people with disabilities means— and PAS is, for these thinkers, a part of it.

The Conversation We Need to Have

So far, we are at an impasse. From a disability studies perspective, there are coherent arguments in favor of PAS and also coherent arguments against it. These views both base their claims on the putative relationship of PAS to the freedom of people with disabilities. It may be possible to resolve this stalemate through some form of argument, but instead I want to highlight what the focus by disability studies scholars on this impasse obscures.

There are disability studies scholars who argue that PAS is an extension of the freedom of disabled people. There are disability studies scholars who argue that PAS is the antithesis of that freedom. But no disability studies scholar claims that either allowing—or for that matter banning—PAS would be sufficient to give disabled people their freedom. On the contrary, PAS is a minor, if contentious, topic in a much broader conversation about what "freedom" for people with disabilities means.

For the most part, this conversation is based in agreement. Disability studies scholars agree that to be free, people with disabilities need access to jobs, to health care, to education, to communal activities, to the voting booth. Do they also need access to PAS? Maybe. Maybe not. When discussing the freedom of people who are disabled, it seems obvious that this is not the most important issue.

And yet, disability studies scholars have not applied this same logic to people who are dying. On the contrary, when disability studies scholars talk about dying people they do so, for the most part, *solely* through the lens of PAS. This has created the false impression—already too widely held in our country—that the right to die is the most important and perhaps the *only* way to talk about freedom at the end of life. This is both unfortunate and unnecessary, since disability studies, more than perhaps any other field, has within it the capacity to expand this conversation's terms.

All it would require is to look at the freedom of dying people the way that disability studies scholars look at the freedom of people with disabilities. Perhaps PAS is an extension of the freedom of dying people. Or maybe it is not. Either way, this matter is peripheral to the topic of freedom itself. There are questions that are bigger and more relevant: How free are dying Americans? And how can we make them freer?

These are questions that we can all ponder, and we can do so without necessarily considering the right to die. In fact, including the right to die in this inquiry might be counterproductive. The topic divides us. Once it is mentioned, it tends to suck the air right out of the room, making it difficult to talk about anything else. By setting it aside—at least for the moment—we might find that there are other things relevant to the freedom of dying people that we might talk about and many matters on which we might agree.

A better starting place than the right to die is hospice, which is the dominant site in America for end-of-life care. From a disability studies perspective, such a site is highly relevant to freedom since, to a great extent, it is in the individual's environment that freedom exists. *How* hospice is relevant to freedom is precisely what I am exploring here.

But there is a problem. Hospice professionals are themselves locked in a heated debate about freedom at the end of life. And this debate—like that of disability studies scholars and our country as a whole—focuses on physician-assisted suicide.

Hospice as Freedom—or Perhaps Its Lack

Since the origins of hospice in America, hospice professionals have been involved in the discussion of freedom at the end of life. Their participation in this conversation has spanned all of the practices considered part of the right to die. But a particular focus, at least since the legalization of the practice in Oregon, has been PAS. For the most part, hospice professionals have been critical of PAS. This critical orientation is, to an extent, a product of the very definition of what hospice does.

As I described above, supporters of PAS argue that dying people suffer incurably because of the incurable nature of their disease. This incurable suffering is the only justification for PAS. After all, if their suffering *could* be cured by nonlethal means, that would seem to be vastly preferable. The result is a necessary linkage in pro-PAS arguments between incurable suffering and terminal disease.

Hospice challenges this linkage at a fundamental level. Hospice is a form of palliative care for dying people. As such, it concedes the impossibility of curing an individual's terminal disease, but it attacks the idea that the suffering that accompanies such a condition is incurable. On the contrary, suffering can be alleviated to a tremendous extent. The entire purpose of hospice is to work toward this alleviation.

This raises a question about those dying individuals who do seek PAS. If the suffering that these people experience could be effectively treated with hospice care, then why would they seek PAS? The answer given by many hospice advocates is that these people's suffering is *not* being effectively treated.[68] They are receiving inadequate end-of-life care.

The result is a distinct view of what causes suicidal ideation among dying individuals. Suicidal ideation in this view is not a natural product of a terminal disease. Nor is it a response to disability oppression. It is rather a response to a lack in hospice itself. If there were better hospice care available, then terminally ill individuals would not suffer so greatly—and therefore they would not want to die.

This argument undermines the idea that PAS is "freedom" in any sense. Rather, the desire for death is a response to a denial of basic health care. This response is rational to the extent that this denial does inflict horrendous suffering. But it is irrational in that it neither recognizes nor alleviates the suffering's actual cause. Advocates for physician-assisted suicide are not primarily pleading for better hospice. What they want instead is their freedom to die.

The resulting view of PAS is not identical to that of disability studies scholars who oppose the practice, but it is highly compatible. Both hospice professionals and disability studies scholars see PAS as a response to social deprivation. Both see it as reinforcing this deprivation. But just as there are disability studies scholars who counter this narrative, there are American hospice professionals who advocate for PAS.

These professionals argue that there are limits to what hospice can do.[69] Hospice workers can spare patients much of the suffering that accompanies dying, but they cannot always spare them all of it. And sometimes, even with good hospice care, dying people suffer a lot. In those cases, it is appropriate for a hospice physician to offer patients the option of PAS. Physician-assisted suicide is consistent with hospice's goal of alleviating patient suffering. It is also consistent with hospice's traditional respect for the patient's freedom of choice. As a result, PAS should not be viewed as the antithesis of hospice but rather as simply one more tool in the hospice physician's medical bag.

This is a good debate. But it suffers from the same flaw as the more general debate about PAS. It views PAS as the sole rubric through which to explore freedom at the end of life. Because of this, it does not consider that individuals in hospice may have their freedom limited by issues that have nothing to do with the right to die. More specifically, it does not consider the possibility that US hospice care itself may be one of those issues. But perhaps it is. This possibility is attested to by hospice professionals themselves. Hospice professionals in America have always been supportive of hospice—and they have understood their support to include criticism of our current hospice system's flaws (see chapter 3).[70] This is true of both professionals who support PAS and those who oppose it. There is thus a broad and refreshing willingness in the hospice community to reflect critically on their own model of care.

Hospice advocates would be aided in their critical reflection by a fuller engagement with the field of disability studies. Disability studies can give hospice proponents a fuller picture of how the US hospice system impacts the freedom of people who are dying. At the same time, an engagement with hospice might help disability studies scholars to further refine their own views. The resulting relationship would be mutually beneficial. It will also be beneficial to us, if we are to have an adequate understanding in America of freedom at the end of life. Such an understanding can only be had by applying a disability studies analysis to the conditions of dying Americans.

Understanding freedom in hospice, in turn, requires tweaking aspects of disability studies. Disability studies is a field that has focused, for the most part, on institutions. Its privileged object of critique is the nursing home. Yet while nursing homes are often sites for the delivery of hospice care, they are not part of the hospice system itself.

Hospice in America is a predominantly home-based benefit. This does not mean that it provides a necessarily liberating environment for the terminally ill. It does mean that studying it requires a different analytic than a standard disability studies approach, which because of its focus on institutions, has generally considered the home to be an inherently liberating space.[71] The resulting bias could be problematic, but it does not have to be. Disability studies scholars do not just call for deinstitutionalization.[72] Rather, they call for deinstitutionalization plus the provision of accessible environments and home-based long-term care. The "home" for them is not by itself enough. A disability studies perspective demands the services necessary to make the home a site where freedom can be enjoyed.

This raises the question of the relationship of hospice to the long-term care necessary to keep dying individuals at home. In America, such care is predominantly provided by the family, as I have mentioned. A disability studies perspective on freedom at the end of life must focus on the relationship between familial caregiving and hospice.

This perspective allows me to return to the topic with which I began this chapter: the gap between hospice requirements and the requisite level of familial care. This gap is no longer a side note in an account of freedom that focuses almost entirely on the right to die. The right to die instead becomes the side note. This is not just a new approach to freedom at the end of life. It is one that is significantly more liberating than its predecessor.

Expanding Freedom, Limiting Debate

Unlike most PAS proponents, Ann Neumann seriously considers the critique raised by disability studies scholars.[73] She dedicates an entire chapter of her book to an exploration of how disability discrimination might impact dying people who seek to end their lives. Nevertheless, other PAS proponents are dismissive. The disability studies critique is, for them, underpinned by paternalism. These critics, including some in the field, argue that disability studies scholars want to make decisions for others and to limit the decisions that people can make.[74] The resulting implication is that disability studies scholars are, in some sense, *against freedom* at the end of life.

This critique is incorrect. In fact, disability studies scholars seek to give dying people *more* choices than they currently have and to remove them from environments that destroy their freedom. They in no sense seek to limit the freedom of dying people. Rather, their goal is to expand freedom in a manner much more radical than that proposed by advocates for PAS.

The death of her father led Neumann to wonder whether he should have been given the option of PAS. This is a fair question—and it is relevant to freedom, even from a disability studies perspective. But it is not the only question. A disability studies approach to dying opens up a range of questions that are not asked by the vast majority of commentators on the right-to-die debate. These questions are, at a minimum, *as* relevant to freedom as the question of whether a dying person would want access to PAS. Indeed, I believe that their relevance is far greater.

Does the person dying want access to higher potency pain medicine?

Does the person dying want access to an inpatient hospice that is closer to their home?

Does the dying person want their home to be made more accessible via interventions such as ramps and fall prevention, so that they can stay in it longer as they become increasingly disabled?

Do they prefer to have their intimate care carried out by a paid professional or by members of their family?

Do they want their children to have to leave their jobs to care for them?

Do they want to be placed in a situation that would—systemically, predictably—make them more likely to inflict physical violence on their children while in a demented state?

Do they want their children to be traumatized not just by their death, but by the *way* that they died?

These are just some of the questions that a disability studies perspective makes possible. The right to die should be one of these questions, but its smallness is conspicuous. Disability studies, then, is a field that expands the questions that we can ask about the end of life. These questions are just as central to the freedom of dying people as that of PAS. Indeed, they are more central. They focus on the very factors that might, conceivably, impel dying people to take their lives. And they would be relevant regardless of whether dying people had any interest in doing so. A disability studies approach thus expands the freedom of dying people and grounds our discussion of this freedom in what matters most.

Whether this approach also expands our debate is debatable. Few people would debate any of the questions that I listed above. Even if they did, these differences of opinion would be due to factors so idiosyncratic and personal that they would not be appropriate for a national discussion. In fact, the questions I listed are not really questions for "debate" in that the answers are already broadly shared.

Thus, these questions do not likely divide us—bioethicists, families, patients, and care providers—into opposing camps. Rather, they are the kinds of questions that could unite us, even if our positions differ on the particular topic of the right to die. They are questions, in a sense, that "limit" debate by creating consensus. But consensus does not in fact limit debate. Instead, it makes it possible to have *better* debates about the topics that really matter. How to construct a hospice system that does not traumatize our children, for example, is a good question, one that we should vigorously discuss. But we cannot have such valuable debates until we set aside the right to die.

I now continue on to a matter that is much more important to freedom at the end of life: the gap, identified in part by Ann Neumann, between the requirements of hospice and the abilities of American families. By examining how this gap came to exist we can better consider how to ameliorate it. Such a question is a matter of freedom at the end of life—and it reveals additional questions that are worthy of our collective discussion.

CHAPTER TWO

Depending on the Family

By the time that Cicely Saunders met David Tasma, it was arguably too late. It was London, England, in 1948, and Tasma was dying of cancer. Having been unable to remain at home, he had been transferred to a hospital.[1] There, he resided in a surgical ward, even though he was not fit for surgery. His nurses attended, to the best of their abilities, to his nausea and his pain.[2] But there seemed little for Tasma to do—except wait for death's arrival.

But Cicely Saunders thought otherwise. Saunders was the social worker assigned to Tasma. Over the course of twenty-five meetings, she learned about his life. He was a Polish Jew who had migrated from the Warsaw ghetto.[3] His family was not present: his mother had died, and his father was either dead or elsewhere. David Tasma was thus not only dying. He was dying alone. Saunders could not prevent his death. But she could, she came to realize, do something: provide him with care and company that would make his remaining time much better than it otherwise would have been.[4]

Saunders and Tasma became quite close. Through their relationship, she discovered something about herself. She wanted to care for people like David Tasma: people who were dying. More than providing care, she wanted to give them a home, a place just for them in a healthcare system that was otherwise hostile. Nineteen years after her initial encounter with Tasma, she accomplished this goal with the opening of St. Christopher's Hospice in London.[5] And thus the modern hospice movement was born: from an act of caring by a relative stranger for a dying man without a family of his own.[6]

The family has always been central to hospice. Hospice began with the premise that even a person without a family should not die alone. But when families are present, it has incorporated them into care to a much greater degree than have other medical specialties. Today, the family is referred to as a "unit" of care, on par with the dying person.[7] As such, family members receive care from the moment their relative enrolls in hospice to even months after their death. But families not only *receive* care. They are also encouraged to *give* it to their dying relatives. This use of familial caregivers has been a feature of the modern hospice movement since its origins.[8] But it has manifested differently depending on where the hospice is located.

This chapter examines the way that family caregiving was incorporated into the first modern hospice organization in the United States: Hospice Inc. To a significant extent, Hospice Inc. is the originator of the hospice system we have today, so by studying it, we can gain a better idea of why we have this system.

The Broken Family of British Hospice Care

The British hospice movement began with the story of a broken family. This breakdown was caused by the Second World War. Over the course of the war, many of David Tasma's family members had been murdered by the Nazis.[9] Those who survived, like Tasma himself, were geographically dislocated, cast about a continent that had been ruined. In this context, Tasma's story was in some ways idiosyncratic, but in others it was representative. Tasma was Jewish and a refugee. But both at home and at the front lines, British families were recovering from breakdowns of their own.

There were 388,000 British people killed during the war.[10] Those who survived had to deal with trauma. English children, for example, had been removed from their families and sent to bomb shelters. British psychoanalysts such as John Bowlby and Donald Winnicott made their careers examining the impact of such disrupted early attachments.[11] Women had worked outside the home during the war, and many were not eager to return to their "traditional" roles as full-time caregivers.[12] And the family's very identity as caregiver for the sick— and the dying—seemed to have been usurped by the establishment of the National Health Service.[13]

This was the British family that Cicely Saunders had inherited when she began to formulate a plan for end-of-life care: a family that was, by most accounts, physically, mentally, emotionally, and culturally in tatters. Such a family did not seem to be one that could care for its dying. And in 1952, a study appeared that provided compelling evidence that it was failing at this task. The study was conducted by the Joint National Cancer Survey Committee of the Marie Curie Memorial Foundation and the Queen's Institute of District Nursing. Researchers visited more than 7,000 cancer patients who were being cared for at home by their relatives. Their findings were grim. Caring for sick relatives inflicted "considerable hardship" on families.[14] Insufficient familial caregiving left the sick suffering from social isolation and untreated physical pain.[15] The reasons for the deficiencies that the study found were debated, but its findings provided ample evidence that British families were unable to care for their dying relatives.[16]

The British hospice movement founded by Saunders was, in part, a response to this evidence. Saunders was critical of the care of dying people in hospitals run by the National Health Service.[17] But she also knew that it would not be possible to return them to their homes. Even families who were willing to provide care lacked the ability to do so; others lacked the willingness. The family was to be nurtured, but it could not provide the basis of British hospice care.

This knowledge influenced Saunders's decision to include the family as a unit of care. Saunders believed that most patients preferred to be cared for by their family members, but she also recognized that for most family members, providing such care was extremely difficult. Thus, a key aspect of hospice would be providing the family with support. This would help family members with their grief and with their caregiving. The need for such support was so great that it infused hospice's very form.

This form was interdisciplinary.[18] Hospice needed to include medical care as well as psychological, social, and spiritual support. Such interdisciplinary care was, in part, a response to the needs of dying patients.[19] But it was also an acknowledgment of the needs of the family. In hospice, family members would themselves receive spiritual and psychosocial care, which would allow them to work through the conflicts they felt about caring for their relative.[20] This support would make them better able to provide care and better able to cope after their relative's death.

For Saunders, the ideal location of hospice delivery was the home. But she recognized that, given the state of British families, home care would not be a feasible option for many dying people. For this reason, among others, she founded St. Christopher's as an inpatient facility. A home hospice service only came two years later in 1969.[21] Even in the inpatient context, Saunders still considered the family to have an essential role.

The limits of British families shaped even Saunders's understanding of terminal disease. She saw death as an event that could heal broken families. Its finality would lead family members to see past grievances as petty. Such disputes would seem minor compared with the loss of a family member forever. In this sense, terminal disease did not destroy the family. It could—and should—unite them. For this reason, Saunders, paraphrasing a patient, referred to cancer as a "bringing-together illness" that united formerly divided families.[22]

But if death was to bring families together, it could only do so in the context of proper care. Hospice would provide this context. Through its supportive care, hospice would make it possible for both patients and families to appreciate the finality of death. It would bring together families that had previously been splintered. Hospice was thus not only a method of caring for patients from broken families, it was also a way of healing the family that had been broken prior to the onset of terminal disease.

If such healing was to happen, the family could not provide the bulk of care. Hospice could not depend on the family. It was the family that would depend on hospice—and, through such dependence, become whole again. Hospice leaders in the United States shared Saunders's desire to improve the situations of dying patients and their families, but their thinking about the family was different, and this difference impacted their model of end-of-life care.

The Supportive Family of US Hospice Care

The generally accepted beginning of the modern US hospice movement was the visit of Cicely Saunders to Yale University in 1963.[23] Though Saunders had not yet founded St. Christopher's, she had been writing for years about the need to develop a new form of end-of-life care, and she gave a talk on the subject during her visit. That talk was attended by Florence Wald, dean of the Yale School of Nursing. Smitten by what she was hearing, Wald decided to examine how Saunders's insights might apply to US end-of-life care.[24]

Wald conducted research over the following years. Based on this research, she argued that there was a need in the United States to develop a specialized form of care for dying people.[25] She formed a network of collaborators and sought to implement this vision. This effort led to the creation of the first modern US hospice, Hospice Inc., in 1971.[26] Wald and her colleagues referred to their care as "hospice" because they considered it a continuation of Saunders's efforts in England. But though they considered the British hospice movement to be a model, they differed from it in important ways.

Like Saunders, US hospice leaders believed that there was no place for dying people in the existing system of hospital care. Hospitals in the United States were oriented around acute care. They had not developed basic resources to attend to the needs of dying people. And the rise of new medical technologies had made it possible to prolong life for a period of time that seemed endless. Patients dying in the hospital context were thus given care that was, at best, ineffective and, at worst, harmful.

British and US hospice leaders differed, however, on the role that the family should play in hospice. For Saunders, the British family was part of the problem. The family was broken, and the 1952 Joint National Cancer Survey Committee study had shown that, as bad as the situation was in hospitals, dying patients were receiving equally insufficient treatment in their homes. The goal of hospice was thus not just to replace the medical system but to repair the family as well. But there was no equivalent of the 1952 study in the US context, and US hospice leaders did not consider deficient familial caretaking to be a major problem. Rather, they thought that the central problem of US end-of-life care was the *removal* of dying people from the familial home.

They understood this removal to be a defining event in the history of end-of-life care. Edward Dobihal, the president of Hospice Inc., wrote in a 1975 pamphlet describing the organization's philosophy: "In primitive and pre-industrial societies, death occurred most often in the home or other familiar surroundings, with little interruption of family, tribal, and community life beyond the ritualized celebrations of life's passage. With our advanced science and technology, we have made death a solitary, mechanized, inhuman, and often gruesome picture."[27] Prior to the advent of the field of medicine, the dying person remained integrated in the family and community; as a result, death formed a part of life and was an expression of self. But "advanced science and technology" separated the dying individual from their family. In the process, it made death into an event that was "solitary, mechanized, inhuman." The separation of death from the family was a historical trauma to which hospice was responding.

But the removal of death from the family was not just an event of the past. It was reenacted in the present. By their very nature as institutions, hospitals and nursing homes removed patients from the familial home. The geographic removal inherent to such facilities was compounded by their internal design. Writing in 1972, hospice leaders noted that treatments in hospitals "too often engross the patient and staff[,] leaving out the family."[28] This exclusion was considered a product of authoritarian doctors and impersonal machines, as well as of restrictive visiting hours and cramped rooms.[29] It was not incidental, but routine. This separation of dying people from their families was thus for hospice leaders a systemic characteristic of US end-of-life care.

Changing this dynamic required shifting the location of care. End-of-life care should not, hospice leaders believed, take place in institutions. It should take place at home. But home care depended on the presence of a supportive family. This was a hospice requirement. All patients, to be enrolled in the home care program, had to have a supportive family member at home.[30] Thus, hospice practice was premised from the beginning on the existence of familial caregiving. Hospice Inc.'s leaders supported this premise because, in general, they assumed that such caregivers existed. They considered the fundamental problem in US end-of-life care to be medicine, not the family. Hospice Inc.'s leaders believed that families would be able to carry out the needed care and would, in general, view it as a privilege rather than a burden.

Like Cicely Saunders, US hospice leaders did recognize that contemporary families had limitations. Such limitations were in large part why they considered the family to be both a provider and a *recipient* of care. Hospice Inc.'s leaders depended on families for care, but they also knew that caring for a dying relative could take a terrible toll. For this reason, families needed access to psychological and spiritual support, which was provided by trained mental health professionals and chaplains, respectively.[31] They also needed aid from volunteers, who could assist them with routine tasks that fell outside of their competence.[32] Indeed, as was the case with the British hospice movement, a recognition of the needs of families was one of the reasons that US leaders formulated hospice as an interdisciplinary treatment modality to begin with.[33]

Hospice Inc.'s leaders also recognized that there were some situations in which no amount of support would be enough to keep patients under familial care. For this reason, they lobbied for the construction of an inpatient unit. This unit would care for two kinds of patients: those whose families could no longer care for them because their condition had progressed and those who had "no supporting persons available outside the Hospice."[34] The former would be short-term patients expected to die relatively soon. The latter would be long-term residents, and US hospice leaders recognized that they would need to receive substantial care outside the home.

But US hospice care was not designed with such patients in mind. Hospice Inc. based its model of care on Florence Wald's "Interdisciplinary Study of the Dying Patient." Carried out between 1969 and 1971, the study examined the extent to which the needs of dying patients could be accommodated within the existing options for US end-of-life care. Based on this research, Hospice Inc.'s leaders determined there was a need to establish a form of end-of-life care separate from the medical system. But a requirement for participation in the study was the presence of a family member who was both "concerned" and "involved" in the patient's care.[35] Thus, patients without familial support were not even included in the conception of US hospice care. They would only be added in after the fundamental tenets of hospice philosophy had already been formed.

To the extent that patients with insufficient familial support were considered, they were viewed as the exception, not the norm. Indeed, Hospice Inc. distinguished itself from other end-of-life care providers not by the quality of their inpatient care but rather by the higher percentage of patients who were able to die at home.[36] When patients died in hospitals or nursing homes, hospice leaders argued that it was often in error: "Many persons with terminal diseases can stay at home much longer than they do now, but they are put into nursing homes because the families think they just can't cope."[37] Home care aided by the family was the goal: "We're not building the [inpatient] hospice to institutionalize our patients. Our aim is to keep them out of institutions, including ours."[38]

The family of the British hospice movement was broken. Its archetypal patient was David Tasma, a man with no family present at all. The family of the US hospice movement, in contrast, was supportive. Its archetypal patient had a family that wanted to care for their loved one but was thwarted in its attempts to do so by the medical system. Images of such families appeared frequently in early hospice literature.[39] They were central to how US hospice leaders understood their movement and justified the need for it to the outside world.

The project of the British hospice movement was repairing the family through end-of-life care. The project of the US hospice movement was repairing end-of-life care through the family. This was a difference of degree. Both hospice movements preferred patients to die at home, and both provided them with assistance in doing so. But compared to its British counterpart, the US hospice movement was much more comfortable *depending* on the family. Over the course of the 1970s, however, the meaning of this familial dependence shifted.

The Family as a Driver of Care

From the very beginning of their work in the early 1970s, the members of the US hospice movement gave the family a central role in end-of-life care. This role was due to their understanding of what ailed the dying patient. Hospice Inc.'s leaders argued that dying Americans suffered from "feeling isolated."[40] This isolation was rooted in a broader denial of death, which hospice leaders considered to be medical, social, and interpersonal. Basing their model on the work of Elisabeth Kübler-Ross, hospice leaders argued that US medicine and society denied the existence and inevitability of death.[41] Since terminally ill individuals were considered reminders of death's existence, they were shunned. Their resulting isolation caused "much of the distress in dying."[42]

Rectifying this situation involved reintegrating the dying individual into society. The entity that hospice leaders relied on to do so was the patient's family. By "family," hospice leaders meant "one or more persons who are involved with and concerned about the patient."[43] The family was thus not primarily a biological unit. Its members were defined by their commitment to the dying person. This commitment was a powerful tool, in part, because such family members knew the patient before they were dying. Familial caretakers had an inherent advantage compared to the hospice team. They *were* the community into which the dying needed to be reintegrated. Hospice care depended on the families because patients themselves depended on the family to, in part, give them their sense of self.

To be sure, patients could not depend on their families to the same extent they might have in decades past. The rise of medicine and its attendant denial of death had weakened the bonds between patients and families. As a result of this weakening, families no longer had a language to talk with their loved ones about death. Attempts by the patient to communicate became "entangled in double talk, denials, white lies and untruths."[44] As a result, the patient "[felt] himself a burden on those around him, unable to contribute and becoming weaker; he sees that he saps their strength as his own diminishes."[45] Leaving patients to their families was not sufficient. Families needed help.

The need for such help was how Hospice Inc.'s leaders justified their form of care. Hospice would provide family members and dying people with the environment necessary for them to come to a shared awareness of death. This awareness was dependent on adequate pain relief, but it transcended what could be provided by medical care. Hospice Inc.'s leaders claimed that they could help both patients and family members reach it. Part of that process entailed empowering the family to care for their dying relative. One goal of hospice was to provide them with the necessary support.

By doing so, hospice would attend to the clinical needs of the family as well. Hospice Inc.'s leaders believed that family members suffered because they wanted to be included in end-of-life care but were prevented from doing so by the structure of US hospitals and nursing homes.[46] But they not only wanted to provide care, they *needed* to do so. Taking part in such care would help families begin the process of grieving for their loved one by allowing them to overcome their denial of the inevitability of their relative's death—and of death in general.[47] Overcoming this denial would make them better caregivers, and by being better caregivers, they would be better able to recover from their eventual loss. Including the family in the care of dying people was thus a way of preventing pathological mourning.[48]

No matter how much care hospice provided, it could not replace the family. The family knew the patient's lifestyle in ways hospice professionals never could, and the family had relationships with the patient that could not be replicated by professional caregivers. For this reason, both the patient and the family would assume "active roles in the decision making processes."[49] By attuning themselves to their patient's lifestyle, hospice professionals could "include this experience of dying and bereavement in [the patient's and family's] life, in their own way."[50] Through such care, dying patients could escape their isolation. Hospice was a vehicle for this reintegration. But the family would, alongside the patient, be the driver of care.

This would be true even in those rare instances when the family could not serve as the primary caregiver. As I discussed earlier, US hospice leaders from the beginning planned to build an inpatient unit for such cases. But the ideal inpatient unit would also include the family in a way that hospitals and nursing homes did not.

The facility as it was originally conceived was to have no restrictive visiting hours. It would contain resources for families to use, such as day care, a chapel, and even a "screaming room" where they could vent their frustrations.[51] It would include the kind of tailored psychological and spiritual care that would be necessary for them to work through their grief and connect with their loved ones.[52] Furthermore, it would be located in an area that was convenient for them to visit.[53] The rooms would be designed with ample space so that families could be "right around the patient," and each visitor would be welcomed as an "active participant" in patient care.[54] Families in the inpatient unit would not be directly caring for their relatives. But they would still be an integral part of care.

Thus, hospice leaders initially depended on the family because they considered it to be significant for clinical care. This vision of the family remained consistent in Hospice Inc. throughout the 1970s. But as the complexities of implementing the organization's vision arose, the family in hospice came to take on a very different meaning.

Paying for It

When Hospice Inc. was incorporated on November 19, 1971, the organization's financial holdings totaled $142.50.[55] Its members were largely faculty members at Yale University. The time they put into the organization was donated. This all-volunteer structure was appropriate for the planning phase of the organization, but it was not feasible when it came to constructing a functioning hospice. Hospice Inc., if it were to exist, would have to find funding.

The first five years of the organization's existence were dominated by costs relating to licensure. In 1971, Hospice Inc. was a nonprofit corporation, but it was not yet licensed as a medical provider. As such, it was not able to provide care. After they had defined Hospice Inc.'s philosophy, the organization's leaders set themselves to the task of obtaining a license. It was a complex and difficult process.

First, hospice leaders had to decide what category of licensure to apply for. They wanted their caretaking model to include both care for patients in a free-standing inpatient institution and outpatient care for patients at home. However, at the time there were no medical licensure categories in the state of Connecticut that offered both caretaking modalities. Hospice Inc.'s leaders were thus faced with a decision: either design a new licensure category specifically for hospice or work within the existing licensure categories for inpatient and outpatient care.[56]

This dilemma was compounded by the deficiencies of the existing licensure categories. As an outpatient institution, Hospice Inc. could be licensed as a home healthcare provider. But home healthcare providers could not provide the level of bereavement services that Hospice Inc.'s leaders desired and were limited in their ability to provide round-the-clock care to patients with terminal illnesses.[57] It was even more difficult to obtain a license as an inpatient unit. Hospice Inc. could have sought licensure as a nursing home, but nursing homes were custodial institutions and therefore not permitted to provide the medical care required by hospice. An alternative was licensure as a "chronic disease hospital." Such institutions were both long term and medical, but they included expensive technological interventions that were not necessary for hospice patients.[58]

In spite of the lack of perfectly fitting licensure categories, Hospice Inc.'s leaders initially sought to work within the existing categories rather than invent a new one. This decision was largely economic. Hospice leaders worried that trying to have a new licensure category approved by the Department of Health would take significantly more time than working within the existing categories.[59] This time would, effectively, be money since increasing rates of inflation would add to the already significant costs of constructing an inpatient facility. As a result, Hospice Inc.'s leaders sought licensure as a home healthcare provider and a chronic disease hospital.

Establishing an outpatient unit proved to be the easier task. Hospice Inc.'s board hired two medical professionals to supervise the home care program: Dr. Sylvia Lack, who came to Hospice Inc. from St. Christopher's Hospice, and Sister Mary Kaye Dunn, an oncology nurse from the Mayo Clinic in Minnesota. When Lack and Dunn arrived in New Haven in April 1973, they encountered the reality that Hospice Inc. was not yet certified by the state to provide outpatient care.[60] In addition, the program was understaffed due to a misunderstanding of the existing licensing procedures by hospice leaders, particularly Florence Wald. But in spite of these delays, the program received certification early in 1974 and began serving patients in May.[61]

Setting up the inpatient center was more difficult. First, Hospice Inc.'s leaders applied to the state of Connecticut to obtain a license to build a forty-four-bed chronic disease hospital.[62] Their application was rejected twice in 1972–1973. The reasons for this rejection were largely political. The state board of health contained a prominent member of the nursing home industry, and he used his influence to argue that nursing homes in the state were already providing sufficient care for dying people. In his view, the new hospice construction was not only unnecessary but also illegal, disqualified under Connecticut's law that healthcare facilities must prove that they are not duplicating existing services.[63]

Overcoming these barriers was costly. First, Hospice Inc. had to do an extensive study to demonstrate that there was a need for its unique form of care. This study required a full-time research staff and took up significant organizational resources without producing any financial returns.[64] In addition, the organization had to hire a political consultant, Dennis Rezendes, to design and implement a strategy to gather the necessary support to obtain a license.[65] Though Rezendes was ultimately successful—Hospice Inc. became licensed as a chronic disease hospital in 1975–the quest for licensure had required an enormous amount of money.[66]

The resources required for licensure were paltry, however, compared to what was required to build the inpatient unit. A central reason that Hospice Inc. had been able to provide outpatient care prior to inpatient care was because it required a much smaller overhead cost. The construction of an inpatient facility would cost, according to Hospice Inc.'s 1973 estimate, $3 million.[67] This figure would be approximately $16 million today.[68] In addition to funding the facility's construction, Hospice Inc. had to pay an architect to design the site.[69] The leaders had to research the area for a town that would be well suited for their needs and then engage in political lobbying to gain the necessary permission to build.[70] Meanwhile, the delay in obtaining licensure was increasing the costs of construction every year due to inflation.[71]

While Hospice Inc. was making progress on licensure and facility construction, its staffing needs grew. In 1971, the organization began with eight staff members, all of whom were volunteering their time.[72] By 1974, the organization had ninety-six members.[73] This growth in staff size coincided with a decrease in staff members volunteering their time. Though Florence Wald continued to provide free services to hospice until 1975, most of Hospice Inc.'s staff were paid professionals.[74]

Paying for their labor was complicated by the lack of clear reimbursement for hospice services. Unlike England, the United States lacked a single-payer healthcare system. Obtaining reimbursement thus required coordinating between diverse funding agencies, including Medicaid, Medicare, and private insurance.[75] Payments were often significantly less than the cost of the services rendered. The resulting frustrations led Hospice Inc.'s leaders to begin in the late 1970s to campaign for the inclusion of hospice in Medicare.[76] Medicare, however, was not a panacea. It had substantial coverage gaps: for example, it would only fund dying patients over the age of sixty-five.[77] But hospice leaders believed that it would provide substantially better coverage than existing alternatives. Nevertheless, Medicare reimbursement would not become a reality for hospice until the early 1980s. In the meantime, Hospice Inc.'s leaders had to struggle to make do.

The move from a philosophical vision to a practicing healthcare organization required an enormous amount of money. And yet, in a Catch-22, Hospice Inc. was not able to make money until it had become a practicing healthcare organization. This situation left Hospice Inc.'s leaders with one path to finance their form of care: fundraising. But in order to raise money effectively, it was necessary to add a new component to the hospice vision.

From Clinically Effective Care to a Method of Cost Saving

Six years prior to the incorporation of Hospice Inc., the US Congress ratified both Medicare and Medicaid.[78] The passage of the Social Security Amendments of 1965 was a watershed in the expansion of the US welfare state. But it also came with a significant increase in governmental expenditures. This increase led to concerns about how to find effective ways to curtail the cost of health care. A particular concern was the care of dying people.[79] End-of-life care was seen as a major driver of costs, particularly among the Medicare population. Furthermore, existing forms of care were considered ineffective and even harmful. For these reasons, lowering the costs of the care of dying people became a key national concern.[80]

In the organization's early years, the leaders of Hospice Inc. were not concerned about the costs of end-of-life care. A desire to cut costs is not mentioned in the foundational documents of Hospice Inc., such as the organization's "philosophy statement."[81] Nor did it appear in the extended conversations that the organization's leaders had with Cicely Saunders about implementing hospice in America.[82] Hospice Inc.'s leaders were concerned about the excessive use of medical technology at the end of life, but only because they considered such technology to be anathema to the appropriate care of dying people. They neither phrased their goals in economic terms nor considered cost reduction to be an essential or even inevitable aspect of their mission.

Indeed, during the period from 1970 to 1972, Hospice Inc.'s leaders did not believe that hospice would be cheaper than existing forms of end-of-life care. In notes from a meeting with the administrators of a nearby hospital, Hospice Inc.'s leaders acknowledged this: "On the basis of comparisons of nursing home and general hospital per patient day costs, we recognize that the per patient day cost in the proposed hospice will not be significantly lower than hospital costs. We must therefore carefully emphasize that the difference between the hospice and hospital is in the type of care, not the cost of care."[83] Thus, at the time of its incorporation, Hospice Inc.'s leaders did not imagine that hospice would reduce the costs of end-of-life care. Rather, they thought that it would redistribute the costs in ways that were more effective. Instead of spending money on heroic interventions and futile technologies, hospice would spend it on palliative, psychosocial, and spiritual care.

But lowering the costs of care *was* a priority for Hospice Inc.'s potential funders. Potential reimbursement from Blue Cross depended on the ability of Hospice Inc. to show that there was "an expected lower per diem rate for care in [hospice] than the prevailing rates in most acute care hospitals."[84] Funding for building and staffing from the Department of Health, Education, and Welfare required Hospice Inc.'s leaders to demonstrate both their clinical efficacy and their skill at "moderating costs."[85] And what Hospice Inc.'s leaders described as the state commission's "obsessions with costs" was a major reason for its reluctance to provide Hospice Inc. with permission to build.[86] Thus, obtaining reimbursement, funding, and even licensure required that hospice be not only a better form of end-of-life care but also "a method of cost saving."[87]

In response to this demand, Hospice Inc.'s leaders staked out a new goal for hospice: reducing "the cost of care for this patient population."[88] The organization began taking account of their costs and arranging them for presentation to external fundraisers. The cost of end-of-life care in a hospital ranged, Hospice Inc. argued, between $125 and $195 a day. Inpatient hospice care, in contrast, would cost only $100.[89] Outpatient care would be even cheaper at $29 a day.[90] All told, hospice leaders estimated that the average cost of hospice would be about "half" of that of hospitals. This cost differential was, they claimed in a letter to Bristol-Myers, a potential funder, "a test that cannot be ignored."[91]

Over the course of the 1970s, US hospice leaders added a new dimension to the language they used to justify hospice. At first, they had argued for hospice based on its improvement in the quality of care compared to other end-of-life treatment options in the US health system. But in order to acquire funding, hospice leaders began to argue that hospice was not only better care, but also more cost effective. Making this rhetoric a reality required redefining the family's role.

The Family as Unpaid Labor

Hospice Inc.'s leaders argued that hospice was, in general, more cost effective than the hospital care of the dying. But not all forms of hospice care were equally cost effective. Outpatient care was approximately $71 less expensive per day than inpatient care—almost a quarter of the price. This cost difference changed the way that hospice leaders thought about the two modalities. Hospice Inc. had previously preferred outpatient to inpatient care because its leaders assumed that by virtue of its care taking place at home, it would do a better job of addressing the social isolation of dying people. Inpatient care was for those rare situations where home care was impossible. By the mid-1970s, Hospice Inc. still privileged outpatient over inpatient care, but now in addition to clinical needs, its reasons for doing so included cost.

This shift in the rationale for outpatient care changed the function of the family. Previously, hospice leaders had preferred familial care for solely clinical reasons, because the family was the unit best suited to assist with the dying person's isolation. But now the family took on another function as a facilitator of cost savings. It could do so because of the unique role that the family played in the provision of outpatient care.

Without familial caregivers, there would be no outpatient hospice care. A family member was the key point person for the hospice team.[92] The family performed routine functions that were necessary for the dying person to be safe in the house. In addition, the family performed essential emotional labor—reintegrating the dying person into society. Hospice Inc.'s leaders had argued from the beginning that the family would have a key role in relieving the emotional and psychological distress of the dying person. Hospice Inc. thus required patients at home to have family members to take care of them. Without such caregivers, patients would presumably need inpatient care—which, at $71 more a day, would nullify much of hospice's cost savings.

But familial caretakers were not only necessary to keep patients in the less expensive outpatient care. They were also a key element of why outpatient care was less expensive to begin with. Many of the tasks carried out by family members could be performed by paid professionals. The assistance with activities of daily living necessary to keep patients safe, for example, could be carried out by a full-time home health provider. A more extensive, interdisciplinary network of professionals could also address, to some extent, the dying person's isolation and attendant psychological and emotional distress. But hospice leaders did not attempt to implement such full-time assistance. Initially, their resistance to doing so was likely based in a valorization of the unique function performed by the family. But now there was a financial motive as well. With more extensive professional support, the affordability of outpatient care would decline.

Such a decline would threaten the existence of hospice itself. Without the ability to demonstrate its utility as a "method of cost savings," Hospice Inc. would never have been licensed. Its outpatient care would not have begun working. Its inpatient unit would never have been built. It would not have been able to find reliable reimbursement for its services. Hospice was only able to come to be when it had demonstrated that it was cheaper than existing alternatives. To do so, it depended on the family to provide the labor necessary for its patients to remain at home. And it needed them to provide this labor without any expectation of financial recompense from Hospice Inc. or anyone else.

Thus, by the end of the 1970s, familial dependence had a new meaning in hospice. It meant not only better clinical care. It also included the cost savings provided by unpaid familial labor. Establishing *both* meanings was necessary for Hospice Inc. to acquire the funds necessary to operate. And, indeed, attempting to establish both meanings of familial dependence simultaneously was not a problem. Familial caregiving could, in theory, be both cheap and clinically effective. But in practice, Hospice Inc.'s leaders grew increasingly concerned that the cost savings of hospice were coming at the detriment of quality of care. The result was a conflict between the two meanings of familial dependence.

The Conflict between Quality and Cost Effectiveness

In 1971, US hospice leaders observed that their model of care was not cheaper than the hospital care of the dying.[93] Rather, hospice was offering *better* services, ones more tailored to the dying patient and their family. But by the late 1970s, Hospice Inc.'s leaders saw the need to make cuts to the services offered in order to be able to market their care to potential funders. These cuts impacted the family's role in both inpatient and outpatient care, but in different ways.

Hospice Inc.'s inpatient unit had initially been designed to welcome the family, but the need to cut costs changed this design. State licensing boards deemed many of the amenities that were to be part of the inpatient unit to be too expensive. Many of these services had been initially designed to allow family members to become more involved in the care of their relatives and to also broaden the range of family members who could do so.[94] By cutting them, Hospice Inc.'s leaders limited the family's involvement in both respects. They also made the inpatient hospice more like the medical facilities that hospice leaders had initially defined themselves in opposition to.

At the same time, requirements for admission to the inpatient unit became stricter. Initially, the main criterion for admission was the inability of the patient to remain at home, regardless of their projected lifespan.[95] But by 1974, the inpatient unit was only for patients who had, on average, three weeks or less to live.[96] The result was a shift in the functioning of the inpatient unit. Now, it was for patients who were dying *imminently*. The official licensure category created in the state of Connecticut for inpatient hospices was "Short-Term Hospitals, Special, Hospice."[97] The criterion for admission was no longer patient need. It was time to death.

By reducing inpatient services, hospice leaders reduced the cost of inpatient care. By reducing hospice's role in long-term caregiving, they shifted care to the less expensive outpatient service. But these cuts made hospice less welcoming to patients with inadequate familial support, and it changed the role of those family members who did want to provide care. The inpatient unit was less welcoming to them too, and inpatient care now had a reduced role in hospice as a whole. But this change could only happen because dying patients were presumably able to remain at home longer with their family's support. Thus, the family had a decreased role in inpatient care, but hospice in general depended on the family more. And because of the new cost-cutting imperatives, the family had fewer resources to carry this burden.

Even though it was dramatically cheaper than inpatient care in either the hospital or hospice, outpatient hospice care also suffered cuts. Funders requested cuts to spiritual, psychosocial, and bereavement care as well as to palliative medicine itself.[98] These reductions made it more likely that family members would find themselves in a situation where they were unequipped to address their relative's suffering and pain. They also limited the assistance that these caregivers received for their own spiritual and emotional struggles. The result was an increase in the work required by families combined with a decrease in the support provided to them.

The irony of this situation was not lost on Hospice Inc.'s leaders, who commented at a board of directors meeting: "One of the most exacerbating [*sic*] realities re reimbursement has been to discover that the system says, 'Keep them at home, in bed, in pain, then we'll pay.' This is antithetical to the Hospice concept of care."[99] Hospice leaders in the United States were sensitive to the impact that economic cuts would have on their patients: transforming the home from a space of freedom into a kind of prison and hospice itself into a form of care that seemed to prolong—perhaps even rationalize—the dying person's pain.

It is also worth noting the other person in the room. The patient kept "at home, in bed, in pain" presumably had a familial caregiver watching over them. This caregiver now lacked the resources to assist their suffering relative. And as a result of that, they might be suffering themselves: anguished and desperate, without any clue of what to do. Hospice leaders in the United States had initially hoped that familial caregiving would be therapeutic for both patients and family. Now it seemed that it was becoming traumatic for all parties concerned.

This predicament was the result of the conflict between the two roles that the family played in US hospice care: a driver of care and a method of cost savings. This conflict became so serious that hospice leaders worried that the care they were providing was not worthy of the hospice name. But they were also concerned that without exacerbating the conflict, there would be no way for hospice to exist.

Family, Not Freedom

As I wrote in the introduction to this book, US hospice leaders believed that the hospice movement was modeled in the tradition of other 1960s liberation movements, specifically the civil rights movement and the women's rights movement. To an extent this is true. Hospice was a critique of existing medical and political authority. But unlike those movements, it did not convert this critique into any call to change that authority. Hospice did not make new demands on medicine nor on the state. It did not call for expanded political rights for the terminally ill—or for anyone else. Rather, what hospice leaders sought was for dying people and their families to be left in peace.

In this sense, hospice was compatible with the emerging movement for what was called "end-of-life decision making" or "freedom" at the end of life. This movement claimed to give dying individuals their freedom, but it formulated freedom solely as a privacy right. This did not entail any action on the part of the state. Rather, it entailed merely that the state get out of the individual's way. The result was an affirmation of what anesthesiologist Henry Beecher called the "right to be left alone."[100] This understanding of freedom as privacy would shape US jurisprudence regarding the rights of patients at the end of life, including the right to refuse life-sustaining treatment.

Such a private conception of freedom was perfectly compatible with the hospice conception of care. Hospice leaders did not argue that dying patients needed more resources in the private sphere. Rather, they claimed that dying people needed fewer resources. This claim was in part a commentary on the inefficient use of resources in US hospitals. But having appropriate hospice care was, hospice leaders acknowledged privately, expensive as well. It was hospice's dependence on the family that made it possible for its leaders to argue that fewer resources would be necessary.

This dependence on the family made hospice fundamentally different from the 1960s liberation struggles. Those movements were all critical of the idea that

the family should be left on its own in the private sphere. Such a private conception of the family had masked the complex ways in which the family could be a
site for the domination of women and African Americans (and African American women in particular).[101] For this reason, the civil rights and women's rights
movements politicized the family while arguing that the family was already political, but in a way that limited the freedom of women and black people. Providing
resources to these populations so that they could escape the limitations of the
private family, if they so chose, was essential to their freedom.[102]

The US hospice movement made no such attempt to politicize the family.
Rather, hospice leaders believed that the problems of US end-of-life care could
be solved by taking the family out of politics: by leaving dying people and their
families alone. Geographer Michael Brown has argued that in this orientation to
the family, the hospice movement ultimately sought to return to an earlier, presumably halcyon era of familial caregiving.[103] Historian Emily Abel has similarly
noted that hospice, rather than attempting to transform existing power structures, sought instead to escape them.[104] Drawing on the work of sociologist Paul
Starr, Abel argues that such escapist movements have historically been co-opted
by the very forces they claim to oppose.[105]

By the end of the 1970s, there is evidence that hospice leaders believed that
this co-optation was taking place. They had to dramatically reduce their vision
of hospice if they wanted to see their project funded; this reduction could lead
to dying people suffering in a manner strikingly similar to that which predomi-
nated in the medicalized facilities that hospice opposed. But US hospice leaders
did not present an alternative to familial caregiving. This raises the question of
what such an alternative vision might have been.

The answer is freedom. The civil rights movement and the women's rights
movement criticized the private freedom of the individual and family in the name
of the public freedom of civil rights. This freedom was not opposed to privacy, and
it was necessary if privacy was to represent freedom at all. Without freedom, the
private family was synonymous with oppression.

Hospice leaders in the United States could have adopted such a freedom-based
model for their care, but doing so would have required fundamentally challenging
their ideology of the family. It would have required acknowledging that there was
no golden age of familial caregiving in America, that the nineteenth-century family was based on the very patriarchy and white supremacy that the civil rights and
women's rights movements had opposed. It would have required acknowledging
that in the 1970s, most American families were dramatically removed from the
task of caring for dying people and that many of them lacked the resources to

do so. It would have required rejecting the fundamental hospice narrative—he hospice family romance—and claiming that the family was not a substitute for freedom.

Hospice leaders in the United States did not make such an argument for freedom. The result was that they were co-opted into the conception of freedom that was emerging at the time with the new political philosophy of neoliberalism. The ensuing relationship between hospice and neoliberalism brought many benefits, but they came with some significant strings attached.

Thus, basing the hospice movement on freedom—not familial dependence—would have allowed hospice leaders to make a stronger claim on the resources they needed. It also would have opened up new political alliances that could have helped them to achieve their goals. These alliances could have been found in two movements that were emerging in the 1970s, which, while different from the hospice movement, had aligned political concerns.

Euthanasia, Freedom, and the Nature of Death

From its origins in England through its development in the United States, the modern hospice movement was opposed to euthanasia. This opposition was a motivating factor for the rise of hospice in the 1960s, and the leaders of Hospice Inc. maintained it consistently throughout the 1970s.[106] In internal documents, they bemoaned reports of suicides by dying people. Such suicides, they argued, were a response to the lack in the United States of appropriate end-of-life care.[107] Hospice, by providing terminally ill people with appropriate care, would work as a form of suicide prevention.

Hospice leaders formally presented their vision in Hospice Inc.'s "Statement on Euthanasia," which was approved by the board of directors in 1976: "Hospice opposes all attempts to legalize, promote, or condone euthanasia . . . which is to cause death by the intentional use of medical technology or by the withholding of ordinary, appropriate, reasonable and prudent medical care. . . . On the other hand, Hospice supports the true use of the term 'death with dignity' . . . meaning to allow death to come naturally to the terminally ill, using appropriate treatment rather than heroic and extraordinary measures to prolong life."[108] In this statement, hospice leaders condemned what bioethicists refer to as "active" euthanasia, which involves directly administering a life-ending substance to a patient. But they also argued that "passive" euthanasia—the removal of life-sustaining treatment—could, in certain circumstances, count as the "intentional" provocation of death. To be valid, such removal of treatment must be accompanied by the provision of appropriate hospice care.[109]

This condemnation of passive euthanasia is significant. Arguments for passive euthanasia sought to differentiate it from active euthanasia on the basis of
a distinction between "killing" and "letting die."[110] According to this distinction,
removing life-sustaining treatment was not actively killing the person, even if
it resulted in death. Instead, it was a way of allowing the person to be killed
not by the medical provider, but by their underlying incurable disease. Since
such a death was caused by disease, it was considered "natural." This concept of
"natural death" has been essential to justifying a distinction between active and
passive euthanasia in US law and bioethics.[111]

These arguments made a particular link between such natural deaths and
individual freedom. Because it only required removing—rather than providing
—treatment, passive euthanasia came to be justified on the basis of the right
to privacy.[112] A natural death, understood as a lack of outside intervention in a
patient's care, thus became synonymous with the idea of freedom at the end of
life. The result was the individualistic conception of freedom known as the right
to be left alone.[113]

But Hospice Inc.'s statement on euthanasia challenged the idea that deaths
due to passive euthanasia were "natural." Simply removing a patient from
life-sustaining treatment did not, hospice leaders claimed, make a death natural.
Rather, for a person to die "naturally," they needed to be provided with appropriate care. It was not enough to just leave them be. The provision of hospice care
was thus inherent to the very nature of death. If care was not provided, then a
death could not be deemed natural. This rethinking of the nature of death was
a powerful challenge to a US end-of-life care system in which the concept of
natural death sometimes obscured an underlying failure to provide appropriate
treatment.

Hospice leaders never took their novel conception of death to its "natural"
conclusion. If the failure to provide appropriate care made a death unnatural, it
followed that death was caused by human intervention: by the lack of appropriate
care. Such human causation of death would seem anathema to a conception of
freedom predicated on privacy rights. Thus, implicit in Hospice Inc.'s "Statement on Euthanasia" was the idea that for someone to be free at the end of life,
it was not enough to remove care. Freedom required that appropriate care be *provided*. This view of freedom could include privacy rights, but such rights were not
in themselves sufficient. It would require a movement for the freedom of dying
people, one that necessarily redefined the relationship between the individual
and the state.

And yet, such a movement never came to pass. Hospice leaders continued to base their arguments on depoliticized calls for economic efficiency, appropriate medical care, or—as in the case of the euthanasia statement—"dignity" and "nature." The US euthanasia movement, in contrast, did claim freedom as its defining political signifier.[114] But its advocates maintained a private conception of freedom that did not make any demands on the state for the provision of appropriate hospice care. The result was a strange phenomenon: two movements on behalf of dying Americans with neither one making any claim on the state to provide dying people with new resources to realize their freedom. Meanwhile, there was a movement emerging that would make claims for precisely such resources. But its focus was not on dying people.

Hospice against Disability Rights?

The disability rights movement began at roughly the same time as the US hospice movement in the late 1960s and early 1970s.[115] It was founded by a wide range of individuals, all of whom had come to the conclusion that people with disabilities were not free in the United States. They were segregated in institutions, barred from access to practically every aspect of society, and discriminated against—sometimes violently—across a range of settings. Rectifying these problems did not require charity, which was the dominant way of thinking about the care of disabled people.[116] It required political rights. Throughout the 1970s and beyond, disability rights leaders worked to secure such rights.

Already at that point in history, the US hospice movement shared numerous potential interests with the disability rights movement. For one, the distinction between chronic disability and terminal illness was always somewhat amorphous. St. Christopher's Hospice in England had housed both chronically disabled and terminally ill people.[117] In America, as historian Emily Abel has shown, what we today would consider the separate categories of people with "chronic disability" and those with "terminal illness" were for the first half of the twentieth century conflated under the rubric of "incurables."[118] The hospice and disability rights movements thus from the beginning cared for populations that to an extent overlapped.

They also had a common enemy: the nursing home industry. Disability rights activists consistently argued that nursing homes were pseudo-carceral institutions that served little purpose other than to segregate disabled people from society.[119] The hospice movement, in turn, had fought the nursing home industry since its inception. Hospice leaders believed that nursing homes were fundamentally inadequate as end-of-life facilities. Indeed, they were effectively unsalvageable; the irreconcilable nature of nursing homes and the end of life was one of the fundamental justifications that US hospice leaders gave for their new modality of care.[120] This new form of care was, as I noted above, opposed—quite successfully for a time—by the nursing home lobby in Connecticut.[121] Beyond this common enemy, the disability rights and hospice movements had a number of shared interests: creating an accessible society, the provision of more extensive long-term care in the home, and the destigmatization of dependence in US political institutions and popular culture.

An alliance between the US disability rights movement and the hospice movement never came to fruition, however. This may have been because of a desire of disability rights activists to distance themselves from the terminally ill. The lumping together of people with disabilities and dying people has been a form of disability discrimination.[122] Given the centrality of labor to the US disability rights movement, it also makes sense that disability rights leaders would not focus on terminally ill people, who are generally too sick to work.[123] Nevertheless, this marginalization of dying people obscured the common interests between hospice and disability rights.

Hospice leaders in the United States also neglected to see those shared interests. But even had they seen them, allying with the disability rights movement would have required changing their approach. The US hospice movement was not a movement for the freedom of dying people. At best, the movement supported attempts to reframe such freedom as the right to privacy. The disability rights movement, in contrast, though supporting privacy rights for people with disabilities, also sought to radicalize them by mandating that the state intervene in US society to promote equality of access. To be sure, disability rights activists emphasized that such interventions would be more cost effective than existing forms of care for disabled people.[124] But the disability rights movement was not primarily oriented to the costs of care. Its goal was securing the rights of disabled people. This required converting them from passive recipients of care to active political subjects.

The US hospice movement never recommended such a conversion with regard to dying Americans. The result was, I argue, a limitation of its ability to make demands on the state. It also made it difficult for hospice leaders to conceive of any mutually beneficial political alliance with the disability rights movement. In a sense, hospice leaders did not understand themselves to be political actors at all, at least not in the same vein as the people fighting for disability rights. This dissonance is best illustrated by the attitude of US hospice leaders toward the Rehabilitation Act of 1973.

The core legislative victory of the disability rights movement in the 1970s was section 504 of the Rehabilitation Act of 1973. The Rehabilitation Act was a response to the increasing population of disabled veterans as a result of the war in Vietnam.[125] The act represented a shift in federal assistance to people with disabilities; this assistance would now encompass not just job training but also measures to improve overall well-being.[126] This shift was based largely in a short paragraph that, in the words of disability studies scholar Lennard Davis, "changed the history of disability rights."[127] Section 504 of the Rehabilitation Act reads:

> No otherwise qualified individual with a disability in the United States, as defined in section 705(20) of this title, shall, solely by reason of her or his disability, be excluded from the participation in, be denied the benefits of, or be subjected to discrimination under any program or activity receiving federal financial assistance.[128]

This section received hardly any notice at the time of the act's passage, and yet it was a major redefinition of the appropriate federal treatment of disabled people. It was, in Davis's words, "the first federal language that clearly and uncompromisingly guaranteed the civil rights of people with disabilities."[129] Modeled on previous civil rights statutes, section 504 redefined "disability" as an identity that could be subject to discrimination and that the federal government had an obligation to protect. The section catalyzed the disability rights movement and was central to the passage almost twenty years later of the Americans with Disabilities Act.[130]

This was not, however, the spirit in which Hospice Inc.'s leaders read the Rehabilitation Act. Their concern was that the act's regulations, if implemented, would be "extremely costly and time consuming."[131] They consulted a lawyer, who sent them an eight-page letter in which he clarified that the act would likely not apply to them. The letter concluded, "I, of course, realize that your members do not discriminate against the handicapped and that their concern with the Regulations is based on the recordkeeping and administrative requirements, as well as the alterations of existing facilities."[132]

I agree with Hospice Inc.'s lawyer that the organization's leaders were not discriminatory against disabled people. Their concern with the burden of the Rehabilitation Act was, in a way, reasonable. By 1977—when they consulted the lawyer—they had spent almost a decade trying to raise funds to build an inpatient facility. The idea of having to alter that facility to make it accessible—thereby increasing its cost—must have been devastating and perhaps even would have made the project financially unfeasible. Since their argument for hospice was based on its cost effectiveness, it is understandable that they recoiled from disability rights, which did require, at a certain point, paying more money.

Yet this reticence is only understandable to a point. The concern of hospice leaders for saving money pitted them against the disability rights movement. But it did not have to be that way. Rather than opposing disability rights, hospice leaders could have seen in the disability rights movement both a model and an ally. Instead of depending on the family, the disability rights movement made demands on the state and did so in the name of the freedom of people with disabilities. There is no compelling reason that a similar claim was not made on behalf of dying people. But the belief among hospice advocates that dying people needed to be returned to the care of their families prevented them from making this connection. The result was a dramatic loss of political capital. Hospice leaders in the United States had placed their bet on the family. This wager would make possible their greatest success—and also undermine it.

The Cost of Hospice's Success

Hospice Inc. was an extremely successful organization. One measure of this success is that by the late 1970s, it no longer occupied a central role in US hospice care. Other hospice organizations, drawing on its model, had sprung up throughout the country. These hospices formed the National Hospice Organization, a lobbying group that, while including some members of Hospice Inc., was not primarily based in that organization.[133] Hospice Inc. had started a new form of care. By the late 1970s, it was just one more practitioner of it. This shift may have been disheartening to some of Hospice Inc.'s early leaders, but it was also an indication of just how effective they had been. That effectiveness was facilitated by their dependence on the family.

But this dependence also raised questions: At what point would the conflict between care and cost savings become too intense? When would the need for cost savings become so great that it cut into the ability of families to provide care, perhaps leaving dying patients in situations as bad or worse than they had been in before? Could hospice's dependence on the family undermine the very success that it had, to a degree, made possible?

These questions were, indeed, troubling to the leaders of Hospice Inc. In 1982, Rosemary Johnson-Hurzeler, the administrator of the organization—which had recently been renamed the Connecticut Hospice—testified before Congress regarding the potential incorporation of hospice into Medicare. Though supportive of Medicare reimbursement in general, Johnson-Hurzeler bemoaned that the bill as then drafted was unnecessarily restrictive of inpatient care. The bill limited inpatient care to 20 percent of a patient's total care; in the view of the Connecticut

Hospice's board, that ratio was unrealistically low. A better ratio would be 50 percent inpatient care to 50 percent outpatient care.[134] Despite Johnson-Hurzeler's suggestion, the bill passed as written. That extra 30 percent of care would fall to American families. Already, US hospice leaders doubted that it was a burden that those families could bear.

CHAPTER THREE

Birth of a Crisis

"Even in a person's dying—*especially in a person's dying*—family and community comprise the proper context for a person's life," writes hospice physician Ira Byock in *The Best Care Possible*.[1] As Emily Abel has pointed out, this view has been a constant in the history of the modern hospice movement.[2] Cicely Saunders, Florence Wald, and contemporary hospice leaders, like Byock, all agree. What they might disagree on is why this context is appropriate and the form that it should take.

In the previous chapter, I examined how the US hospice movement came to depend on familial caregiving. In this chapter, I examine the culmination of this process: the passage of the Medicare Hospice Benefit. Passed in 1982, the MHB incorporated hospice into the US Medicare system.[3] This dramatically increased the scope of US hospice care, making it possible for hospice providers to reach individuals throughout the country who previously did not have access to their services.[4] But the benefit also defined "hospice" in a manner that placed a high burden of care on the family members of dying individuals.

I argue that in general US families are not positioned to carry that burden. Even at the time of the MHB's passage, US hospice leaders believed that there was a mismatch between what the benefit required of familial caregivers and what they would be able to provide. This initial mismatch has widened over the almost four decades since that passage. The result has been the creation of a crisis that systemically undermines the delivery of US hospice care.

Why US Hospice Leaders Wanted the Medicare Hospice Benefit

The push for the incorporation of hospice into Medicare came from organizations like Hospice Inc.: hospices from around the United States that were struggling to be reimbursed for their services.[5] Without adequate reimbursement, the hospices would not acquire the capital necessary to run their existing programs, much less to expand. The process of seeking reimbursement locally was burdensome, however, and inconsistent reimbursement came at the cost of an enormous expenditure of resources by hospice organizations that were already underfunded.

In part as a response to this predicament, members of hospices from around the country began to meet in the late 1970s with the purpose of developing a consistent and systemic model of US hospice care.[6] Such a model would make them well positioned to advocate for reimbursement from the US government. A federal system of reimbursement would be a much more efficient way of supporting hospice services than attempting to fight various local battles. It would give hospice an immediate and wide-ranging legitimacy. And it would ease the burden on local hospices, which would be able to focus on providing care.

As a vehicle for such a federal reimbursement system, hospice leaders turned to Medicare. Because it was national in scope, Medicare would circumvent the need to haggle with state authorities. Hospice leaders did recognize some drawbacks to Medicare affiliation.[7] Dennis Rezendes, for example, was concerned that tying hospice to Medicare would exclude terminally ill individuals who were under sixty-five years of age.[8] But it was too good an opportunity to pass up. Becoming part of Medicare, however, required hospice leaders to make their case to constituencies that, while sharing their desire for better end-of-life care, were also motivated by a growing desire to reduce costs.

Forging a Political Consensus

The Medicare Hospice Benefit was passed during the presidency of Ronald Reagan. A key goal of Reagan's economic policy was to decrease the size of government by cutting various social service programs. This context would not seem to be amenable to the passage of a substantial expansion of healthcare entitlements to the terminally ill. Yet Republican and Democratic leaders were anxious about the seemingly excessive costs of US end-of-life care.[9]

Hospice leaders responded to this anxiety by promoting hospice as a primarily home-based benefit. In making this argument, hospice leaders were aided by —and explicitly drew on—the popularity of deinstitutionalization as a strategy for both minimizing costs and improving care.[10] Incorporating hospice into Medicare thus seemed to be cheaper, more clinically effective, and, at a basic level, more just. These arguments allowed hospice leaders to appeal to legislators on both sides of the aisle.[11] They could do so without self-contradiction because of their belief that care should be returned to the family: the hospice family romance (see chapter 2). Nevertheless, the MHB differed from the vision of hospice leaders in how it understood the *proportion* of care to be provided at home by the family, as opposed to in hospice facilities by trained professionals. This question of proportion, seemingly minor in the abstract, was contentious from the beginning and grew more significant with time.

Shifting Care onto the Family

The MHB defines hospice as an interdisciplinary form of treatment for patients who are "terminally ill."[12] This definition of hospice was—and, in general, remains—relatively uncontroversial. Much more controversial was the way the MHB transformed the services that were included under the "hospice" banner.

The first part of this transformation was the definition of hospice as a primarily outpatient treatment modality. The benefit mandates that of the care provided by any particular hospice, 80 percent has to be outpatient care, carried out either at home or in a non-hospice facility, such as a nursing home. Only 20 percent can be inpatient care housed in a hospice institution.[13] For US hospice leaders, this limitation of inpatient care was significant and abrupt.

Hospice leaders in the United States had imagined a less extensive role for inpatient care than their British counterparts offered, but they still considered it important. Indeed, the majority of Hospice Inc.'s fundraising in the 1970s was to build an inpatient center. The MHB gave such centers a very small role. They would be short-term facilities whose primary goal was to deal with emergency situations. If they were used for longer than a few days, hospices would not be reimbursed for the cost of care. As a result, the benefit strongly disincentivized hospices from providing long-term inpatient care.

The MHB did not provide long-term care to patients in the outpatient context either. Instead, the patient's long-term care needs were presumably to be met by the patient's family.[14] Such needs include assistance with basic activities of daily living (ADLs), such as bathing, clothing, feeding, safety, and daily hygienic maintenance. More fundamentally, such assistance entails monitoring the patient daily and nightly to ensure that they are safe. The benefit only allows for twenty-four-hour care in the case of an emergency; while it allows for home health aide services to assist patients with ADLs, it limits the extent of such services to a part-time basis.[15] The benefit does require that hospices provide some volunteer labor to address the additional companionship needs of patients, but these volunteers are restricted in the activities they can perform.[16] Thus, the benefit's combined emergency care, CNA (certified nurse assistant) visits, and volunteer services do not amount to comprehensive long-term care. Rather, they *support* the patient's family, who provide most of the patient's long-term care and receive no economic reimbursement to do so.

This reliance on unpaid familial labor is such a central aspect of hospice policy that it has remained virtually unchanged after almost forty years, even as several other aspects of the MHB have changed dramatically.[17] But this lack of change should not be mistaken for an affirmation of the feasibility of the benefit's structure. Indeed, even at the time of the benefit's passage, US hospice leaders were aware that it created a bigger burden on families than was advisable for them, for hospice professionals, and for dying people.

The Mismatch

The discomfort that US hospice leaders felt with the MHB was expressed by Rosemary Johnson-Hurzeler, whose comments on the benefit's ratio of inpatient to outpatient care were mentioned at the conclusion of chapter 2. Here, I quote her extensively in order to provide a fuller context with regard to the restricted aspects of the benefit, as well as the rationale that hospice leaders saw for this restriction:

> The proposed legislation contains the requirement that no patient receive more than 20% of their care days in an inpatient setting after that patient is accepted into the hospice system. The experience of the Connecticut Hospice indicates that this requirement is unrealistic. Physicians in Connecticut have prescribed inpatient hospice care days for their patients which comprise 50% of all care days. . . . The mix of inpatient and home care days experienced by the same group was directed by physicians and care providers whose only consideration was the optimal care for each patient. . . . Based on these results, we recommend . . . a 50:50 ratio of home care to inpatient days.[18]

Even in 1982, when the MHB was being passed, US hospice leaders were concerned that the bill's limitations on inpatient care were too restrictive. Rather than an 80:20 outpatient to inpatient ratio, Johnson-Hurzeler recommended an even split: 50:50.

Johnson-Hurzeler did not mention the "family" specifically. But the implications of her comments for familial caregivers can be inferred. By raising the percentage of hospice care that would be delivered in an outpatient context, the MHB increased the amount of care that would have to be provided by familial caregivers. Johnson-Hurzeler's claim that the benefit's outpatient ratio was too high was, in part, a statement about the ability of familial caregivers to adequately address their dying relative's needs. It expressed a concern that there was a disparity between the degree to which the MHB depended on familial caregiving and the amount of care that US families could provide.

Her statement implies the explanation for this mismatch. Johnson-Hurzeler's 50:50 ratio was determined "by physicians and care providers whose only consideration was the optimal care for each patient." The 80:20 ratio of the MHB was, by contrast, dictated by concerns that were presumably *not* those of providing the best care possible. Rather, hospice care was being incorporated into Medicare with the goal of reducing the federal government's financing of US end-of-life care.

Health policy scholar Vincent Mor's 1987 study, *Hospice Care Systems*, gives a fuller picture of how broadly these concerns were shared.[19] As quoted by Mor, hospice professionals Michael Preodor and Sally Owen-Still wrote that the MHB was passed "on the basis of its purported cost savings to the Medicare programs, with little consideration of its effects on the moral and ethical issues in the care of the terminally ill."[20] Sociologist Donald Gibson interpreted the benefit's underlying message to be "that nontreatment for the severely ill is an acceptable way to reduce expenditures."[21] Such views confirm Abel's argument that "to many advocates of the hospice benefit, relatives appear to have represented primarily a cheap form of labor."[22]

The MHB's design thus created a mismatch between what the US hospice system would give familial caregivers and what those caregivers needed. This disparity was a product of the need to cut costs. But it was not just that. It was also created by the way in which US hospice leaders had long imagined the family to be.

What Hospice Leaders Got Wrong

By the time the MHB was passed, US families were generally removed from caring for their dying relatives. The rise of modern medicine in the late nineteenth and early twentieth centuries had taken dying people from their familial homes. They were cared for, instead, in hospitals.[23] Due to the discovery of the germ theory, there was great optimism about the ability to cure these patients. But when such remedies never materialized, the "incurables" were often left unattended in hospital wards, locked up in derelict institutions, or thrown out to the streets.[24]

Hospice had emerged in response to this horrific situation. Hospice leaders in the United States were aware of this state of things, and they were also aware that families were removed from the care of their dying kin. But what they did not consider was that the removal of US families from the care of the dying was not *just* a response to changes in US medicine. It was also a response to changes in family life.

These changes had made US families less able to provide care to their dying relatives. They also made them less *willing* to do so and, in fact, decreased the willingness of dying people to receive familial care. While there was merit in the hospice critique of hospital-based end-of-life care, it was not possible to simply return care to the family. Indeed, the "family" had never quite existed in the terms that US hospice leaders thought.

Reconsidering the Golden Age of US End-of-Life Care

During the mid-nineteenth century, US citizens defined themselves largely through their membership in a family.[25] Such strong familial identification was a product of economic necessity.[26] Individuals depended on the labor of their family members in order to survive. This dependence was based on strong gender roles: men worked outside the home, while women worked inside the home and were caregivers. The result was the presence, in the home, of reliable caregivers for the dying. But such caregiving was carried out in part due to economic necessity, and it depended on a highly restrictive conception of women's identity.[27]

Further, in the mid-nineteenth century, individuals generally died suddenly.[28] They usually did not require prolonged end-of-life care, and the care they did require was not expected to meet a professional standard. Indeed, there was no standardized medical profession.[29] In this context, the role of the familial caregiver was not to dramatically reduce the dying individual's pain; such pain reduction was impossible prior to the advent of anesthesiology. Rather, the role of the caregiver was to tend to the dying person's body as ably as possible while bearing witness, preferably in the company of a religious advisor, to their transition to the afterlife.[30] This primarily religious standard of care made family caregiving relatively accessible.

The broad lay population that could freely participate in caring for their dying relatives was almost entirely white, however. The United States prior to the advent of modern medicine was a country defined to a significant extent by its dependence on the labor of enslaved people and the violent expropriation of Native Americans' land. Slavery ripped black families apart, separating them from their relatives.[31] Native Americans were massacred in a genocide carried out by the US government.[32] Despite such circumstances, both African Americans and Native Americans did find ways to care for their dying relatives, and they also redefined the family, in part out of necessity, in largely nonbiological terms.[33] But the deaths of their relatives and their ability to care for and mourn them were to a significant degree shaped by their exposure to routine racist violence.

This racist violence supported many white families, including those who did not participate in it directly. The labor of enslaved people was essential to the sustenance of white family life in the South. Even in the North, slavery played a central part in the economy that facilitated unity among white families.[34] And the ability of white families to care for their loved ones was based, in part, on the economic gains created by the Native American genocide.[35] Thus, the United States, during the mid-nineteenth century, was characterized by a racist double standard in familial caregiving. The ability of whites to care for their dying relatives was to a substantial degree premised on the violent destruction of black and Native American families.

There was thus no golden age of US end-of-life care. Prior to the rise of medicine, the American family was not idyllic. It was a unit tightly bound by economic necessity, patriarchal gender roles, white supremacy, and a low standard of care. To a degree, it featured stable familial caregiving for dying people, but it did so at the cost of basic values that many of us now take for granted: women's rights, racial equality, and medical competence. Over the course of the twentieth century, these values increasingly manifested in the American social fabric. The result was momentous social progress. But the conception of the family that emerged from this progress posed difficulties for the vision of care advanced by US hospice leaders.

From the Family to the State

The rise of modern medicine coincided with the development of industrialization, which transformed the mid- to late nineteenth-century family structure.[36] Previously, the family had been held together, in part, by its members' economic interdependence. But with industrialization, it became possible to obtain the goods previously provided by the family in mass quantities. Industrialization, however, did not just give family members more options. It also, to a degree, forced them to shift the site of their labor from the home to the factory. This shift—which was at once economic and geographic—led to the breakdown of the preindustrial family. This disintegration made it more possible for the members of the family to see themselves as distinct from—and in opposition to—their relatives. This created a new kind of person: the individual.[37]

Prior to industrialization, individual identities had been subsumed in the prescribed roles of the family. Now, it became increasingly possible for individuals to imagine themselves as entities apart. The result was a weakening of the bonds that had characterized the nineteenth-century family. For many, this erosion was liberating. But it also entailed a shift in the meaning of family. The mid-nineteenth-century family had been characterized largely by a shared sense of obligation to biological kin. In the twentieth-century family, to a greater degree than before, individuals had the freedom to choose.[38]

As the century progressed, individuals increasingly chose families far away from the ones in which they had grown up. The result was a dramatic increase in internal migration, the process by which individuals move away from their childhood homes and biological families.[39] The causes for such internal migration were both economic and personal: individuals left home, in part, to acquire a better job—or any job at all—and, in part, because they enjoyed the freedom of living farther away from their relatives. The United States has generally had a higher degree of internal migration than other developed countries.[40] American internal migration has been particularly significant because of the country's relatively large size.

Women were one group that benefited from this enhanced mobility. They now found increasing opportunities to work independently and to earn their own sustenance.[41] At the same time, the development of birth control in the late 1950s made it possible for women to no longer be defined by their role as mothers.[42] Such changes allowed women to achieve a level of social and economic capital that was greater than had previously been the case. This capital was gained, to an extent, by leaving the labor of familial caregiving behind.[43]

This shift was accompanied by the declining significance of marriage in American life. Divorce rates increased dramatically over the twentieth century.[44] At present, 40–50 percent of marriages end in divorce.[45] This increase in divorce was due to a number of factors, including the rise of no-fault divorces, the decline of religion, and the decreasing significance of marriage in US life.[46] While these effects have been liberating in many ways, they also have left divorced people with less access to familial caregiving. Divorced people are more likely to live alone and at some distance from their relatives. Children of divorced families may have more conflicted relationships with their parents, which can make them feel fewer obligations to care for them.[47]

There are also fewer children to care for parents. The US fertility rate has been in steady decline since World War II and is currently at its lowest point on record.[48] While in 1800, a typical white woman had approximately seven children, that number is now fewer than two.[49] There are thus fewer children to care for their parents, and those children who do care likely do so with a greater burden. At the same time that birthrates have declined, the aging population has increased. Due to advances in medicine, individuals now live longer overall and for a longer period of time with some significant disability.[50] This demographic shift in the distribution of aging has created a situation in which a higher percentage of the population at any given time is dying.[51] All of this has increased the burden on individual familial caregivers.

Those who do provide care are expected to do so at a much higher standard than in the nineteenth century. By the mid-twentieth century, a "good death" was no longer defined in theological terms. Rather, it was defined in medical terms, as a death in the absence of pain and suffering.[52] This new conception of a good death changed the role of familial caretakers. To provide their loved ones with a good death, caretakers were expected to keep them relatively pain-free. And yet mitigating pain—including psychological suffering—at the end of life requires more than dedication. It also requires professional competence, which many familial caregivers lack.

Thus, the twentieth century witnessed a breakdown of the caregiving nucleus that had characterized the nineteenth-century family. This disintegration was due to the increasing amount of liberty that individuals had to shape their own lives in relative independence from their families. Individual identity was no longer prescribed by the family, and family members—particularly women—were no longer bound by obligation to care for each other. This was a liberating development in human history and meant a shift in how familial caregiving was defined.

In response to these developments, familial caregiving became an increasingly professionalized activity. By the mid-twentieth century, for example, women caregivers understood their role not as providing primary care, but rather as managing the different professional caregivers who provided services to their dying relatives.[53] This trend continued throughout the twentieth century with the rise of the nursing home and home health industries.[54] These industries replaced the familial caregiver, but only in a sense. Family members were still involved in the care of their relatives, but they were no longer the primary caregivers.

This professionalization, with increasing frequency, came at the request of dying patients themselves. Over the course of the twentieth century, elderly and dying individuals began to prefer to live independently from their relatives—specifically from their children—and to receive care from professionals.[55] This situation is referred to as "intimacy at a distance."[56] It stems from a desire on the part of the disabled or dying person not to burden their family members. It may also be due to a desire to not have their families see them in a state of debility. By the end of the twentieth century, caregiving was increasingly seen by dying people as something they would prefer to have carried out by professionals rather than by their families.[57]

Professional caregiving services are extremely expensive, and this increase in their role also increased the role that the state played in end-of-life care. In part to subsidize these services, President Lyndon Johnson signed into law the Social Security Amendments of 1965, which included Medicare and Medicaid.[58] In addition, the Social Security Amendments contained various provisions that benefited family caregivers and patients needing long-term care.[59] Due to Social Security benefits, familial caregivers would be better able to afford to continue working while caring for their dying loved ones. At the same time, through other Great Society programs aimed at ameliorating poverty and improving housing, caregivers who did not work outside the home would have greater resources to care for their dying relatives at home.[60] The dramatic expansion of the US welfare state in the 1960s worked, in part, to respond to the changes in the family that had occurred over the course of the early to mid-twentieth century.

Another expansion of the state that aided familial caregiving was the passage of the Civil Rights Act of 1964.[61] Though slavery had been abolished in 1865, African Americans continued to live with various forms of state-sponsored racism throughout the first half of the twentieth century.[62] African Americans were to a substantial degree excluded from the biggest expansions of the welfare state in the twentieth century: the New Deal.[63] Formal and informal residential segregation made it difficult for black people to acquire basic medical services.[64] And the tremendous obstacles to resource accumulation that were a result of segregation most likely made it difficult for African Americans to care for their dying relatives.[65]

African Americans responded to this white racism by continuing the formation of nonbiological kinship networks.[66] By expanding the pool of familial caregivers to include individuals who were nonbiological "family," they also created an expansive space for caregiving in black communities. Such flexible caregiving networks had helped black families to cope before the Civil Rights Act, and they continued to do so after.[67]

The professionalization of end-of-life care impacted black families differently than white ones. The paid caregiving labor of professional long-term care and home health workers is disproportionately carried out by women of color.[68] Such professional caregivers have been essential to helping predominantly white families cope with end-of-life care. But their labor for white people who are dying means that they have been less able to care for their own family members.[69] Since their work is not, in general, well paid, professional caregivers are unlikely to be able to afford to contract the labor of others. By plugging a gap in caregiving among predominantly white families, another hole is created in the families of nonwhite professional caregivers.

Thus, over the course of the twentieth century, the state came to subsidize and, in some cases, replace the role of the family in end-of-life care. Such subsidization came in the form of the expansion of the social safety net via benefits such as welfare, Medicare, Medicaid, and Social Security. Although such benefits were not received equally, they were helpful to some people, given the extent to which families were no longer prepared to provide end-of-life care. But even these small, significant improvements would be substantially rolled back as part of a larger shift in views about the role of government—a shift in which US hospice leaders played a part.

The Medicare Hospice Benefit and the Origins of US Neoliberalism

In the 1970s, the United States became the site for a major rethinking of the relationship between the family and the state. This reevaluation occurred under the auspices of an economic and political philosophy known as "neoliberalism."[70] Neoliberalism postulates that the ability of individuals to choose among available options in the marketplace is the essence of freedom. At the same time, such freedom comes at the expense of state power. The less power the state has to regulate the market, the freer the individual. Thus, neoliberalism construes an inverse relationship between individual freedom and state power, and it sides with individual freedom, believing it to be the highest social good. For this reason, neoliberalism is oriented toward replacing public services with private, market-based ones.

Though based in the individual, neoliberalism also places a strong emphasis on the family. As the sociologist Melinda Cooper has argued, the family, for neoliberals, operates as a support network for the individual during times when they cannot participate as a free subject in the marketplace.[71] Such times include when one is a child, during periods of illness, and at the end of life. When an individual is, as a result of a terminal disease, unable to enjoy freedom to the same degree previously possible, familial caregiving creates the foundation for individual freedom.

But such caregiving must not be supported by the state. In neoliberalism, state support is considered to be antithetical to familial caregiving. The extension of the welfare state, it is argued, undermines the ability and willingness of family members to provide care. The erosion of such bonds is a threat to individual freedom, and it is also a corrosion of the nature of the family. In this sense, Cooper argues, neoliberalism depends on a particular conception of family values, one in which caregiving relationships in the private sphere form the basis of what it means to be a "family."[72]

The US hospice movement, emerging in the 1970s, did not begin as part of this neoliberal revolution. Hospice leaders did not originally intend for the family's role in hospice to be to reduce the cost of state expenditures. But their belief in a nostalgic return to the "private" family of the nineteenth century cohered with the emerging neoliberal philosophy. It was because of its fit with neoliberalism that US hospice care was able to succeed to the degree it did. This co-optation of hospice by neoliberals, in turn, played a fundamental role in the expansion of neoliberalism on the national stage.

Cooper argues that the first site for the implementation of neoliberal policies began in the early 1970s with Governor Ronald Reagan's cuts to California's welfare program Aid to Families with Dependent Children.[73] As the historian Marisa Chappell has noted, these cuts could not be justified on a purely economic basis, since much more costly programs were left untouched.[74] Their basis, rather, was the fear that dependence on welfare eroded familial responsibility. Reagan's California reforms were the model for attempts at federal welfare reform throughout the 1970s and '80s. But Cooper argues that it was not until the Clinton administration's welfare reform efforts in the 1990s that "Governor Reagan's dream of a fully federalized system of familial responsibility" was realized.[75]

Though Cooper is correct about US government policy regarding early family life, the Reagan administration did succeed at implementing a federal program of familial responsibility at life's end: the Medicare Hospice Benefit. The benefit aimed to shrink the size of federal government expenditures by displacing care from the state onto the family. To do so, it implicitly promoted an ethic of familial responsibility to dying people. In this move from state support to a "traditional" model of familial caregiving, the MHB advanced the development of American neoliberalism.

This development was present in the benefit's moving of caregiving responsibilities from state-subsidized professionals to the private family. But it was particularly evident in the *degree* to which these caregiving responsibilities were transferred. The neoliberal philosophy underpinning the benefit was responsible for the mismatch that hospice leaders saw between the burden of care placed on American families and the amount of care that these families could provide. Though the MHB was set up to depend on the family, the degree of this familial dependence thwarted the ability of American families to provide the necessary care. In this sense, the Medicare Hospice Benefit was set up to fail on its own terms.

But the benefit not only epitomized the small government, pro-market ideology that is indicative of neoliberalism. It also set the wheels in motion for a series of other neoliberal reforms. These reforms have often been framed in terms of their advantages for families—and sometimes for family caregivers in particular. But in reality they undercut the social support necessary for effective caregiving, and they place both caregivers and dying individuals in positions of strain that are both unnecessary and immense. The result has been a transition from a mismatch to a crisis.

From Reaganomics to the Housing Crisis

The passage of the MHB coincided with the beginning of a period of dramatic cutbacks to social services. The next four US presidents—Reagan, George H. W. Bush, Bill Clinton, and George W. Bush—shared the belief that federal social welfare programs had to be scaled back.[76] Such government cutbacks have led to an increasing burden being placed on US families both in general and at the end of life.

The first serious shift came shortly after the MHB's passage with the Social Security Amendments of 1983. As described by sociologist Sandra Levitsky, the amendments created limits on the length of time a patient with a particular diagnosis could be hospitalized while receiving Medicare or Medicaid. Hospitals that did not comply with this limit were financially penalized, which led them to discharge patients earlier. Such discharges, in turn, led to patients at home being, on the whole, sicker than they had been prior to the amendments' passage.[77] The result has been that familial caregivers now have to provide care earlier than they did at the time of the MHB's passage, and they need to do so with a higher degree of technical capacity than had previously been the case.

Families also provide care with significantly fewer opportunities for financial assistance from the federal government. Between 1994 and 2012, the amount of government funds spent on welfare dramatically decreased. Whereas 14.2 million Americans in 1994 had been eligible for welfare, in 2012 only 4.6 million were—a decrease of 68 percent.[78] And due to inflation, the welfare benefits individuals did receive were less substantive than before. For example, it was reported in 2016 that the Temporary Assistance for Needy Families block grant, which was initiated with Clinton's 1996 welfare reform, had remained stagnant at $16.5 billion annually for the entire twenty years of its existence. Its benefits have lost more than one-third of their value.[79] At the same time that the value of welfare decreased, the eligibility requirements became more stringent.[80]

Welfare has thus become both less valuable and harder to obtain, even as it has become more necessary. Social scientists H. Luke Shaefer and Kathryn Edin have found that since the passage of welfare reform, there has been a dramatic increase in extreme poverty: households living on less than $2 in daily cash income per person. The number of households in this predicament increased 159 percent: from 636,000 in 1996 to 1.65 million in mid-2011.[81] Meanwhile, in 1996, welfare benefits were received by 68 out of 100 poor families with children. By 2014, that number had declined to 23 out of 100 poor families.[82] The amount of state support this population receives is less than at any point since the mid-1990s, and the work requirements of Clinton's welfare reform place familial caregivers in the difficult situation of having to choose between caring for their relatives or imperiling their benefits.[83]

Those who continue to work face another problem: the lack of paid familial leave. The 1993 Family and Medical Leave Act requires that businesses with more than fifty employees grant unpaid leave when it is needed for familial caregiving.[84] But the act has significant restrictions. By mandating only leave without pay, "the government," as sociologist Evelyn Nakano Glenn has argued, "accommodates care rather than fully supporting it."[85] And by exempting companies with fewer than fifty employees, the act does not mandate coverage for more than half of the workforce. Unpaid leave is thus, for many, both inadequate and inaccessible.

In theory, individuals unable to take paid familial leave should be able to contract for long-term care for their loved ones. In practice, this is extremely difficult. Since the late 1980s the cost of long-term care has increased substantially. In 1996, the average cost of one year of nursing home care was $40,000.[86] By 2016, that average cost was $100,000—an increase of 150 percent.[87] During that same period, the real median household income in the United States went from approximately $53,000 in 1996 to $56,000 in 2015—an increase of less than 6 percent.[88] In other words, in 1996 the cost of a year of nursing home care was 75 percent of the median household income. Now, it is more than 175 percent. Professional home care is even more expensive: round-the-clock home care averages $175,000 a year.[89]

As privately funding long-term care has become unfeasible, the difficulties of receiving publicly funded long-term care have increased. While the Reagan administration was expanding the government funding of US hospice care, it was curtailing the funding of long-term care.[90] At present, Medicare pays for at most 100 days of rehabilitation, which is not in general relevant for terminally ill patients.[91] Most long-term care is paid for by Medicaid.[92] But Medicaid requires that the assets of the beneficiary be no more than $2,000.[93] Most individuals in need of long-term care do not qualify and thus are faced with a decision about receiving appropriate care, significantly depleting their finances, or asking their family members for help.[94]

This lack of long-term care damages familial caregiving. Families in poverty frequently live unstable lives. They struggle for the basics, including food, housing, and health care. In such an environment, the ability of family members to care for dying relatives is severely compromised. Family members working long hours to make ends meet do not have the time to spend with their dying relatives. And if they do have the time, they often lack the material resources necessary to care for them.[95] Even when families receive the MHB, caring for dying people still comes with substantial costs.[96]

The lack of appropriate social support for end-of-life care is compounded by the effects of living in poverty. Poor families frequently live in neighborhoods that, ironically, significantly raise their cost of living.[97] Such neighborhoods often lack ready access to grocery stores and healthy food.[98] Dying individuals and their caregivers thus need to travel farther to obtain sustenance. This requires time (to travel) and economic resources (to afford transportation and food). But such areas frequently lack accessible public transportation.[99] These problems are significant in urban contexts, and poor communities in rural areas face similar obstacles.[100]

Already bad, this situation dramatically worsened with the recession and housing crisis of 2007–2009. The Great Recession increased the US poverty rate from 12.5 percent in 2007 to 15 percent in 2011, leaving more than 45 million Americans in poverty.[101] The recession did not just affect the poor. Middle-class families lost approximately 23 percent of their wealth,[102] which damaged the ability of individuals to provide care. The recession created situations in which people had less money to afford basic goods, much less paid assistance. It made those individuals who had jobs have to work longer hours, away from their dying relatives. And it broke up families through increased suicide rates and compounded health problems.[103]

The crisis had a particularly negative impact on the site where US hospice care is designed to take place: the home. Ten million Americans lost their homes as a result of the recession.[104] More than two-thirds of the families whose homes were foreclosed on will not be homeowners again.[105] The US home ownership rate thus is down to its lowest level in more than fifty years.[106] The situation for renters is similarly grim. Since 2010, rental prices have risen at nearly twice the rate of average hourly wages. As a result, one in four US renters use half of their income to pay their housing costs. This leaves working Americans—2.3 million people—on the brink of financial collapse and homelessness.[107] These citizens have no place to care for their relatives, and the toll of foreclosure and eviction on the familial bonds necessary for caregiving is intense.[108]

Thus, the almost forty years since the MHB's passage have witnessed reductions in the social services that are essential to both dying people and their caregivers. These cutbacks have become even more harmful in the wake of the Great Recession, which damaged not only the economic resources and vocational aspirations of millions of Americans, but also the core site of hospice care delivery and the familial bonds necessary for its success. This has devastated both the families and the home environments necessary for US hospice care. This devastation is widespread, but it has a particularly harsh impact on individuals of marginalized racial groups.

Systemic Racism at the End of Life

Since the early twentieth century, racist housing discrimination has been a dominant force in American life. This discrimination has been levied against people of color in general, but it has primarily targeted African Americans.[109] Through discriminatory policies at the level of federal, state, and local governments—as well as informal acts of bias by realtors, property owners, and banks—African Americans have been disproportionately segregated in neighborhoods with significantly less wealth than their white counterparts. For lower-class black people, racist housing discrimination compounds the problems associated with poverty. But middle- and upper-class black people also suffer the negative effects of such bias, including higher costs of living and increased crime rates.[110] And the persistence of discrimination makes it difficult for African Americans and other people of color to leave such neighborhoods.[111]

Ultimately, these discriminatory practices target the home. The median net worth of white households is thirteen times greater than that of African Americans.[112] These depressed home values negatively affect all other aspects of life, hindering black people's upward mobility and making it more difficult to leave neighborhoods struggling with the effects of racism.[113] This housing discrimination was amplified by the housing crisis. African Americans and Latinos lost their homes due to foreclosure at significantly higher rates than whites. Blacks and Latinos were both targets of the loans that precipitated the crisis, and they were the biggest victims of what came afterward.[114]

Racial bias adds significant barriers to familial caretaking. African Americans of lower and middle socioeconomic status often live in neighborhoods that are more likely to lack food access and public transportation.[115] These areas are also likely to have higher crime rates than white neighborhoods.[116] Although the causes of crime in urban black communities are complicated, there is ample evidence that they are influenced by the pervasive lack of opportunities due to discrimination.[117] Further, pervasively lower home values have given African Americans less economic capital to be upwardly mobile.[118] As a result, African American families suffer from a disproportionate lack of the services necessary to sustain long-term end-of-life care.

At the same time, kinship bonds in African American communities have been fragmented due to the rise of mass incarceration. Beginning in the early 1970s, the US prison population dramatically expanded, climbing from less than 200,000 people in 1970 to more than 1.5 million in 2014.[119] This increase in incarceration, which has disproportionately impacted African Americans, was heightened by the Reagan administration's "war on drugs."[120] But its causes are complex, related both to federal, state, and local policies and to attitudes about crime in the black community itself.[121] Though African Americans make up only 13 percent of the US population, they account for 35.8 percent of those in prison.[122] Mass incarceration has broken up African American families, hindered their access to resources, and diluted socially cohesive groups that used to be protective in times of crisis.[123]

Housing discrimination, poverty, and mass incarceration have taken a significant toll on the familial organizations and resources that African American communities depend on for the delivery of hospice care. To the extent that the MHB depends on familial caregiver support—and does not address these racial inequalities—it leaves African American families in discriminated-against areas in situations where they are unable to benefit from hospice services. Such bias also has negatively impacted other nonwhite groups, leading to the creation of a hospice system that enforces systemic discrimination in end-of-life care.

Thus, since the MHB's passage, a number of events—outside of hospice— occurred that have further heightened the level of care required of familial caregivers, while limiting the resources available to assist them in providing it. These changes have been accompanied by changes internal to hospice that have further increased the caregiving burden placed on American families.

From Medicare to Obamacare

The president's rhetoric notwithstanding, the Reagan administration did not cut US healthcare expenditures. Rather, it redirected them. While government expenditures on health care had previously been focused on the nonprofit sector, Reagan incentivized public investment in for-profit institutions. This was part of his administration's larger shift toward the privatization of public resources.[124] The MHB was part of this change. It not only funded existing hospice organizations, but also incentivized the creation of a new entity: the for-profit hospice.[125]

This shift to the public remuneration of private, for-profit corporations dramatically changed the economic structure of US hospice care. At the time of the

MHB's passage, there were practically no for-profit hospices.[126] The industry was entirely dominated by nonprofit and government hospices.[127] But by 1992, 13 percent of Medicare-certified hospices were for profit.[128] This grew to 47 percent by 2002. At present, more than 60 percent of US hospices are for profit.[129] According to the Medicare Payment Advisory Commission (MedPAC), for-profit providers have accounted "almost entirely" for the growth in the hospice industry since 2002.[130] The industry share of for-profit hospices, if these trends continue, is likely to grow larger.

For-profit hospices have a different financial structure than nonprofit hospices. Nonprofit hospices do not have shareholders. Their earnings must be reinvested in their business. For-profit hospice organizations, in contrast, must be financially profitable for their shareholders if they are to stay viable. They are thus incentivized to enroll patients that they are better able to profit from.[131] Which patients fit this category—and which do not—depends on the reimbursement structure of the MHB.

Under the MHB, hospices are paid a flat per diem rate on each patient. In theory, this would lead them to treat all patients equally. But even on a flat rate, all patients are not equally cost effective. The highest costs of care occur at the beginning of hospice treatment—when the patient is enrolling—and at the end, when they are dying. As a result, hospices make the most money in the middle of service, when the patient has already been enrolled but is not yet actively dying.[132] Because of this, hospices have an economic incentive to enroll patients with longer disease trajectories.

The result has been a shift in the disease patterns of patients admitted to hospice. When the MHB began in 1982, approximately 95 percent of hospice patients were dying of cancer.[133] But cancer patients do not have long disease trajectories in hospice. Hospice requires that they give up the chemotherapeutic and targeted biological treatments that constitute much of American cancer care. As a result, cancer patients do not generally arrive for services until very late in their illness, and they die, on average, after a little more than two weeks in hospice.[134] Patients with non-cancer diagnoses have longer lengths of stay: on average, forty-three days for dementia and twenty-three for other non-cancer diagnoses.[135] This makes them more profitable and has led to these patients being selectively recruited by for-profit hospices.[136] Due to this selective recruitment, for-profit hospices enroll a disproportionate number of patients with non-cancer diagnoses.[137] In part as a result of this incentive structure, the number of hospice patients with non-cancer diagnoses has substantially grown.[138]

This increase of patients with non-cancer diagnoses is welcome. They need end-of-life care too. But patients with non-cancer diagnoses require more labor from familial caregivers than cancer patients do. They live for longer periods of time. As a result, they require family members to be present for longer periods. This can require significant sacrifices. Family caregivers providing long-term care frequently have to take time off work.[139] There also is an increased chance that, over that caregiving period, they may experience some form of disability or other condition that impedes their ability to provide care.[140] And the economic burden of providing familial caregiving is significant.[141] The epidemiological shift in hospice to dying patients with more long-term diagnoses intensifies these problems.

At the same time, hospice services are not fully supportive for patients with more long-term diagnoses. Hospice was designed in the United States to care for cancer patients. They served as the major patient population on which the hospice model of care was based. This model is insufficient, however, for the needs of patients with longer-term diagnoses.[142] These diagnoses can include significant cognitive problems—such as Alzheimer's disease and dementia—and physical disabilities. Hospice does not include services designed for these populations. The result can be difficulties in the delivery of care.[143]

The shift to a for-profit model of hospice has had negative implications for patients with the most severe conditions. Patients with more significant medical needs are in general less likely to be admitted to for-profit hospices.[144] Once admitted, they are more likely to be denied treatments that are effective but expensive.[145] They also on average receive less continuing care in the home context than they would in a nonprofit counterpart. For-profit hospices are 22 percent less likely to dispatch a nurse to see patients during the last two weeks of life.[146] They are less responsive at precisely the time when patients and families most need help, and they limit the type of help they are willing to provide.

The MHB requires spiritual care and social work, but requirements for this care are so general that many hospices offer only minimal levels of spiritual counseling or psychosocial support.[147] These hospices promote themselves "as providing holistic care when, in fact, many [do] not support active involvement of nonmedical professionals."[148] This marginalization of nonmedical services is compounded by the deficiencies in social work and chaplaincy education in the training of professionals who provide care at the end of life.[149] Consequently, these services are not sufficiently offered and, even when offered, often are not adequate to the patient's and family's needs. This leaves familial caregivers with a greater burden of nonmedical care.

When family members cannot cope, the US hospice system provides only a minimal safety net for them. Under the MHB's reimbursement structure, it is difficult to run a financially viable inpatient hospice. As a result, only one in five hospices offers inpatient care.[150] Hospice care does include a component designed to give a rest—known as "respite"—to familial caregivers. But due to the limited number of inpatient hospices, this respite care has to take place in either a nursing home or a hospital. Furthermore, it can be difficult to find nursing homes and hospitals that will take these patients at the Medicare reimbursement rate of $100 per day.[151] This suggests—in the words of health economists Haiden Huskamp, Melinda Beeuwkes Buntin, Virginia Wang, and Joseph P. Newhouse— that "the respite per diem does not reflect the marginal costs of treating respite patients."[152] This discrepancy impedes the ability of caregivers to obtain relief.

The Affordable Care Act (ACA) does contain provisions that ease this familial burden. MedPAC—the advisory body established by the ACA to oversee hospice —recommended that hospice be made available to individuals who continue to receive curative interventions. This recommendation—which at the end of 2018 was undergoing a test demonstration—will perhaps allow more dying patients to get involved in hospice earlier, thus making supportive services available to family members earlier.[153] MedPAC has also recommended changing the reimbursement structure of hospice so that the per diem is not flat, but higher at the beginning and at the end of care.[154] The Centers for Medicare and Medicaid Services have duly revised the payment guidelines, in part to discourage longer stays, while also increasing the funding available during the last seven days of life.[155]

Even if they are helpful, the interventions suggested by the MedPAC board are not targeted at easing the burdens of familial caretakers. Rather, the primary goal is eliminating fraud.[156] Various major US hospice corporations have been found guilty of systematically enrolling patients before they are technically "terminally ill."[157] But the focus on fraud ignores the fact that the patients enrolled "prematurely" often do benefit from, and even need, hospice care. Ultimately, by using fraud as the primary lens to view the federal regulation of hospice care, the MedPAC board wrongly implies that the care that dying people in the United States receive is *too much*. But this conclusion does not consider the shifts in hospice epidemiology and treatment that have been inaugurated under the increasingly for-profit model of US hospice care. Although the ACA originally included provisions to increase long-term care support to familial caregivers, these were left out of the final bill.[158] As a result, the ACA does not address the trend in hospice toward increasingly burdening families.

Since the passage of the Medicare Hospice Benefit, US hospice care has come to depend increasingly on the support of familial caretakers. At the same time, the benefit gives them less support than had originally been planned. This two-pronged situation in itself is troubling. But it is catastrophic when we acknowledge that the family that the MHB depends on is for the most part not really there.

Crisis

I have argued that the Medicare Hospice Benefit relies on a familial support network that, even at the time of its passage, was overextended. In the almost forty years since, the gap between the capabilities of US families and hospice requirements has grown. Contemporary families are in general far removed from the task of caring for dying people. They are being asked to carry out tasks that they have little or no experience in, for relatives about whom they often have complex and ambivalent feelings. In the best of circumstances, this would be difficult.

But many US families are not living in the best of circumstances. Their economic capital has been substantially depleted. They are either unemployed, underemployed, or working too much, with no paid leave. And the home is more tenuous than it has been in decades. Families need support, but they have less than they did in the early 1980s. Since the housing collapse, we are facing a situation that can only be defined as a crisis, in which the gap between the demands made on familial caregivers and their ability to meet them is so great as to imperil the functioning of US hospice care.

Evidence of this crisis abounds. It can be found in both the increasing number of hospice patients cared for in inpatient facilities—such as nursing homes and assisted living facilities—and the increasing number of patients and family members who prefer care to take place in such institutional settings.[159] It can be found in the burnout and compassion fatigue of familial caregivers and hospice staff, both of whom are faced with patients who have greater needs than they can provide.[160] It can be found in the increasingly limited enrollment policies of US hospices, 12 percent of which do not accept patients without familial caregivers.[161] It can be found in investigations revealing that 18 percent of US hospices—serving 50,000 patients—provide the dying and their families with "very little care" in the period immediately before death.[162]

Evidence of this crisis also can be found in the research of physician Joan Teno. She found that during 2000–2009, transitions between different care settings increased by 50 percent during the last ninety days of life.[163] Though more people are dying at home, they are spending less time at home in the weeks prior to death and more time moving between care settings, such as hospitals and nursing homes. Such transitions are indicative of the lack of a fixed location for dying individuals and suggest that home caregivers are increasingly unable to meet the needs of their dying family members. It also suggests that there are not alternative institutions available in the United States that can house them. The result is a dramatic lack of stability for dying people at the very end of their lives.

In response to this crisis, the nursing home has reemerged as a site for the delivery of end-of-life care. But the US hospice movement was a response to the failure of nursing homes to adequately care for dying people. Regardless of that initial problem, due to the structure of the US hospice system, the number of Americans dying in nursing homes has significantly increased, doubling between 1999 and 2006.[164]

Placing dying patients in nursing homes is a response to the lack of sufficient caregiving in the home environment. Nursing homes are not facilities for dying people, but they provide custodial care to patients while hospices deliver end-of-life care. As I explain further in chapter 4, such coordinated care is inefficient and ineffective—perhaps irredeemably so. That it even exists—much less is growing exponentially—is evidence of a serious problem. Indeed, the usage of nursing homes at the end of life highlights the extent to which the crisis in US hospice care is inextricable from a broader crisis in long-term care. The aging of the US population has created a significant need for long-term care. But the availability of such care has decreased due to a shortage of home healthcare workers and a significant drop in the number of nursing homes.[165]

Even if sufficient locations of care existed, there is currently no financing method that would make this care readily available. Indeed, as Sandra Levitsky points out, the US welfare state largely dates back to a period when the country's long-term care needs were much smaller than they are today.[166] This is a problem since US hospice care depends on professional long-term care to alleviate the burden on families. But right now, the US long-term care system is itself highly dependent on the family.

This makes the issue of familial dependence far more widespread—and serious —than just a problem of hospice. Familial caregivers do not just care for dying people. They care for their disabled relatives long before they begin to be "dying" —and they continue caring for each other after as well. The burden on caregivers is thus even higher than I have depicted here.

This is particularly the case because individuals do not in general end up on hospice until it is far too late. Indeed, hospice begins for dying Americans, on average, in the last two weeks of their life.[167] This is far too short a time for patients to receive adequate end-of-life care. The cause of this problem is in part how we have organized hospice. But it is also a problem of the healthcare system as a whole. It is a product of what Sharon Kaufman has shown to be the incentives in Medicare to give dying people "curative" treatments that make them ineligible for hospice.[168] Such incentives could be counteracted by Medicare reform. But they could also be challenged—as both the MedPAC board and legal scholar Kathy Cerminara have suggested—by changing Medicare so that curative interventions and hospice are not pitted in opposition.[169]

And yet, *just* making hospice more accessible to dying people is not enough. Indeed, as I have argued, long stays on hospice increase the burden of caregiving to a degree that is unsustainable for many family members. That so few people even receive hospice until it is too late also increases that burden. The problems are both the lack of hospice accessibility *and* the lack of services once hospice is accessible. These issues go well beyond the purview of individual hospice providers or even our hospice system, but they collude to create a crisis in US hospice care.

The crisis can be found in stories like that of Ying Tai Choi.[170] An eighty-five-year-old woman, Choi was abandoned by her hospice nurse shortly before her death. Her daughter, Ching Cheung, had to comfort her alone. Although lacking the training to do so, Cheung tried giving her mother "a few drops of water," but understandably felt helpless. Her mother died an hour later—under hospice service but without professional support.

Such cases of abandonment have been the focus of several journalistic exposés: the *Washington Post* series "Business of Dying" by Peter Whoriskey and Dan Keating; "'No One Is Coming': Hospice Patients Abandoned at Death's Door" by JoNel Aleccia and Melissa Bailey in *Kaiser Health News*; and "Hospice in Crisis" by Joanne Kenen in *Politico*.[171] Though different in some respects, these exposés all emphasize the substantial gap between what hospice asks familial caregivers to do and what they are reasonably able to provide.

Aleccia and Bailey, for example, provide evidence of this mismatch with numerous stories that parallel that of Choi. Robert Martin, Leo Fuerstenberg, James Ingle, and Leanne Mills were all abandoned by hospice in their hour of need; this neglect hurt them and haunted their caregivers for long after. The extent of such abandonment is detailed in a retrospective study of more than 600,000 Medicare hospice patients, 12 percent of whom died without seeing a skilled professional in the last two days of their lives—precisely the time when they and their families most required professional help.[172] Government inspection reports collected by the Centers for Medicare and Medicaid Services provide a picture of the problem's severity. Based on an analysis of 20,000 of these reports, Aleccia and Bailey note that "missed visits and neglect are common for patients dying at home."[173]

Since 2012, families or caregivers filed more than 3,200 complaints with state officials. This number is significant, but it is in all likelihood a severe underestimation of the current state of affairs. Hospice experts say that many families may be "too traumatized" to file formal reports.[174] As Joan Teno put it, the reports that we do have are from only the most rare and extreme cases: "people who got upset enough to complain."[175]

The hospices that abandoned these patients should be held accountable. But the root cause of this neglect is not the actions of any individual hospice. It is the mismatch between the capacities of familial caregivers and the assistance that the US hospice system is willing to provide. Countering this mismatch requires changing the US hospice system as a whole.

This has been recognized by the Institute of Medicine (IOM), a nonprofit organization affiliated with the National Academy of Sciences. The IOM's purpose is to provide evidence-based recommendations for American health policy. It addressed end-of-life policy in its report *Dying in America*.[176]

The report was written by a committee of twenty-one of our country's most distinguished experts on end-of-life care. These experts note that familial caregivers in the US hospice system face "enormous burdens"—"physical, emotional, practical and financial."[177] In the context of these burdens, they argue that "a major reorientation of Medicare and Medicaid is needed to craft a system of care that is properly designed to address the central needs of nearly all Americans nearing the end of life."[178]

A "major reorientation of Medicare and Medicaid" is necessary to address the needs of "nearly all Americans nearing the end of life." This quotation indicates the presence of what can only be called a crisis. The IOM's report offers much that illustrates this dire situation and deepens our understanding of it. It also provides a wealth of helpful suggestions as to what must be done to alleviate it.

Such suggestions are well worth taking because without dramatic action, this crisis *will* get worse. The demographic shifts that I have detailed in this chapter are intensifying. There will be more dying people and fewer family members to take care of them.[179] There will also be fewer long-term care facilities where dying people can be cared for and fewer adequate funding mechanisms to support this care.[180] Unless there is dramatic national action of the sort the IOM recommends, the present crisis of US hospice care will reach a catastrophic zenith.

It does not have to turn out this way. But to prevent this escalation, we need a coherent understanding of why this situation emerged, which is what I have provided over these last two chapters. The current crisis of US hospice care could be described as having origins in the 80:20 ratio of outpatient to inpatient care or, more broadly, in the neoliberal attack on the welfare state. But these explanations, though essential, do not grasp the crisis's underlying root. This root is freedom—or, more specifically the lack thereof.

In the MHB, dying people are treated as sufferers to be cared for or as cost-drivers to be contained. But they are not treated as political subjects whose freedom the state has an obligation to secure. There is no obligation on the part of the federal government to provide them with care, no attempt to write them into the larger narrative of freedom in America. There is no argument being made for the freedom of dying people or even any theory about what such freedom would mean. With regard to the question of freedom, the Medicare Hospice Benefit declares itself to be irrelevant.

This irrelevance is of a piece with the larger logic of neoliberalism itself. As political theorist Wendy Brown has argued, neoliberalism operates by *de*politicization.[181] It redefines freedom—and other political issues—as questions of economic management. This takes freedom out of the public domain, where its meaning can be contested. Neoliberalism makes freedom the purview of a class of professional technocrats. This is harmful with respect to the individual issues these technocrats mean to address. Worse, it harms democracy itself.

The MHB epitomizes both these harms. Rather than defining dying people as political beings, it describes them in terms that are medical and economic. It establishes no state obligation to secure their freedom. And it takes the debate about the need for such an obligation out of the public domain. The basing of US hospice care on familial caregiving is a by-product of this depoliticization. Had our hospice system been designed with the freedom of dying people in mind, we might have avoided the crisis we currently face.

CHAPTER FOUR

What Happens to Dying People When Love Is Not Enough

Raúl Acosta was dying. He had dementia and Parkinson's. And now lung cancer. None of this was shocking in a man of ninety-plus years. But, shocking or not, they made his life hard. He had difficulty talking, difficulty in being understood, difficulty swallowing, difficulty bathing and brushing and moving, difficulty turning himself in bed. He spoke no English, had little money, and lived in a suburb of Atlanta known for its gigantic memorial to the Confederate dead. For these—and perhaps a few other—reasons he might have been expected to die alone, in pain, too unknown to even be forgotten. And yet when I visited, he was safely cushioned, munching on a banana in a room whose curtains were layered with light.

It was Marta who made it possible. Marta, his daughter, one of three, who was caring for him until the end. She had been doing it for six years, ever since he had fallen in New York. She had quit her job selling real estate and moved him to Georgia. Now, she spent her days formulating ways to make him fit into her world, and herself fit into his. The hospice physician had thought Raúl needed to be tube-fed, but Marta designed meals that were easily chewable, cutting up his food into pieces small enough for him to swallow. She read to him from the Bible, devised innovative ways to get him the medicine he needed, and had conversations with him that no other person could understand. She did it all while being a mother to two children, a wife, a sister, and a dedicated friend.

"He's my father." She shrugged when I asked her about it. He had cared for her when she was a child, and now she was doing the same for him.

She did it with the help of hospice. Hospice sent her a home health aide who, twice a week, bathed her father. Marta would have done it herself, but Raúl was a Jehovah's Witness, and due to religious reasons he preferred to be bathed by a stranger. Hospice provided medication, some of which was administered by hospice nurses, some of which Marta administered herself. Hospice also provided a chaplain who, once every week or two, came and prayed with them. Finally, hospice provided a volunteer who sat with her father for a few hours once a week, so that Marta could do chores in the house and run errands outside.

This support from hospice was helpful. But it was only *support*. Marta—not the hospice team—was the one who took care of her father. She stayed with him day and night. She figured out how to feed him and then fed him. She took the time to listen to what he was saying and knew enough about him to make even the most seemingly nonsensical conversations make sense. She took him up the stairs and down the stairs, brought her whole family together around him, and she was there, with as many of them as could be gathered, on the day that he finally died.

Given his condition and the world we live in, Raúl Acosta had no right to expect a good death, but a good death was what he got. In part, this was due to hospice. Hospice lightened the load and provided medicine and supplies—such as his bed—that made life easier for both Raúl and Marta Acosta. But her father's good death was mainly the work of Marta. Without her support, his fate would have been far worse.

It is easy to get misty-eyed when thinking about cases like this. This is a beautiful story, one that reminds us that even in the direst of circumstances—dementia! cancer! Parkinson's!—a good death is possible. We celebrate caregivers like Marta as examples of familial dedication, of the ability of hospice to allow patients to die at home, and of the ability to rescue—and even elevate—human dignity in the midst of seemingly inevitable suffering. Celebration is certainly warranted, but we should not be tricked into thinking that such caregiving is the norm.

There was nothing normal about Marta's care. She provided it due to a reason that is foreign to many Americans in the twenty-first century: a commitment to her father so strong that she was willing to abandon her professional life in its entirety. And she could only make this commitment because she had a level of material resources, interpersonal support, and physical and mental health that many others lack. Her husband's income as a mechanic was enough to support her family. The neighborhood where they lived was affordable, was safe, and had ready access to quality grocery stores and good public schools. She was also supported by the state. Her father was on Medicare and received both Social Security and veteran's benefits. Without this material support, Marta would not have been able to provide care over even a short period—much less six years.

Further, she might not have been able to continue, even with her level of dedication and resources, if her father's condition had been worse. Marta's father had extremely significant medical conditions, conditions that would make home care impossible in many circumstances. But if Raúl Acosta had Alzheimer's disease, for example, rather than "mere" dementia, then it is unlikely that Marta Acosta would have been able to continue caring for him in her home. Marta should serve as an example of what exceptional familial caregiving can accomplish. This example should not, however, create the impression that familial caregiving—even of an exceptional kind—will be enough.

Marta should be commended for what she is: a hero. But we should not design a hospice system with the assumption that heroes are the norm. Most people do not have the resources or the will to make heroic sacrifices. And even if they did, it is not reasonable to expect them to do so. Marta Acosta is the ideal caregiver that, to some degree, we should all aspire to be. But we have designed our hospice system with two assumptions: that most people can be like her and that if they were like her, it would be enough. Both these assumptions are wrong.

They also reinforce the social expectations that we have set for people in general and women in particular. I am comfortable calling the care that Marta provided for her father "heroic." But I am not sure that it is necessarily more heroic than the exertions of a woman who, rather than sacrifice her life for a dying parent, chooses to work instead. Such a woman is a hero in her own right—bucking centuries of patriarchal values that have consigned her to the role of caregiver. Valorizing the heroism of the working woman—fighting a system designed to keep her in her place—does not entail denigrating the work of someone like Marta. But valorizing Marta should not require us to denigrate women who choose not to be caregivers.

What we should denigrate is a public policy structure that makes the choice of caring or working a zero-sum game. The lack of paid familial leave requires people who want to be primary caregivers to forfeit their jobs and career aspirations in order to care for their loved ones. The lack of adequate long-term care financing—and even adequate long-term care—means that people who do "choose" to work are forced to place their relatives in situations that they themselves suspect are inadequate or even harmful. The result can be feelings of guilt and depression.[1] In this sense, the US health system and the larger economy are set up in a way that at once forces people, especially women, to choose while giving them no good choice at all.

This was true of Marta as well. Though Marta chose to give up her career, she was forced into this choice by the sharp divide between her family values and the design of the US hospice system and welfare state. Had there been more support for paid familial leave, more long-term care support, and even more robust hospice services, she might not have needed to sacrifice her career to care for her father. Though she relished providing such care, the extreme circumstances in which she provided it did force her to make several sacrifices that imperiled not only her own well-being, but also that of her family. The average familial caregiver forgoes $304,000 in wages and benefits over their lifetime.[2] My guess is that Marta gave up a lot more. That she did so is an admirable reflection of her will to care and a despairing indictment of the lack of such will in US public policy. In this sense, Marta Acosta is not just a hero. She is also a victim. And such victimhood is part and parcel of the "choices" that our public policy apparatus forces caregivers—primarily women—to make throughout the lifespan, but particularly at the end of life.

The focus of this chapter, however, is not the effects of the US hospice design on primary caregivers. My focus here is its effects on dying people themselves. I specifically examine what happens to patients who do not have caregivers like Marta—caregivers who are able to be adequate. "Adequate" may seem like an underwhelming term to describe the heroism of someone like Marta. But that is my point. In the US hospice system, caregivers are forced to become heroes if they want to be adequate. The hospice system requires their contribution in order to function: it is a form of care that supports but does not replace the familial caregiver.

But when adequate familial caregiving is lacking, the benefits of hospice are significantly limited. The result is a failure in the delivery of basic health services —but it is more than a service failure. It destroys the very freedom of dying patients. This destruction is systemic and pervasive, and the problem is not just medical, but political. It will continue as long as the US hospice system is dependent on familial caregiving rather than providing political freedom.

I examine this destruction through an ethnographic study of a facility that I refer to as "Amberview Hospice." Before doing so, I explain why I am using ethnography to study the relationship between freedom and familial caregiving in US hospice care.

The Uses of Ethnography

Ethnography is a method of empirical research that is based on qualitative interviews and systematic observation. Since it is usually rooted in particular settings, ethnography has been criticized for not being generalizable. As my goal here is to illustrate problems in US hospice care as a whole, such a method might seem inappropriately narrow in its scope. But this is not the case because of the nature of the US hospice system.

Amberview Hospice, which I discuss here, is a local institution, but its structure is determined by Medicare, which funds the vast majority of US hospice services. Amberview is a good window into the overall hospice system because its structure epitomizes at a basic level that of every other hospice in the country. Indeed, the observations that I make are not only generalizable; they have largely already been generalized. Copious research by quantitative scientists has attested to the extent of the various problems that I identify here (see also chapter 3).

Ethnography is an *interpretive* method. What it gives up in terms of its ability to generalize from data, it gains in its ability to evaluate it. Such interpretation ideally examines the relationships between the individuals studied, the local communities in which they are enmeshed, and the society in which they participate. In this sense, ethnographic interpretation is unusually flexible and wide-ranging. Such flexibility is necessary for two related aspects of this book.

First, I describe and define a category that I refer to as "patients with inadequate familial support." This category is new.[3] Though it intersects with a number of existing sociological categories—such as race, socioeconomic status, disability, marital status—it does not clearly map onto any of them. It involves multiple factors that are mediated through the biological aspects of terminal illness, resist quantification, and would likely be missed by a purely quantitative approach.[4] Constructing this category thus requires a method that is exploratory, analytical, and synthetic, capable of creating new classifications from observation. Ethnography is appropriate for this task.

Second, I examine the impact of such inadequate familial support on dying people. This requires another work of interpretation: creating a conceptual framework that grasps the impact of diverse stimuli on an individual. The framework I have chosen is freedom, and ethnography provides a means of defining it and then analyzing its applicability to the circumstances of particular dying individuals and of "dying people" as a population. Ultimately, through interpretation, ethnography provides a means of relating freedom and inadequate familial support. Since this book represents a first attempt to create and relate these categories within the ambit of US hospice care, my method is necessarily exploratory. With its relatively open means of gathering data, ethnography is appropriate for such exploration.

Ethnography is also particularly well suited for the literary power that my task requires. It is one thing to write that someone is "not free," but unless that statement is accompanied by a strong illustration of what "freedom" means, it is almost worthless. Such a description, in turn, should carry with it a certain amount of affect. It should not just present a person who is lacking freedom, but also explain *why* they are unfree and what the lack of freedom *feels* like: what it is like to be crushed by your own body and an entire society at the same time.

Affecting literary depictions are necessary if we are to productively reorient our national conversations about freedom at the end of life. Such conversations have in general not been guided by quantitative data. For example, the number of people who have sought out physician-assisted suicide is, as PAS supporters acknowledge, extremely small relative to the general population of dying people.[5] But PAS has dominated national headlines in part because it weds a powerful concept—freedom—to highly poignant individual stories. The US debate about freedom at the end of life has thus centered around a few central figures, including Brittany Maynard, Terri Schiavo, Karen Quinlan, and Nancy Cruzan.

We might respond to this situation by attempting to deemphasize individual stories altogether, instead opting for a quantitative approach that is more "rational." The stories I give here are a more accurate statistical representation of what dying in America is like than that which is generally showcased in our assisted-suicide debate. But statistics are not enough, nor should they be. The people I mentioned above have catalyzed us because their stories speak to us personally, as individuals, and politically, as members of a nation-state that claims to share certain values. These stories *are* important.

The problem is that they are not as important as is generally taken to be the case. Placing them in perspective requires presenting new stories of freedom at the end of life. Such stories can and indeed must catalyze us at our deepest level, speaking to our hopes and fears as individuals and as a people. By doing so, they can provide a perspective that is more representative of what dying in America currently is, and they can motivate us to transform this current state into a collectively shared vision of what dying *should be*. Ethnography, because of its literary power, because of its ability to analyze the individual from a comprehensive perspective is an essential tool to reorient our national debate.[6]

General Structure of Amberview Hospice

Amberview Hospice—a pseudonym—is an Atlanta branch of the Amberview Hospice Corporation, a major provider of hospice services throughout the country. The parent company is a for-profit corporation, and this for-profit structure is consistent in all of the organization's branches. These branches vary greatly in size and patient demographics, but they all comply with Medicare regulations. As a result of this compliance, while Amberview has many characteristics that are particular to its metro Atlanta area, it also mirrors the broader structure of other branches of the Amberview Hospice Corporation as well as Amberview's competitors throughout the United States.

Since the Medicare Hospice Benefit mandates that hospice be primarily an outpatient benefit, the vast majority of Amberview's clinical staff is oriented toward outpatient care. This outpatient staff is divided into two teams. As stipulated in the MHB, each team is interdisciplinary, which means that the structure of each team is a manifestation of the holistic orientation of hospice, encompassing, in theory, the medical, psychosocial, and spiritual dimensions of care.[7] The team's members each represent one of these dimensions. Each team is led by a medical director, who is a trained physician, and a patient care manager (PCM), who is a registered nurse. The medical director prescribes medications and care plans and ensures that each patient meets hospice eligibility requirements. The PCM manages the administration of medications through two case managers, who are also registered nurses. They are joined by the assistant to the patient care manager, who does paperwork to ensure that the hospice is appropriately reimbursed by its payers for each patient. Together, the case managers, the medical director, and the PCM make up each team's medical staff.

This medical staff is complemented by one chaplain, who oversees spiritual care for patients, families, and, occasionally, hospice staff. Psychosocial care is carried out by a social worker, who oversees placement, discharge planning, and, occasionally, counseling. In addition, both teams' meetings are attended by the hospice's bereavement coordinator and volunteer coordinator. In total, the team contains nine members: a medical director, a PCM, two case managers, a chaplain, a social worker, the volunteer coordinator, the bereavement coordinator, and an assistant to the PCM.

In addition to this team, Amberview includes several professionals who, though not attending team meetings, provide clinical care. Such individuals include critical care nurses, who care for patients who are actively dying—meaning they will die within a few days—as well as certified nurse assistants (CNAs) and home health aides (HHAs), who visit patients up to three times a week to provide assistance with activities of daily living. Finally, as stipulated in the MHB, the hospice includes a staff of volunteers that is sufficient to account for 5 percent of the organization's total patient care hours.[8] Though volunteers do not generally attend team meetings, they are discussed at meetings as quasi professionals who can be requested to serve patients who need companionship.

Amberview also features a number of staff members concerned with nonclinical aspects of the organization's functioning, including two admissions people, who recruit patients for the hospice. The staff also includes a financial manager, who oversees the hospice's financial operations, a medical records coordinator, and an administrative assistant. Though not participating in clinical care directly, these staff frequently pop into meetings to update team members on a variety of issues, including new admissions, missing paperwork, and financial pressures. These nonclinical and clinical members make up the totality of Amberview's outpatient staff.

Outpatient services are complemented by Amberview's inpatient facility. That Amberview has such a facility makes it a rarity among hospice providers in the United States, where, as I mentioned above, four out of five hospices do not offer inpatient services.[9] Amberview's facility is equipped to handle twelve patients, though its census dropped to as low as four during the time that I was conducting research. Since inpatient services comprise a significantly smaller portion of the hospice's care, the inpatient center features only one clinical team. This team is, like the outpatient teams, interdisciplinary, composed of a medical director, one or two registered nurses, an office manager, a social worker, and a chaplain. In addition to these members, who work solely in the inpatient setting, inpatient meetings are also attended by the hospice's volunteer coordinator. Finally, team meetings are supervised by the manager of the inpatient facility, who is a nurse and who performs a function similar to that of the PCM in the outpatient setting.

The hospice's caretaking in both settings is overseen by the executive director (ED). The ED performs a variety of functions, including ensuring that the hospice is taking in a sufficient number of patients, monitoring and supporting the activities of team members, and helping to troubleshoot with patients who require services that are outside of those normally provided by the hospice. Such patients could include those who require home care that is not reimbursed by Medicare (including additional CNA visits), patients and family members who might be considered dangerous, and nonfunded patients whom the hospice is continuing to treat. Ultimately, the ED is responsible for communication between the local branch and the national office. Such communication ensures that the hospice is meeting the national office's stipulations for patient care, profitability, and organizational efficiency.

This structure coheres with that of other hospices throughout the United States. Amberview is primarily an outpatient facility that provides holistic, interdisciplinary care to terminally ill patients. This care is provided to patients from the metro Atlanta area and, as Amberview's staff explained to me repeatedly, is meant to "support," not supplant, the patient's primary caretakers. As a primarily outpatient facility working toward the administration of supportive, interdisciplinary end-of-life care to terminally ill patients, Amberview is structurally identical to many hospices in the country.

To examine how Amberview's overarching structure configures its practice of hospice care, I studied the facility during the six-month period from May 2012 through November 2012. This fieldwork consisted of thirty-one interviews with Amberview's staff in both the inpatient and outpatient facilities, as well as the hospice's corporate office. In addition, I made daily observations of inpatient or outpatient care and attended the weekly staff meetings of the inpatient team and the outpatient Team 2. My focus was how the Medicare Hospice Benefit's dependence on familial caregiving impacted Amberview's provision of patient care.

Patients with Inadequate Familial Caregivers

One way of thinking of the structure of US hospice care is as an exchange. In exchange for some hospice care funded by the state, the family members of the dying person take care of certain patient needs that otherwise might require state funding. This exchange has made it possible to extend hospice care to the enormous number of dying people who have benefited from hospice's incorporation into Medicare. But it has also created a population that is systematically underserved: terminally ill patients who lack an adequate level of familial caregiving to sustain hospice care.

As I noted in the introduction, the use of the word "inadequate" is not a commentary on the effort put forth by caregivers nor on their moral worth or love for the dying person. I take as a given that every dying person I discuss in this chapter had people who loved them and who "cared" on some level for them as they were dying. But this love was frequently not enough. Inadequate familial caregiving is what emerges from this space between love and labor.

Inadequate caregiving frequently is created by factors that are not directly related to existing family dynamics. Such factors can be biological—based in the severity of the dying person's disease or the limiting nature of a caregiver's own ailments—or sociological, due to structural factors that are ultimately outside of the family's control. Even when the limitations are directly due to issues relating to familial bonds, the failure of familial caregiving should not create a negative judgment of the caregiver. They often have perfectly good reasons—albeit personal, idiosyncratic ones—for not fulfilling the dying person's needs.

In this sense, the term "inadequate familial caregiving" is a placeholder for any number of factors that can go wrong in hospice care. Why use it at all then? I do so because of the role played in the US hospice system by familial caregiving. The "family," in hospice, is presumed to act in a way that can alleviate problems that are, in reality, well beyond its control. The label "inadequate familial caregiving" thus tells us very little about a particular family and much more about the expectations that we have placed on all families at the end of life. These expectations are not, I believe, ethical or realistic, and they are not conducive to the freedom of dying people.

In order to explain why this is the case, it is necessary to examine the level of familial care required to sustain a terminally ill patient until the time of their death. Such care will depend on the nature and severity of the terminally ill person's condition. For example, a person with chronic obstructive pulmonary disease (COPD) may have significant difficulties in getting to the bathroom, while an individual with dementia may be able to move to the bathroom but is unable to recognize the need to perform routine activities of self-care. Because they are dying, most hospice patients have extremely significant conditions that limit their ability to perform basic activities of daily living and to comply with their medication schedule. They require an enormous amount of care. Indeed, almost by definition, dying individuals require more care than anyone else in the US health system.

The difficulties in caring for them are compounded because dying people are rarely "just" dying. They frequently have preexisting comorbid diseases and disabilities. Comorbidities can be lifelong conditions that, though not immediately related to a patient's terminal diagnosis, significantly complicate it. For example, a patient with pancreatic cancer may not be able to walk as a result of a lower extremity amputation dating to the Vietnam War. Comorbidities can also be related to mental health. The ability of an individual with Parkinson's disease to take their medications may be adversely impacted by the chronic depression that they have experienced on and off for ten years. The presence of such comorbidities in hospice patients at Amberview provided the justification for a saying that was used by several different staff members over the course of team meetings: "The end of life does not begin at the end of life."

This adage applies to the presence of not only comorbidities among patients, but also illnesses and disabilities in their familial caretakers. While Amberview's staff did not treat such conditions themselves, these disorders had a direct—and potentially devastating—impact on the provision of hospice care. For example, Maya, whom I mentioned in this book's introduction, was unable to provide her terminally ill husband with consistent care because she had breast cancer; she was absent from the home while receiving treatment and, even while at home, was often too tired to sufficiently carry out the physically grueling labor of caring for his needs. In another case, an elderly man with a heart condition and lower back problems could not perform the daily labor of assisting his wife into the wheelchair that was necessary for her to move. Neither his wife's wheelchair use nor the man's own coronary and lumbar problems would be classified as terminal conditions, but both impeded the delivery of end-of-life care. In one extreme situation, a father and son—both with a history of opioid addiction—were dying in hospice at the same time.

In addition to such diagnosed conditions, dysfunctional family dynamics also hindered the provision of Amberview's hospice care. In one team meeting, hospice staff discussed a patient whose wife was routinely forgetting to give him his pain medication. The PCM claimed that such "forgetting" was a manifestation of the aggression that the wife felt toward her husband, whom the PCM characterized as "a guy who was probably very controlling and dominating to [the wife] earlier in life." Whether it was conscious or unconscious, the wife's noncompliance was thus a form of payback for her husband's treatment of her. While I did not observe patient care in this case specifically, the PCM's scenario provides an example of how dysfunctional family dynamics subvert care delivery. In such cases, the hospice's interdisciplinary team must either address these noxious familial relations before they actively harm the patient or have the patient removed from the home.

While many comorbidities are unrelated to the end of life, terminal diseases are prolific generators of comorbid conditions. At Amberview, nearly every patient had, in addition to the terminal diagnosis necessary to admit them, a series of comorbid conditions most likely related to their disease. One man had been admitted to hospice for "failure to thrive" but also had significant recent hearing loss. An eighty-seven-year-old woman with dementia had significant lower extremity bruising as a result of a fall that had occurred in her own house. In addition to disease-related accidents, terminal conditions like cancer, COPD, and dementia, though often localized in a particular region of the body, have effects that impinge on the body's ability to function as a whole. The disabling nature of such conditions makes it difficult for hospice patients to care for themselves, while also hindering their family's capacity to attend to them.

Moreover, the rapidly escalating nature of such conditions may outpace the means or the ability of the terminally ill individual to make their home accessible. A person who becomes unable to walk over a matter of weeks may become trapped in a house with stairs. Compounding these problems with accessibility internal to an individual's own environment are problems particular to their local surroundings. The city of Atlanta, for example, is geographically very spread out.[10] Its public transportation network, MARTA, though relatively accessible to people with disabilities, has limited coverage.[11] As a result of this lack of accessible transportation, it was extremely difficult for Amberview's patients—who in general were too disabled to drive themselves—to attain basic necessities.

With their rapidly escalating terminal conditions coupled with the lack of accessible housing and transportation, terminally ill patients at Amberview generally required a high level of care. This care had an important medical dimension: these patients generally required extensive pain control as well as treatment for neurological conditions like dementia. But in order to be successful, this medical treatment had to occur in a context that was responsive to the activities of daily living. While Amberview could provide assistance with such activities on a part-time basis, it was not reimbursed for daily assistance nor for providing patients with a sitter. Without assistance from Medicare, the high cost of home health care for such activities—approximately $300 a day, according to an Amberview social worker—was prohibitive for most Amberview patients, who were generally individuals of middle or lower socioeconomic status. As a result, most Amberview patients had to depend on their family members for full-time care that included companionship and assistance with activities of daily living.

There were several obstacles to the provision of such familial care. First, many patients lacked family members who lived in sufficient proximity to provide them with routine care. Second, even if family members were present, the emotional dynamics of familial relationships often impeded the provision of care. Caretakers who were—for either valid or invalid reasons—upset at their terminally ill relatives were reluctant to provide them with necessary care. Third, even if caretakers were committed to providing care, they might be economically unable to do so. If a caretaker needed to work a full-time job, for example, they may have left their terminally ill relative at home in a potentially precarious position. Finally, if a person had sufficient economic resources so that they could provide care themselves—or even hire a full-time sitter—the progressive nature of terminal illness placed significant strains on their mental, emotional, and physical resources.

The Medicare Hospice Benefit presumes—and implicitly requires—the presence of familial caregivers that have adequate physical, mental, and emotional abilities to provide care for a dying loved one; they must also have the financial resources either to not have to work or to pay for a full-time caretaker out of pocket. When such a caregiver is present—as was the case for Marta and Raúl Acosta, described above—the benefit works well. But due to the historical shifts I discussed in chapter 3, they are often lacking. This lack has a devastating effect on terminally ill patients.

Steven's Case

When I first walked into Steven's apartment, all I saw were paper plates and pills. Or rather, paper plates *filled* with pills. They were a range of diverse shapes and colors: capsules, circles, and even diamonds in blue and green, red and yellow. Amid such resplendent litter, there was also more quotidian trash: withered sweatshirts, microwavable ravioli trays—their insides long dried out—and tissues with dark stains of ominous origin. There was a twin bed rendered unusable and effectively invisible by the clothing, books, pill bottles, and even paintings atop it; there was a sink filled with dirty dishes and a small safe lying open on the floor, its exposed interior displaying a few dollars and more half-empty bottles of pills.

Steven had bipolar disorder. He was fifty-four years old, white, and divorced, a former construction worker and former amphetamine addict. He lived in a facility run by a nationally recognized addiction recovery organization. This "facility" was, in reality, a long, two-story building of studio apartments whose size and level of maintenance mirrored that of a seedy motel. This complex was located in an area of the city that was not only unsafe, but extremely inaccessible: a residential neighborhood with limited sidewalks, where the closest supermarket was more than a mile away. The neighborhood had been subjected to housing discrimination—redlining—and, partially as a result, had a high crime rate. Steven had been mugged one day while walking back from the market. He had stopped going after that, but only partially because of the robbery. It had become too hard for him to make the trip.

Two years before I met him, Steven had been diagnosed with cancer of the throat, and he had been on hospice service for a year and a half. The disease was terminal, but it was uncertain when exactly it would kill him. In the meantime, his main concern was not the cancer but his stomach. Steven had terrible ulcers, which, he argued, were due to his chronic back pain. Because of his work in construction, he had suffered routine back injuries since the 1980s. He had addressed these back injuries by taking pain medications, which had eroded his stomach lining, giving him ulcers and acid reflux. His stomach condition caused him constant pain and, coupled with his throat cancer, made it extremely difficult for him to ingest food. As a result, he ate only a limited range of microwavable foods—mainly beef ravioli and chicken pot pie. But even when he was able to obtain and prepare such foods, he could take down only a small amount, often leaving the premeasured portions more than half uneaten.

Steven lived alone. He had been divorced a long time ago and never remarried. He subsisted entirely on Social Security Disability payments. Though he was under sixty-five, he had been disabled for more than two years—thus making him eligible for Medicare, which paid for the hospice care that he had been receiving for the previous year and a half. During his time as a hospice patient, Steven had developed close relationships with several Amberview staffers. "Have you met Steven yet?" one Amberview social worker had asked me in the middle of an interview. "I love Steven." She was not alone. Steven was well loved by his attending social worker, chaplain, and nurse. And, indeed, he was easy to love: chatty, energetic, cheerily self-deprecating, genuine, and somewhat naïve. People enjoyed his company and wanted to help him out.

And Steven needed help. Although Medicare covered his hospice care, he lacked a local caregiver. He had long been estranged from his wife. His two brothers lived on the other side of the country. His daughter lived in New York and had a young child at home. In part, Steven's distance from his family may have been the result of his own actions. As he readily admitted, he was no saint, and a lifetime of addiction, mental illness, and psychological trauma had led him to, if not completely burn, then at least deeply singe, many of his bridges. But regardless of the cause, he was now alone in a small apartment without transportation. He had access to all of the resources that Amberview Hospice could provide: high-level pain medications and visits from nurses, chaplains, social workers, and volunteers. Though these visits were frequent, the amount of time that Steven spent with hospice personnel was around fifteen hours a week. For the most part, he was alone.

Steven's situation in a residential facility for recovering addicts was highly problematic. The facility's other residents had, by his account, stolen his drugs on two occasions. Such drugs included both the psychiatric medications for his bipolar disorder and the high-intensity pain medication given to him by hospice. Due to his psychiatric condition, he was incapable of adequately organizing and hiding his medications and also unable to defend himself from robbery. Amberview Hospice attempted to help him prevent theft by providing a locked pillbox, but he frequently forgot to use it. In the meantime, the outpatient psychiatric care he received from a local nonprofit, while helpful, was having only a limited impact because it depended on his ability to comply with medication regimens. But for Steven—bipolar, terminally ill, in constant pain and anxiety—such compliance proved impossible.

Steven's only reprieve from the pain, anxiety, and isolation he experienced at home were his trips to Amberview's inpatient unit. While Steven's condition was not significant enough to qualify him for general inpatient care, he was able to visit the inpatient facility for five days a month through the Medicare Hospice Benefit's allowance for respite care. Such care is designed to benefit familial caregivers, but since Steven was his own caregiver, his respite care was, in a sort of paradox, giving him respite from himself.

Regardless, he was happy. At the inpatient facility, he received regular meals delivered to his room. Having been a patient for a year and a half, he knew the cook well, and she prepared special meals that he would be able to eat. He also knew and was well liked by the inpatient facility's nurses, social worker, and chaplain. He socialized regularly with these staff and with volunteer visitors. In addition, the facility had even, well-maintained floors, which, unlike those of his apartment, he could walk on freely, without tripping over a pile of junk. Steven's respite visits to Amberview's inpatient unit provided him with the care that his home environment lacked. Nevertheless, each month, after five days of comfort and care, he had to return to his pill-littered apartment.

Both the quirkiness of Steven's personality and the desperation of his situation manifested in his dying wish: to donate his body to science. In what would be the final weeks of his life, Steven spoke enthusiastically to me about his desire to give his remains to a body donation service. This desire was, in part, motivated by his intellectual curiosity. But beyond this, there was also a financial motivation. Steven did not have the money to pay for his own burial. In exchange for receiving his body, the donation service would cremate him and send his ashes to his daughter. This solution was welcomed by Steven—who was happy to save his daughter the cost of the funeral.

Though I was perturbed by the economic situation that prompted Steven's desire, there was also something inspiring, almost heartwarming about it. Steven *really* wanted to donate his body to science. He showed me the pamphlet several times when I visited, excitedly explaining both the physical procedures to be performed on him and the memorial rituals that would follow. The prospect of donating his body to science seemed to give him a sense of control that was lacking in every other aspect of his life.

One Sunday, Steven woke up with a searing pain in his gut. He called for an ambulance and was taken to the nearest hospital. There, the doctors discovered that his cancer had spread to his stomach. Over the course of an operation, he began to lose a large amount of blood. While he had signed a DNR (do not resuscitate) order that prohibited life-saving procedures, after the surgery the doctors asked if he wanted to rescind it in order to receive a transfusion. Thinking that he was saving his life, Steven agreed. He received the transfusion but died hours afterward. Unfortunately, as a result of this transfusion, he was no longer eligible to donate his body to science.[12]

Invisible Abandonment

In *Vita: Life in a Zone of Social Abandonment*, anthropologist João Biehl examines the aftermath of the Brazilian government's decision to deinstitutionalize care for the mentally ill.[13] This deinstitutionalization was accompanied by two related factors: first, drastic cuts to the social services needed to support the mentally ill in local communities, and second, a dramatic increase in the use of pharmaceuticals in Brazilian public health approaches to psychiatry. As a result, mentally ill individuals were entrusted to the care of family members who had neither the economic resources nor the professional skills to care for them. Overwhelmed family members responded to this situation by drugging their relatives to sedation, then leaving them, at first in the home and then in ramshackle, informal facilities that were equally deficient.

Biehl uses the term "zone of social abandonment" to refer to such facilities.[14] But his study highlights that abandonment is not confined to such institutions. It can also exist in the home. Indeed, as neoliberal policy makers attempt to dramatically decrease the size of health spending, the primary site of abandonment has perhaps shifted from institutions to the home. This is dramatically different than the abandonment of the "total institutions" that Erving Goffman chronicled in his studies of asylums and penitentiaries.[15] Though such institutions persist, abandonment in the current context does not require their centralized structure. Rather, neoliberal abandonment is diffuse in its organization, spread throughout individual homes that from the outside may look quite innocuous. It is invisible in part because it exists potentially everywhere you look.

Steven's case highlights the presence of abandonment in the US hospice system. This abandonment was not the result of negligence on the part of Amberview Hospice. On the contrary, he was receiving hospice care from highly trained professionals who, because of their long-term relationship with him, cared for him deeply and knew him well. And yet, because the full-time provision of care depends on the presence of adequate familial caregiving in the private sphere, Steven was abandoned. He did not have familial caregivers who were adequate to support him, and the hospice organization's ability to provide appropriate care was limited by the same regulations that permitted it to provide Steven with interdisciplinary end-of-life care in the first place.

Without familial caregivers, Steven did not receive his medical care. His drugs were stolen, lost, or forgotten. He lacked assistance with the basic activities of hygiene and environmental cleanliness. While he could prepare his own food, when his stockpile of frozen meals began to dwindle, he lived with uncertainty about when someone could pick up another batch from the store. When he did die, it was not at home but in an emergency room, bleeding out among strangers, most likely without knowing that he was losing the one wish he had held onto in the preceding weeks. It was not a good death. But it was also not a fluke.

Steven died because of the design of the Medicare Hospice Benefit. Because the benefit does not provide long-term care for patients receiving hospice, it thrusts the burden of care onto the patients themselves and their family members. When patients like Steven lack appropriate support, they are left abandoned in their own homes. In many ways, Steven represents an extreme version of such abandonment. He had no local caregivers, was poor and mentally ill, and lived in a dangerous area with little access to food. But to varying degrees, abandonment was common among Amberview's patients.

Hospice physician and bioethicist Timothy Quill has argued that "nonabandonment" represents the fundamental principle of the hospice physician. For Quill, nonabandonment is "a concept exemplified in a continuous caring partnership between physician and patient."[16] The provision of continuous care is necessary, in part, due to the grueling nature of the dying process. But Quill notes that the need for continuous care is also a function of changes in the US health system, in which "managed care systems and competitive market approaches to cost containment" have made it difficult for physicians to stay with their patients.[17] Such disruptive forces make the provision of continuous care particularly necessary for the patient's physical and psychological health.

I concur with Quill's analysis of the impact of neoliberal health reforms on the doctor-patient relationship and with his postulation of nonabandonment as a bedrock hospice principle. But I am skeptical that containing this principle to the doctor-patient relationship will be sufficient to address the current state of US hospice care. The US hospice system is, as I have argued, geared to the abandonment of patients with insufficient familial support. The hospice clinicians that attended to Steven were very dedicated, as were all the members of their interdisciplinary team. But their professional dedication to nonabandonment was ultimately not enough.

The limits of such dedication become clear when one considers the principal alternative available in the US health system to Steven's abandonment in the home: the nursing home.

Plugging Gaps, Creating Holes

As I described in the introduction, nursing homes are long-term inpatient facilities for people with disabilities.[18] They are designed to provide room, board, and assistance with activities of daily living (ADLs) to chronically disabled patients who are no longer able to live at home. Such ADLs include feeding, bathing, clothing, and daily hygienic maintenance. Skilled nursing facilities are nursing homes that, in addition to helping with ADLs, provide skilled nursing care. In the US healthcare system, this includes the provision of antibiotics, IV fluids, and feeding tubes, as well as rehabilitative services designed to help individuals regain lost functionality and, ideally, return to life in their own homes.[19] Thus, while regular nursing home services provide assistance with ADLs, skilled services are specifically *medical* treatments.

Skilled and unskilled nursing home services have different payment structures in the US health system. Skilled nursing services can be reimbursed via either Medicare Part A, Medicaid, or private insurance, or they can be paid out of pocket. Unskilled nursing home services can only be reimbursed through Medicaid or private payer; Medicare does not contain a long-term care benefit that will pay for them. Overall, both skilled nursing services and regular nursing home services are expensive. In 2012, a semiprivate room in a nursing home cost, on average, more than $81,000 per year.[20] Due to the extremely high costs of nursing home care, approximately two-thirds of nursing home patients pay for their care through Medicaid.[21]

In general, terminally ill patients who lack sufficient familial support are placed in nursing homes. There, they receive assistance with activities of daily living, but because nursing homes specialize in care for disabled people, they are not equipped to provide end-of-life care. This deficiency is remedied, in theory, by pairing inpatient nursing home care for ADLs with the provision of outpatient hospice care. Thus, the nursing home replaces, to a degree, the patient's familial caregiver. This environment ostensibly facilitates the provision of hospice's medical, spiritual, and psychosocial care. By coordinating hospice and nursing home care, the US healthcare system theoretically plugs the gap created by the needs of terminally ill patients without sufficient familial support. But in practice, this solution is as bad—if not worse—than the problem itself.

"Like a Hamster in a Wheel"

Interviews with Amberview staff members at various levels—case managers, medical team directors, PCMs, and senior executives at the national corporate office—revealed the provision of hospice care in nursing home settings to be one of the organization's central problems. This problem is rooted in a basic incompatibility between hospices and nursing homes in each treatment modality's orientation toward death. While hospice care is organized to bring patients to a comfortable death, nursing home care is organized to prevent death at practically all costs. This distinction arises from the diagnostic categories in which each institution specializes. Nursing homes care for chronically disabled individuals —maintaining them and possibly rehabilitating them—while hospices are designed for terminally ill patients for whom death is both imminent and inevitable. Consequently, hospices and nursing homes are designed to treat conditions that are not simply distinct, but opposed.

The opposition between hospice and nursing home care is best illustrated by the reimbursement structure of Medicare. Part A is available to pay for *either* hospice care *or* skilled nursing care. It will not pay for both. As a result, hospice and skilled nursing providers are in direct competition for the same pool of money. Other authors have noted that this direct economic conflict significantly impedes patient care. For example, a team of investigators at the University of California, San Francisco, argued that the conflict over Medicare funding between hospice and nursing providers leads to nursing home patients not receiving sufficient palliative care.[22] Nursing home staff may be untrained to provide such care, but they are also disincentivized from doing so by Medicare guidelines. At the same time, patients may be reluctant to abandon skilled nursing interventions that they believe could improve their quality of life as well as lengthen their lifespan. The result is that patients are denied—or incentivized to refuse—palliative interventions that might otherwise benefit them.

This economic and medical conflict produces a larger cultural conflict between nursing home and hospice providers. In various interviews and during my observations of outpatient team meetings, hospice providers complained that their palliative interventions were regarded with suspicion by nursing home staff. Such staff considered hospice to be "giving up" on patients who might be eligible for rehabilitation or, at the very least, able to live for long periods of time with mechanical assistance. Hospice staff, in turn, suspected that nursing home providers maintained patients through "artificial" means like feeding tubes and ventilation largely in order to extract more money from them. Their organization around distinct diagnostic categories—"terminal illness" and "chronic disability" —produces a conflict between hospices and nursing homes that is at once medical, economic, and cultural.

This situation subverts the delivery of hospice care in the nursing home setting. Nursing home providers are either reluctant or unable to prescribe some of the medicines essential to palliative care, such as high-intensity pain medication, anti-anxiety medication, and anti-psychotics. Because they lack training and, at times, a belief in the validity of such interventions, nursing home providers often administer medications irregularly. At outpatient staff meetings, hospice team members repeatedly emphasized the need to "educate" nursing home personnel on various aspects of patient care, including the administration of Roxanol and other high-potency pain medications, fall protection, and turning bedbound patients, and more generally on getting "comfortable with death." Through their educational interventions, hospice staff tried to minimize the negative impact of the nursing home's conflicting organizational culture.

Nursing home employees are relatively poorly paid while negotiating high caseloads under stressful circumstances. This combination has been found to lead to high turnover rates among nursing home staff.[23] For Amberview's staff, this high turnover transformed "education" from an occasional practice to a full-time aspect of providing hospice care in the nursing home setting. The constant pedagogical interventions were considered by team members to be a necessary but inefficient use of time, as they only marginally helped to stem the tide of service failures. The result was that hospice staff members were left feeling, in the words of Dr. Evelynn Sewell, an Amberview medical director, "like a hamster in a wheel."

Resistance to the provision of hospice medications in the nursing home setting is more than a matter of education. It is a direct result of the regulations governing medical treatment in the nursing home. As Dr. Sewell explained:

> They have so many different regulations about what they can do with their medications. Some of them have a pharmacy they can access twenty-four hours. Some of them don't. So if [you] need pain medication or some other symptom medication in the middle of the night, you may be out of luck. Sometimes they'll allow you to have what we call a "comfort kit" in the . . . nursing home. . . . But then it has to be assigned to that one patient. So that you now have a comfort kit that may have the morphine, or Ativan, or Haldol that [you] may need, but suppose it happens to another patient, unexpectedly. . . . That other patient has to wait.

Sewell highlighted how the limitations of nursing homes in prescribing high-intensity pain medication or anti-psychotics leads to routine problems in the delivery of hospice care. These problems stem from the difficulty of addressing unexpected complications at the end of life in long-term care facilities that are not designed to provide end-of-life care.

Nursing home regulations designed to help chronically disabled patients can, in the context of end-of-life care, have dramatically different results. For example, nursing home staff must document that they are feeding patients. Regulations that mandate feeding emerged as necessary responses to the previous neglect of chronically disabled patients in the nursing home setting.[24] But in the hospice context, mandatory feedings can be disastrous when nursing home staff provide feeding tubes to patients in whom cessation of appetite is, in Sewell's words, "a natural part of the disease progress." The tubes can lead to patient aspiration and unnecessarily prolong the dying process in patients whose bodies cannot process the nourishment they receive. Although there are regulations through which mandatory feeding can be discontinued, Sewell emphasized that the high caseloads of nursing home staff regularly preclude such regulations from being followed. Consequently, regulatory solutions to the coordination of hospice and nursing home care only superficially mitigate the more fundamental conflict between these two treatment modalities.

To account for the structural difficulties in coordinating hospice and nursing home care, hospice professionals adopt standardized routines. Dr. Sewell explained the rationale and method of such standardization:

> What we do [in hospice] is often to use medications PRN—"as needed"—[and], well, you can't do that in a nursing home. Because one nurse on one shift may think that pain looks like one thing. And one nurse on another shift may think that pain looks like [another] thing. And they may not medicate the patient. So sometimes we sit down and we go, "Okay, well let's make a happy medium. Let's give it to them just twice a day so that we know they get some medication in them." You know, that's not the way to practice good medicine and good care for the patient. But it's almost like we've accepted that as being the way to do it, because of the fact that there really is no other easy way to get around the system.

The standardization of pain medication described by Sewell is a response not to the patient's pain, but to a nursing home context that makes "good" medical care impossible. Similar problems with unnecessary standardization can manifest with other medications, such as the psychiatric medications used to address anxiety. The result is the potential undertreatment or overtreatment of a patient's pain and suffering, as well as the waste of expensive medications. But such risks are necessary, in Sewell's view, to avoid the greater danger of allowing terminally ill patients to stay in a nursing facility with limited resources to palliate them.

The divided economic structure of Medicare Part A not only impedes the delivery of hospice services, but also leads patients to leave hospice in order to receive skilled nursing care. Mr. Mark Riglin, a patient care manager at Amberview, claimed that such structural departures were his "biggest problem" with the Medicare Hospice Benefit:

> You can be [in a nursing home] on hospice. You can be dying. And nursing homes will call the family [who will say,] "Oh, send them to the hospital." So now they're

a hospice patient, they're DNR, but now they're at the hospital. But now they'll say, "Well, while he's here, we'll let him be treated." And I say to them, "Well, you have two choices. You can either have him come off hospice, and Medicare will cover the hospital bill. Or you can have him stay on hospice, and you'll be responsible for the hospital bill." So you can imagine what most people decide to do. So when they leave the hospital and they go back to the nursing home, even if they have a hospice order, the nursing home will say, "[He] need[s] IV antibiotics, we're going to skill him." I can't admit a patient who's being skilled, even though they're dying.

Riglin laid out what, in his experience, is a routine pathway by which termi-nally ill nursing home patients are transferred from hospice to skilled nursing care. When patients begin to actively die, the nursing home contacts the family, who—believing that they are saving their family member's life—override their DNR and send them to the hospital, revoking hospice so that Medicare covers the hospital bill. When their family member returns to the nursing home, they are then "skilled." As "skilled" patients, they cannot, according to Medicare guide-lines, be enrolled in hospice care. Consequently, although they are terminally ill and hospice eligible, they must forsake hospice services. As a result of this, terminally ill patients may experience untreated pain at the end of life.

Such untreated pain in the nursing home setting is not happenstance. It is, as the Institute of Medicine has noted, a by-product of the competing incentive structures of hospice and nursing providers.[25] The result of the competing incen-tive structures, as Riglin recounted, can be fatal:

> Literally, they can skill you to death. I had a patient who was actively dying, and they were sent to the hospital. [The] nursing home should have called hospice, but didn't. "My bad," [the nursing home staff said]. [The] hospital gives them a round of antibiot-ics [and] discharges them back to the nursing home with ten days of IV antibiotics. . . . This happens a lot. You get a doctor in a nursing home who will write an order for hospice. And yet still they will skill them. "Oh, well, you can admit them after the hundred days [of reimbursable skilled care] are passed, if [they haven't] expired." And a lot of times they will die while they are being skilled.

By the expression "skilled to death," Riglin means that patients will "die while they are being skilled." And yet, it is possible to understand being "skilled to death" in another sense as well. Studies have shown that the administration of palliative care can lengthen a patient's lifespan by between one and three months.[26] By denying patients palliative care, the provision of skilled nursing home care can itself shorten their lives. This shortening is not inherent to skilled nursing care, but rather results from the conflict between hospice and skilled nursing care in Medicare Part A.

Mary's Case

Mary was a patient of Amberview Hospice. She was eighty-two years old and had been admitted to hospice with Parkinson's disease and advanced dementia. This combination of dementia and Parkinson's had made it impossible for her husband—who was also in his early eighties—to care for her. As a result, she had been placed in an Atlanta facility that I anonymize as Sunny Day Nursing Home.

Mary had family members that, though unable to care for her personally, were very supportive. The Sunny Day home was only five miles from her house, and her husband visited her almost every evening. She had several grandchildren living in the area, who visited her two or three times a month. Most important, Mary had a son who lived nearby and who visited her several times a week. During these visits, Mary's son not only kept her company—serving as an invaluable connection between her life inside the nursing home and her life outside of it—but also advocated for her with both hospice and nursing home staff. Thus, though Mary's familial support had not been sufficient for her to continue home care, she was in an optimal position compared to the nursing home patients who lacked familial advocates. Nevertheless, even this advocacy was insufficient to assure Mary the delivery of adequate long-term or end-of-life care.

I first heard about Mary in an outpatient team meeting, where she was described as having a cough so serious that the hospice staff would have to "manage it like [a] symptom, just like pain." In fact, the attending caseworker reported that Mary was in "significant pain." However, because the nursing home staff was—for reasons not clearly explained—reluctant to give her highly potent pain medication, she was only receiving Tylenol. The hospice medical director had left a message with the nurse on duty about giving oxycodone to Mary, but had yet to receive a response. The patient care manager gave a weary chuckle and asked the hospice nurses whether the facility was a "place where they can split a pill." In other words, was the nursing home capable of administering medication with a basic level of competence?

As it turned out, it was not. Mary encountered repeated difficulties in receiving both her pain medication and her dementia care. Over the following weeks, the nursing home staff failed several times to provide her medications at the regularly scheduled hours. This failure persisted despite the presence of Mary's son as a strong patient advocate. He was in a hard position. He had to hunt down nursing home personnel, who seemed to change every other day and who—

even when consistent—were so busy that they didn't have time to talk; at the same time, he had to talk by phone with hospice personnel, who only visited his mother at Sunny Day around twice a week. The process was at once exhausting and futile. Mary endured untreated pain, and her son's final months with his mother were lost in bureaucracy.

While Mary was at Sunny Day, the nursing home had an outbreak of pneumonia. Mary became sick, as did several other patients. Though she recovered from the pneumonia, the experience was traumatizing for both her and her son. In addition, she fell several times at the nursing home. Though she did not break any bones, her bruises were painful and—when coupled with her dementia and the nursing home's lack of skill with pain medication—left Mary in a state of both pain and persistent confusion. During a later team meeting, the hospice staff reported that, in addition to these falls, Mary's "arms [were] tearing from where [the nursing home nurses] pull[ed] her."

Though much of Mary's mistreatment was the fault of the nursing home, Amberview Hospice's care for her was also lacking. The deficiencies in this care were highlighted during my own weekly visits with her. I found that though Mary had dementia, she was animated and coherent and had a memory that, though occasionally spotty, could be quite sharp. But I did not find my perception of Mary to be echoed in the descriptions of her at hospice team meetings. There, Mary was discussed as if she were a nonperson. She "occasionally will speak a word," one PCM commented in a somewhat judgmental tone, and was "completely unable to make [her] needs known." When I initially heard this description, my inclination was to assume that Mary's condition had significantly deteriorated since my last visit. But I found no evidence of such a decline when I saw her a few days later. We watched the James Bond movie *Goldfinger* and talked at length about the virtues and defects of the various actors who played Bond.

The gap between my perception and the PCM's was largely a result of both the amount and the quality of the time that we spent with Mary. The PCM visited Mary only once or perhaps twice a month. Such visits were oriented toward the management of Mary's pain. They did not include lengthy conversations on other topics and were most likely short, since the PCM had to visit several other patients in the facility. With such short, focused visits, it was easy to conclude that Mary was unable to communicate. She was not the most efficient talker and may not have immediately understood the PCM's inquiries about her pain. Perhaps the PCM had just caught her at a bad moment. Whatever the circumstances, because the PCM and other hospice nursing staff saw Mary for only brief, medically oriented visits in a non-hospice setting, they were not positioned to have an understanding of her as a person. They saw her largely as a vehicle for terminal disease. Such incomplete practices of patient care were characteristic of the attempts to coordinate hospice and nursing home care that I observed.

The Fragmentation of the Patient

Mary's scenario epitomized what Dr. Ruth Oberlin, one of the Amberview corporation's board members, referred to as the "fragmentation of the patient." Oberlin was commenting on how hospice patients in nursing homes are pulled in two different directions by their long-term and end-of-life providers. This fragmentation was embodied in the service failures and inefficiencies that Amberview staff experienced in their dealings with various local nursing homes. The conflicting incentive structures of hospice and nursing home providers made it difficult for hospice to collaborate with nursing homes and frequently placed these two forms of medical care at odds.

This fragmentation is not only figurative. Both in discussions with Amberview team members and in my own observations of patient care in the nursing home setting, I witnessed nursing home patients whose bodies were bruised from repeated falls, who suffered from untreated pain, and who endured bedsores due to a lack of proper turning by the nursing staff. The skin of Mary's arms was, in the words of Amberview's staff, "tearing from where they pull[ed] her." Her torn body was a literal manifestation of the conflict between hospice and nursing providers. It was not a result of a biological process, nor was it an isolated service failure; it was a product of the underlying structure of the US healthcare system.

Indeed, the fragmentary nature of this system is well known. Commentators frequently point out its negative effects, including poor coordination of services and excessive costs. Such effects are, as the Institute of Medicine notes, pervasive at the end of life.[27] Because of this system, though hospice is the dominant form of end-of-life care in America, terminally ill patients frequently have more than one healthcare provider when they are dying. Steven, for example, was seeing mental health providers in addition to his hospice team. But often lost in discussions of the systemic costs of fragmentation is its effect on the patient. A fragmentary healthcare system fragments patients systematically, tearing them in multiple directions at once. Being subjected to such routine violence was the fate of Mary in her final days.

Fragmentation is different from the abandonment that, I argue, is characteristic of the provision of hospice to patients without sufficient familial support in the home care setting. That abandonment is a product of the ways in which the lack of long-term care in the US hospice system has subverted the provision of end-of-life care. Fragmentation, in contrast, is a result of the simultaneous provision of both caretaking modalities. Fragmented patients receive hospice and nursing home care. And yet, because these forms of care are, in the US healthcare system, structurally opposed, their provision pulls the patient apart.

The Destruction of Freedom

In this chapter, I have described two patients with inadequate familial support in US hospice care. Steven was left abandoned in his own home. Mary's body was torn apart by health service providers with conflicting conceptions of care. Though these are individuals, their situations are not unique to them. Their experiences were a product of the way that we have organized hospice care. In the US hospice system, patients with inadequate familial support are either abandoned at home or fragmented in the context of the nursing home or some other inpatient facility like assisted living, which was not designed with the care of dying people in mind (see the afterword). The outcome is a failure in the delivery of relevant health services.

But it is not *just* a failure of health service delivery. It is a destruction of the freedom of dying patients to control their lives. Dying patients without sufficient familial support have no such control. At a basic level they are at the mercy of their own bodies. But this inability to control their bodies is itself, to a significant degree, a product of the failure of society to provide them with the resources necessary to do so. Such resources would include, in this context, the delivery of hospice and long-term care. Without them, patients experience unnecessary pain and suffering and find themselves without essential—and available—resources to control their lives. The provision of appropriate care is not external to the freedom of the dying patient. It is the very means through which such freedom is realized.

But health service delivery is only a starting point for freedom at the end of life. Such freedom is not just medical but social as well. Terminally ill people without adequate familial support are segregated. For those in nursing homes, such segregation is institutional. They are placed in facilities they cannot leave, which deny them the basic resources necessary to interact with the broader world. Those in home care experience segregation as well. Steven, for example, had no means to leave his home. His segregation was a product of various factors in US society: urban zoning, untreated disabilities, pain, a lack of public transportation, and a lack of resources. Though not "institutional," Steven's segregation was every bit as limiting as the segregation experienced by nursing home inhabitants. In this sense, patients with insufficient familial support are stripped of a fundamental freedom: access to society.

This destruction of freedom is rendered invisible, however, by the way freedom at the end of life is typically viewed. From the perspective of the current definition of freedom at the end of life, Steven was free when he died because he controlled his own medical decisions. Given that definition, there is not a question of whether or how his freedom might have been impinged on. The only way this question could be raised was if doctors had overruled his desire to receive a transfusion. From the perspective of this definition of freedom, the best that could be done for future Stevens would be to put in place a procedure that could better protect against patients making life-changing medical decisions too hastily. But the only thing that seems to matter in the current system is who made the decision that caused Steven's death.

There is no consideration of how Steven might have been given other options. Debates in the United States about freedom at the end of life do not take into account what anthropologist Sharon Kaufman has called the "ethical frame."[28] For Kaufman, the ethical frame refers to the range of choices made available to patients by the structure of US health policy and Medicare in particular. Debates about freedom at the end of life take the limited range of options as a given. As a result, they do not raise the question of whether or how we might expand the choices available to patients like Steven and Mary. An expansion of options would not just give them the freedom to choose. It would allow them to choose freedom.

An apt analogy has been proposed by political theorist Wendy Brown, who writes that to become realized, democratic values such as "inclusion" and "participation" must be accompanied by "modest control over setting parameters and constraints and by the capacity to decide fundamental values and directions."[29] Without such abilities, our values cannot be said to be "democratic any more than providing a death row inmate with choices about the method of execution offers the inmate freedom."[30]

To compare dying individuals in the US hospice system to inmates on death row might seem harsh. And it is. But the lives of people like Steven and Mary are extremely harsh. Steven and Mary had what economists Milton Friedman and Rose Friedman referred to as the "freedom to choose."[31] But none of the choices available to them could give them freedom in the sense of control over their own lives. On the contrary, the limited "choices" before them were a grim confirmation that they had already lost their freedom and that they would not, given their current circumstances, be able to ever get it back.

Steven had his freedom stripped long before he made his "choice" to have a blood transfusion. He had his freedom stripped when he was drowning among his pill-filled paper plates. He had his freedom stripped when he was shunted off in a neighborhood where he was routinely robbed both at home and in the streets. He had his freedom stripped when his moments of pain-free existence lasted less than the time it took to microwave a pot pie. He had his freedom stripped when he was sent from the inpatient hospice to a home that he well knew—everyone knew—was unfit for human life at any stage, especially when the person in question was too vulnerable to do much of anything but die.

Both the months prior to Steven's death and the final day of his life illustrate the problem with the current conception of freedom at the end of life. This conception is not too *expansive* because it potentially allows individuals to end their lives with medical assistance. It is in reality too *narrow* because it only defines freedom based on the final decision that individuals make. It does not consider the state that they were in prior to making that decision. It does not take into account how, long before they decide to die—or not—their control over their lives may be erased by a hospice system that is not designed for people like them and by a society that does everything possible to keep them out of sight. The problem with our current view of freedom at the end of life is not that we are pushing it to its limit. It is that we limit it so grossly that it makes freedom for most dying people impossible.

This gross limitation has been the basis of our national conversations about what to do at the end of life. These conversations claim an aura of gravitas. And they are important, concerning as they do matters of life and death. But to the extent that they focus only on one particular hypothetical action—physician-assisted suicide—undertaken by an extremely small portion of the dying population, these conversations are profoundly unserious. They do not bring us closer to the reality of death. They impede our acknowledgment of the vicious ways in which Americans die. In its current form, US hospice care can, at its best, serve as a palliative to this cruelty, a measure of comfort in a system that tears the dying apart. But right now, the conditions of this country are not those in which the current US hospice system can in general fulfill this role.

If this phenomenon were marginal, it would still be a problem. Even if the numbers of patients without sufficient familial support were relatively small, their existence in a state of systemic unfreedom would require an immediate response. It would be a humanitarian problem, an ethical problem, and an intellectual problem. And it would be an American problem, calling into question basic assumptions about our end-of-life care system and, more fundamentally, about the country's commitment to the freedom of its citizens.

But this is not a marginal phenomenon. In chapter 3, I argued that the gap between the requirements of US hospice care and the capacities of familial care-givers is so large that it has to be called a crisis. Steven and Mary are examples of what happens to dying individuals in that gap. Their situations, in many ways, could not have been more different. Steven lived in a lower-class, blighted neigh-borhood that had a high crime rate and basic resource deprivation. Mary lived a middle-class life in the suburbs. Steven's family was scattered around the coun-try. Mary's husband was still present in her life, and her son was actively involved in every aspect of her care. Mary seemed to have much more familial support than Steven, but it was still not enough. She was dying in an institution that was not made to care for people like her. And as terminal disease broke down her body, the care she received tore her apart.

Steven and Mary had enormous differences in their socioeconomic status, familial support, and degree of marginalization in US society. But in the end these differences did not impact what happened to them in US hospice care. In both cases, they lost their freedom. The breadth of their differences illustrates the breadth of the crisis. The crisis of freedom in US hospice care impacts most demographic groups throughout US society, including groups that might be iso-lated from social precariousness in many other ways. This is because of the fe-rocity of dying, the strain it puts on (often already weakened) familial bonds, and the expensive, often ineffective nature of the long-term care on which patients with insufficient familial support often depend. This crisis does not impact di-vergent demographic groups equally, but in a US society fragmented by many vectors, its impact on the freedom of dying people is broad.

Hospice in the United States does not have to be this way. There are alterna-tives to the current arrangement, and they carry a richer, more expansive vision of what it means to be free.

CHAPTER FIVE

Caring across the American
Political Divide

There are few who would say that Pilar Martínez died a good death. But in many ways her death was much better than we would have been inclined to expect.

Martínez was thirty-eight years old when I met her. For the previous two years, she had been living with her husband, Pablo, in a small house in Conyers, Georgia, a predominantly Latino suburb of Atlanta. Pilar and Pablo were originally from Nicaragua, and they were both in the United States illegally. Pablo had moved to the Atlanta area six years prior to work in construction. When Pilar had come to the United States one year later, she had gone north to Boston, where she lived with her sister and worked as a cook in a number of small restaurants. After two years of that, she found work in construction in Alabama, where she stayed for an additional two years.

The first sign that something was wrong with Pilar came shortly after her arrival in Alabama. One day on the job, she experienced a shooting pain in her back. The pain was so strong that she needed to be sent to the emergency room. There, a physician examined her and concluded that it was likely a muscular problem induced by her work in construction. After all, she was an extremely slight woman—weighing 120 pounds—engaged in arduous physical labor day after day. She rested, took pain killers, and was able to return to work later that week. A few months later, she experienced a relapse and returned to the emergency room, this time in a different hospital since she was working at another site. After examining both her and the medical records, the doctor looked at her and asked a question that she would remember for the rest of her life: "You don't know?"

Pilar Martínez had spinal cancer. Though it had not metastasized at that point, it would be fatal if she were not treated. But treatment was impossible for her. As an undocumented immigrant, she had no healthcare coverage. At the same time, she and her husband had so little money that private pay was not an option, and it was inconceivable for her to take time off work. After all, the only reason that they were in this country was because they needed to make money. This money was not for their own benefit. It was for the two daughters and one son whom Pilar had left back home in Nicaragua under the care of her mother.

Pilar Martínez had come to the United States to make a better life for her children. There was no way she was going to be interrupted now.

Pilar held out for as long as she possibly could. She moved to Atlanta to live, finally, with her husband and began work cleaning recently picked tomatoes. It was a long workday, but the labor was much less intense than in construction. She was able to continue working in this setting for a number of months until her back pain resurfaced, and she was forced to go to the emergency room again. There, they found that the cancer had metastasized throughout her body. They sent her to Amberview Hospice, where Pilar stayed for most of the nine months prior to her death.

Amberview Hospice did not make any money on the care of Pilar Martínez. On the contrary, it likely lost a significant amount. She was "on service" for several months. Much of this time was spent receiving home care. To be sure, home care is relatively inexpensive, but it still costs money. Furthermore, Pilar was only on home care for part of the time. She spent an extraordinary amount of time on inpatient care: three months. The entirety of these services was provided by the Amberview Hospice Corporation for free.

In chapter 4, I was quite critical of the structure of US hospice care. While this critique is valid, it needs to be counterbalanced with an awareness that there are not only problems in our contemporary hospice arrangement. There are also solutions. These solutions may exist in partial form. They may need to be developed, even made into something new. But they are starting points for the transformation of the US hospice system into one that provides dying people with a level of care and of freedom that we all should expect.

One starting point is the extremely high level of charitable care given by hospice providers. This charity is, in part, required. The Medicare Hospice Benefit obligates hospices to treat patients who cannot afford to pay.[1] In this sense, there is a systemic necessity for hospices to provide charity care. But the level of charitable care given by Amberview Hospice cannot *just* be explained by the need to follow Medicare requirements. Although hospices do have to provide some charitable care, there are many ways that they can minimize or forgo such obligations to patients in need. Pilar, for example, could have been forced to remain at home, where the financial drain on Amberview would have been far less substantial. But Amberview Hospice—or, more specifically, its parent company, the Amberview Hospice Corporation—did not skimp. It gave Pilar three months of high-quality inpatient care and did so for reasons beyond regulatory requirements or financial gain. The organization's board had made a commitment to serving patients in need.

This commitment extended to the staff of Amberview's Atlanta branch, who loved Pilar. This was true of everyone, from the organization's medical directors to its janitors, including social workers, nurses, chaplains, and volunteers. While Pablo was away working long days, Pilar was rarely alone. She only spoke Spanish, but staff who knew no words but *hola* tried to create a common language, which bridged any communicative divide. When she became too sick to talk much at all, volunteers sat with her as she slept, knitting, studying, or watching TV as her chest wheezed up and down. They started a fund to garner the money to fly her back to Nicaragua. She was still hoping, up until the very end, that she might be with her children when she died.

This hope never came to fruition. But though Amberview's staff could not make it happen, they—and the larger organization—did practically everything else. This charity highlights the immense kindness of the people working in hospice—professionals who, in general, forgo significant earnings in order to be able to provide end-of-life care—as well as the beneficial, productive aspects of our country's hospice design. To the degree that it encourages these aspects, the Medicare Hospice Benefit should be celebrated. But this celebration should not obscure the limits of hospice charity nor that charity in the US hospice system is the exception rather than the rule.

Even Amberview's charity eventually ran out. The cost of Pilar's inpatient treatment grew too high. As a result, the hospice had to look for a place to discharge her to. This place had to be an appropriate end-of-life care facility. It also had to be willing to accept a patient who could not afford to pay and who would continue to have significant medical expenses. In the US hospice system, there are few organizations that are willing or able to do that. But fortunately for both Pilar and the Amberview social worker assigned to her case, there is in the Atlanta area one institution that, though not technically a hospice, was perfect for the job.

That institution is Our Lady of Perpetual Help Home.[2] Our Lady, as it is known to locals, cares for patients who, like Pilar Martínez, lack the familial caregiving necessary to receive hospice care. The facility can provide this care because of its financial structure. Charity is the exception in the US hospice system, but Our Lady is a fundamentally charitable institution. It operates only on donations, without accepting payment from Medicare or patients themselves. As a result, it does not have to abide by Medicare regulations that prohibit facilities from combining long-term and end-of-life care. The home can thus offer two caregiving modalities that are normally kept separate and can care for patients who have nowhere else to turn.

In this sense, Our Lady provides a solution to the crisis of US hospice care. It cares for patients who would otherwise be stripped of their freedom. In the process, it provides them with care that is not only "adequate" but effectively *emancipatory*, giving them a far greater degree of liberty than had previously been the case. The basis for this emancipatory form of end-of-life care is, in part, the facility's charitable financial structure. But this structure is itself underpinned by the home's Catholic theology. Our Lady of Perpetual Help Home is thus an end-of-life facility that promotes freedom at the end of life because of its Catholic religious foundation.

Nevertheless, the very Catholicism that enables Our Lady's care limits the extent to which its model can be implemented in a religiously pluralistic US society. On a local level, the home is very helpful. But it only provides a starting point to resolving the crisis of freedom in US hospice care. Going beyond this starting point requires forming a diverse political coalition that cuts across the right-to-die debate and the larger culture wars of which it is a part. The collaboration between Amberview Hospice and Our Lady in the care of patients like Pilar Martínez provides a model for the kind of politics we need. Our Lady's high level of care is a model for what these politics can achieve.

Our Lady of Perpetual Help Home

As I discussed in chapter 4, in the US healthcare system, hospice care is defined as an outpatient benefit, delivered almost entirely to patients at home. This outpatient delivery structure presumes that the patient's long-term care needs will be addressed by their familial caregivers. When patients lack sufficient familial support to meet these needs, they are sent to nursing homes. Nursing homes, however, though meeting the patient's long-term care needs, cannot provide end-of-life care. Terminally ill patients in the nursing home setting must continue to receive hospice care on an outpatient basis. But hospices and nursing homes have conflicting organizational cultures. The conflict between these treatment modalities results in routine failures in the delivery of care and, ultimately, the destruction of the freedom of the dying patient.

Atlanta's Our Lady of Perpetual Help Home provides a different way of organizing end-of-life care. It merges the qualities of a nursing home with those of a hospice. Like a nursing home, it provides long-term care with a focus on the activities of daily living. Like a hospice, it provides a range of holistic end-of-life treatments, including medical, spiritual, and psychosocial interventions. Rather than understanding these treatment modalities as conflicting, Our Lady's staff consider them to be complementary. Long-term care facilitates the delivery of end-of-life care, while successful end-of-life care can increase the duration of the patient's final days. By synthesizing these disparate treatment modalities, Our Lady represents an anomaly in the US healthcare system: a long-term inpatient facility designed for dying people.

Our Lady is operated by approximately twelve nuns in the home at a given time. These sisters are all nurses, both licensed practical nurses and registered nurses. They range from forty to ninety years of age, with most in their fifties and sixties. The nuns preside over a healthcare facility that features one doctor and one social worker—both of whom work part time—and approximately ten male nurses. Both the facility's architecture and its division of labor are gender-segregated. On the first floor, male nurses care for male patients. The second floor houses female patients, who are cared for directly by the sisters. The nuns do regularly visit with the male patients, and the sister serving as the nursing coordinator oversees care on both floors. In addition, there are a receptionist, janitors, groundskeepers, and an events coordinator, who schedules daily activities in the home. These forty-odd staff are responsible for the care of the home's approximately twenty to twenty-five patients.

To be admitted to Our Lady, patients must meet three criteria. First, they must have a diagnosis of terminal cancer. Second, they must have sworn off all life-saving medical interventions, such as chemotherapy. Third, they must show proof that they are unable to pay for their care or find immediate placement in another end-of-life facility. Such proof is generally provided not by the patients themselves, but rather by the social worker at the institution that refers them to Our Lady. It can include financial statements as well as general explanations of why Our Lady's services are needed. Once admitted, patients who were previously not able to find care in any facility are, ironically, able receive end-of-life care that is virtually unavailable to even the most resource-rich patients in the healthcare system.

Our Lady's avoidance of the payment structures governing US health care makes the home extremely valuable to Atlanta end-of-life providers. Local hospices and hospitals rely on the home to care for patients whom they cannot easily accommodate in their own institutions. Such difficulties in accommodation may stem from a variety of factors, including a patient's lacking Medicaid or the independent means to pay for nursing home care, a lack of available beds at nursing facilities, or a patient's unwillingness to enter a nursing home. In theory, these patients could be cared for at a hospice's own inpatient facility. But the vast majority of hospices do not have inpatient facilities. Even if they do, Medicare reimbursement hampers their ability to provide care without taking a financial loss.

Both Medicaid and Medicare regulations disincentivize hospices from accommodating patients without sufficient economic resources and familial support. Area social workers refer patients to Our Lady to care for these patients and to spare their own institutions the cost of unreimbursed care.

Social workers do not, however, send patients to Our Lady just because the facility will take them. They also believe that at Our Lady patients will receive care that is superior to that which they would otherwise receive at a nursing home. One social worker noted that for cancer patients with inadequate familial support, her "first choice" was to place them at Our Lady. She clarified her opinion: "These nursing homes, some are less desirable. Have you been in them? [They're] disgusting. . . . [Our Lady's patients] get great care, and they're a hospice. They provide all the pain and symptom control a patient needs."

Though this social worker referred to Our Lady as a "hospice," technically this is not the case. The facility is licensed as a nursing home. Though they only care for dying patients, the sisters have elected to forgo seeking licensure as a hospice. In part, their reason for doing so is that hospice licensure is unnecessary. As a charitable institution, they would not benefit from Medicare reimbursement. But it is also true that if Our Lady were a hospice, the home would not be able to provide its unique form of long-term inpatient care. Area social workers may still see Our Lady as a hospice—and, in a sense, they are correct—but the irony is that it can only serve as one by refusing to be a "hospice" by the letter of the law.

Institutionalizing Integration

To gain a better understanding of Our Lady's care, I spent fifteen months conducting ethnographic research in the home. I visited the facility weekly, spending between six and eight hours per visit. I talked with patients and staff, participated in leisure activities, and observed the care of more than forty patients. In addition to interviews with the home's staff, I interviewed eight terminally ill patients about the circumstances through which they came to the home and the care they received. This combination of interviews and observations forms the basis of my analysis of Our Lady's practice of end-of-life care.

The first thing provided by Our Lady of Perpetual Help Home to dying patients is stability. Once patients arrive at the home, they know that they will be able to stay there until they die. While in theory, hospice patients should know that they will die at home, such security eludes patients who do not have adequate familial support. Those patients are constantly at the risk of being moved—from home to an inpatient facility, hospital, or nursing home and perhaps back. Such shifts create anxiety in patients regarding where they are going and who will be paying the bill. At Our Lady, terminally ill patients can focus on making their remaining time as meaningful as possible.

They are aided in doing so by the home's staffing structure. At any given time, there is at least one trained nurse available for every three patients in the home. This high staff-patient ratio means that staff at Our Lady are able to spend more time with each patient than those at either nursing homes or hospices. This freedom allows them to better tend to each patient's needs and creates a less stressful working environment. This reduced stress leads to a decline in staff turnover. Whereas nursing homes have extremely high staff turnover rates, the medical staff at Our Lady were consistent during the entire time of my ethnography— and had been for years.[3]

Each patient is assigned to one regular nurse, who attends to their daily needs of feeding, bathing, and other hygiene. This relationship generally lasts from the patient's admission until their death—a period of days, months, or even years. Because of the stability of these relationships, each nurse knows the needs of their patients very well. They are able to respond to patients' needs rapidly as they change over time. And in this response, they are able to draw on both long-term care and palliative medicine. The result is the highly effective delivery of end-of-life care.

Because of the favorable staff-patient ratio, the staff have time to spend with patients beyond caregiving. Such time can be spent in private conversations or watching daytime television shows, such as *Walker, Texas Ranger*. Staff have the time to participate in the home's regularly scheduled events, including movies, Bible study, barbeques, Nintendo Wii sessions, and bingo. Such shared moments of leisure provide opportunities for staff members to relate with patients in a capacity other than as medical professionals. They are not adversarial or superior figures, but rather confidantes, fellow travelers, or even friends.

This leisure time is dependent on the effective delivery of end-of-life care. Without adequate pain and symptom management and long-term care, it would be impossible for patients to have fun. But this effective end-of-life care, in turn, draws on the relationships that form during leisure time. For example, a nurse changing a patient's dressings may go back and forth with them about the merits of a quarterback whom they both watched play the day before. This conversation transforms the delivery of long-term care into another means of hanging out. The patient becomes more receptive to receiving care because they are not *only* receiving care. They are debating with a friend about something that they are both interested in. Leisure time is thus not wasted time. It facilitates the delivery of end-of-life care.

Patients at Our Lady are also encouraged to socialize among themselves. One site of socialization is the smoking lounge. The home features one designated smoking lounge on each floor because Our Lady's patients are not allowed to smoke in their rooms. Each smoking lounge is adjacent to the floor's regular lounge, separated from it by a glass window and door. When smoking patients congregate in a communal space, relationships are fostered between patients who, outside of Our Lady, would likely never have interacted at all.

Consider the patients who were known as Three Musketeers. The Three Musketeers were women, all in their sixties, who were dying of cancer. One woman was a white drug addict who had recently watched her daughter die in hospice. Another was a white divorcée who had previously worked as a schoolteacher. The last was a recently widowed African American woman whose son worked for the FBI. These women came from different racial, socioeconomic, and professional backgrounds. And yet they congregated every afternoon for several hours to smoke cigarettes and talk about the day's events, their respective familial problems, the issues that they were having in Our Lady, and, occasionally, their thoughts and feelings about dying. Though a smoking lounge might not seem to be a health-promoting space, at Our Lady it provided a venue for the formation of nourishing personal relationships that would have otherwise been difficult to cultivate.

Such new friendships complement the relationships that Our Lady's patients continue to have with their families. In theory, familial relationships might seem to be diminished because patients are no longer living at home. In practice, the opposite is more often true. Prior to their relative's enrollment at Our Lady, these familial caregivers were so preoccupied with attending to their loved one's basic needs that they had little left for emotional connection. By attending to these needs, Our Lady's staff allow family members to bond with their relatives in ways that were not possible before.

Patients are also encouraged to reinsert themselves into the world beyond the home's walls. Members of the community visit Our Lady's patients routinely: volunteers, church groups, grade school students, high school football teams, and even high-end restaurateurs. Patients who are able also can leave the home, whether through informal trips with family and friends or through excursions scheduled by the home's event planner. Both visitors to the home and visits outside its walls remind Our Lady's patients that even though they are dying, they continue to be valued members of society.

Our Lady of Perpetual Help Home is an institution. But its patients are not segregated. On the contrary, the facility takes patients out of previously segregated contexts—the home or the nursing home—and integrates them into a vibrant community that allows them to reengage the world. In this sense, Our Lady does not provide its patients with access into society. It remakes society to better fit them.

More Freedom

The impact of Our Lady of Perpetual Help Home on its patients can be described in various ways. It is medical, in that it improves their symptoms and pain relief and in many cases extends their lives. It is social, in that it allows them to become part of a community built for them. It is psychological, in that it provides them with an ability to reorient their lives and confront their dying on terms that are amenable to them. But it is also *political*: Our Lady of Perpetual Help Home increases the freedom of dying people.

The home takes patients whose freedom has been destroyed and restores—even enhances—it. At Our Lady, patients are able to receive end-of-life care that, at a basic level, is appropriate to their needs. But they are also able to participate in a community. How they choose to engage this community is up to them. If they want to watch television with others they can, but they are also free to smoke outside and watch the birds. In either case, the home gives them the resources to live as they want with the life that they have left. Prior to entering, they had no options.

As a result, patients at Our Lady are much freer than they were prior to their arrival at the home. Through its integrated form of long-term end-of-life care, the home gives them much better treatment options than would otherwise be available to them in the US hospice system. It provides them with a much wider range of choices in terms of how they want to live the remainder of their life. It takes them out of a segregated environment and into one that, though institutional, is integrated into society—and, in turn, integrates society into it. How Our Lady's residents want to engage this richness is their decision. That they have the option of engaging it makes them much freer than they would have been otherwise.

For the home's patients, this freedom is not just a philosophical construct. It is a lived experience, something that they feel. Often, this feeling is one of relief: they no longer have to worry if the pain medication will come. At other times, it is one of joy: watching the World Series, playing bingo, drinking a beer, or chatting about the Korean War. And, at other times, it can be one of sorrow and frustration: dying is perhaps an inevitably sad experience. Our Lady of Perpetual Help Home does not deny this sadness. By taking care of the needs of patients, it allows them to feel it more acutely, if they so choose. It is difficult to mourn the loss of your own life if you find yourself fending off robbers or struggling to choke down a piece of bread.

The range of emotions that Our Lady allows its patients to feel is an indicator of their freedom. The affective range of someone in traumatizing circumstances is severely restricted.[4] But amid all the different emotions that patients at Our Lady feel, there was one that I found to be a constant: gratitude. All the home's patients with whom I spoke were grateful to be at Our Lady. They may not have liked every aspect of the home, but they saw it as a significant improvement over their prior living arrangements. And they felt an enormous debt to its workers for giving them the kind of care that no one else would. This gratitude was itself a way of recognizing the freedom they felt.

At times, the home's patients even identified this freedom as such. A patient I call Tim described the difference between Our Lady and the other facilities where he had received care:

> [At Our Lady] they don't do what many places do—that is to say, they order you about. And this place doesn't. And to that extent you have more freedom and feel freer. . . . The feeling of freedom this place engenders is better than the places I've been to before—the hospital and the rehabilitation place for the muscular drills. . . . The hospital used one of my arms for a needle trial of some new nurses. . . . And that was not fun. . . . The hospital did that, not the rehabilitation people, who . . . let me go my own way with a wheelchair, which I enjoyed. So it was somewhat freer, but you always had the feeling that you could be told what to do, and the feeling that this place engenders is so much freer by not giving you that feeling that I enjoy being here considerably more than being at the other places.

While hospitals and rehabilitation centers had inhibited Tim's freedom through their rigid schedules, Our Lady gave him more freedom simply by allowing him to live as he saw fit. But the home did not *just* get out of his way. Prior to his arrival at Our Lady, Tim was bedbound at home. Our Lady provided him with the care necessary so that he could enjoy his freedom and then gave him an environment in which he could realize it. The result was a feeling of liberation that, though unique for him, was common among the patients I met.

Simon's Case

When I met Simon, he was forty-eight years old. He had worked in the airline industry in Florida for more than ten years, but when the financial crisis hit in 2008, he was laid off. He lived alone at the time, but decided to move to Missouri to be near his first wife, with whom he was still close. There, he found work at a pet store but began feeling a pain in his left arm. During a severe episode, he went to the emergency room, where physicians found a tumor in his lung so large that it was breaking his ribs.

Simon paid for his chemotherapy and radiation through a combination of Medicaid and charitable donations. But when there was no remission, his doctor recommended hospice. Since Simon's ex-wife could not take care of him full time, Simon moved to his brother's house in Atlanta. He began home hospice care, while his brother and niece provided him with assistance with the activities of daily living. This care was sufficient until his brother found work as a trucker, a job that required that he spend long stretches of time away from home. Simon's niece cared for him in his brother's absence, but in the fall of 2011, she left for college. As a result, Simon was left alone in the house.

Simon soon deteriorated. His brother's house had a lot of stairs, and he fell several times. At the same time, the suburban Atlanta neighborhood isolated him. He went weeks with little more than sporadic face-to-face interactions with his hospice caretakers, whose work largely consisted of providing him with pain medication, which he would later administer himself. Simon became depressed. He slept as much as fourteen hours a day and largely stopped eating. He experienced for the first time significant cognitive impairments, including a general lack of awareness and short-term memory loss.

Simon and his brother decided that he needed to be transferred to an inpatient facility. But his hospice lacked such a facility, and it would have taken weeks to overcome the financial and bureaucratic obstacles to his being placed in a nursing home. As an alternative, Simon's social worker suggested he apply for admission to Our Lady of Perpetual Help Home. Simon applied and was granted entry to the home within a week's time.

After entering, his quality of life and condition significantly improved. He resumed sleeping eight hours a night and eating regularly. He had daily opportunities for socialization with the home's patients, nuns, and nurses, and he was able move freely in the institution, which is completely accessible. He had regular visits from family and friends, as well as volunteers. He stayed there for nine months—outlasting his initial prognosis by almost a year—and though the home did not cure him of cancer, it gave him the opportunity to live out the final months of his life in relative calm with high-level medical care, a stable environment, and regular socializing.

Prior to his arrival at Our Lady, Simon could, in a sense, have "chosen" his medical treatment options: either his brother's house or a nursing home. Whichever one he chose, he would have spent his final days in almost total constraint.

At home, he could not move around without falling. At a nursing home, even if he was not physically mistreated, he would have been cut off from the entire world. Choosing between these options is not freedom. It is choosing how one prefers to be deprived of it.

Our Lady gave Simon real choices. Which form of pain medication did he prefer? What was the best way for him to be washed? Would he like to watch television or see the birds? Did he feel like talking in the smoking lounge, or would he rather stay in his room and read? These choices may seem trivial. But Simon had been robbed of them just months before.

Simon himself had no doubt that he was freer at Our Lady than he had been at home. He had been at death's door, with nothing left to lose and nothing to gain by going on. He described feeling like a "commodity": he felt that his hospice was just providing basic services to him in order to make a profit. Now he felt like a "person" again. When he agreed to be interviewed for my research, he did so with a caveat: "Sure, but if you ever write anything negative about these people, I'll come find you and kick your ass."

In his feeling of freedom, Simon was much like Tim and the other patients I talked to at Our Lady. But this very basic sense of freedom remains hidden in our current discussion of "freedom" at the end of life.

The Right to Die Is Not the Only Path to Freedom

I have argued that Simon's arrival at Our Lady of Perpetual Help Home increased his freedom. This is not a difficult argument to make. The facility gave him more control over his life in practically every sense. It would thus seem self-evident that it increased his freedom at the end of life. After all, the very premise of our discussion of freedom at the end of life is the individual's self-control.

But our usual discussion does not have much to say about Simon's situation. The reason is simple. Although Our Lady expanded Simon's freedom at the end of life, it did not do so by giving him the "freedom to die." In the current framework, it is only via such an opportunity that Simon's freedom could be extended. It is worth considering the implications of this analysis for Simon's life.

Prior to his enrollment in Our Lady of Perpetual Help Home, Simon was a patient in the US hospice system. He was constrained to his home environment, where he had no freedom. The alternative within this system was for him to move to a nursing home. But there, it is likely that his freedom would have been constrained equally, or even more so. Thus, the only freedom that Simon had available to him in US hospice care was the freedom to decide how not to be free.

Physician-assisted suicide would have given him another option: death. It is possible that he might have perceived this as an improvement over his situation. Indeed, it is easy to understand how death might be preferable to virtual imprisonment, be it in a forgotten corner of a nursing home or a forgotten floor in his brother's house. We can debate whether it is a good thing that patients have this option available to them. It is more difficult to debate that it should be the *only* option.

This, however, is the premise of our current conversation about freedom at the end of life. This debate does not consider whether Simon should have access to better fall prevention or public transportation or meal options or long-term care. It only considers whether or not he should have the freedom to die. But even if Simon had this freedom, there would be nothing free about his actual dying. Prior to his enrollment at Our Lady, Simon lived in an environment that destroyed his freedom. This type of destruction does not even register in a conversation that only examines the right to die.

The result is a debate that is premised on the maintenance of the status quo. This status quo bias is true of both proponents and opponents of PAS. Proponents of PAS would want Simon to have the option of PAS. Opponents would not. But neither would, in general, have much to say about the *non*fatal options available to him in the US hospice system. Rather, both would take for granted that this system is not of primary importance to the question of freedom at the end of life. Indeed, this is why both proponents and opponents of physician-assisted suicide recommend that dying patients receive hospice care.[5] For proponents, such a recommendation attests that the dying did not make their decision in response to a failure of end-of-life services. For opponents, the hope is that with appropriate hospice care, terminally ill patients will not want PAS. There is merit to these positions, but they both assume that existing US hospice options are liberating.

The existing options, however, are not liberating for patients who lack sufficient familial support. Such patients live in environments in which their freedom is constrained. This was true for Simon prior to his arrival at Our Lady, just as it was true for Steven and Mary, whom I profiled in chapter 4. It was regularly true for the patients at Amberview Hospice. There is a crisis of freedom in US hospice care.

Legalizing physician-assisted suicide will not solve this crisis. But banning it will not either. Rather, the solution is providing patients who have inadequate familial support with options that are genuinely liberating. For Simon and the other residents, Our Lady of Perpetual Help Home does just that—but not by providing more hospice care. Our Lady offers liberating options by *challenging* the existing arrangement of US hospice care, providing an alternative model of caretaking that is more appropriate to the needs of the patients it serves.

Our Lady can mount this challenge because of its unique payment structure. But this raises a question: *Why* does Our Lady function according to a financial incentive structure that differs radically from other medical institutions in the US healthcare system? Understanding this incentive structure entails studying the order of nuns that operates Our Lady: the Hawthorne Dominicans.

Rose Hawthorne Lathrop and the Hawthorne Dominicans

Our Lady of Perpetual Help Home is run by the Dominican Sisters of Hawthorne, an order of nuns that was founded in 1900 by Rose Hawthorne Lathrop, the youngest daughter of American novelist Nathaniel Hawthorne. Raised a Unitarian, Lathrop converted to Catholicism at the age of forty in 1891.[6] This conversion was a formative moment in Lathrop's life, and it eventually led her in 1896 to leave her husband, become a nun, and consecrate her life to the charitable labor of caring for the cancerous poor.[7]

Renting a small apartment on Manhattan's Lower East Side, Lathrop placed an advertisement in the *New York Times*, in which she invited all cancer patients in need of treatment to come to her for free care.[8] Such patients were particularly in need of care since at the time—shortly after the discovery of germ theory—cancer patients were shunned by physicians as being both incurable and contagious.[9] Nevertheless, Lathrop cared for them, at first by herself and then later with the aid of a group of female followers. In 1906, these women succeeded in gaining official recognition from the Catholic Church and joined the Dominican order.[10]

Lathrop believed that dying patients should receive the same level of care regardless of their ability to pay. This belief led her to reject monetary remuneration in her facility for the dying. Receiving payment for services, she believed, would lead to favoring paying patients over their nonpaying counterparts.[11] Such a two-tiered system was the root of the very exclusion of the cancerous poor that her home was designed to counteract. Nevertheless, while rejecting payment, she accepted donations, and it is on such a charitable economy that Hawthorne facilities have operated ever since.

With the help of many donors, the Hawthorne Dominicans underwent a remarkable expansion. Over the twentieth century, they opened up seven nursing homes in the United States and one in Kenya. In recent years, the sisters have scaled back their activities, closing their Kenyan location and four of the US homes. As members of the order explained to me, this downsizing occurred due to decreased recruitment and older members passing away.

At present, there are three active Hawthorne Dominican facilities: Rosary Hill Home, located just outside of Manhattan; Sacred Heart Home in Philadelphia; and Atlanta's Our Lady of Perpetual Help Home. These all provide long-term, charitable end-of-life care for patients who have no other feasible options for end-of-life care.

In what follows, I draw on conversations with four members of the Hawthorne Dominicans—all of whom were at the time working at Our Lady—and one of the order's priests in order to reconstruct their religious worldview. Though my account is mainly drawn from these conversations, when possible I provide citations of relevant passages from the Catechism of the Catholic Church.[12] Together, these interviews and textual sources provide a picture of end-of-life care grounded in a particular and powerful understanding of death.

Death, Works, Resurrection

As Catholics, the sisters of Our Lady of Perpetual Help Home believe that the universe was created by a being they call God. God's chief characteristic is having created something from nothing. He is invisible, yet present in all that exists. God created humans in his own image and gave them free will. Adam and Eve, the first humans, used this free will to betray God. As a result of this original sin, God condemned all of humankind to a condition of sinfulness.[13]

Nevertheless, though angry at humans, God also loves them. Because of this love, he sent them his son, Jesus Christ. Christ, in the Catholic understanding solidified after the First Council of Nicaea, is equally God and human.[14] As a human, Christ was capable of free will and also capable of death. To atone for humanity's original sin, he gave himself up to die on the cross. And yet, three days after his death, Christ was resurrected. If his death proved his humanity, then his resurrection from death asserted his divinity. By having faith in Christ, humans can share in this resurrection and overcome, at least partially, their own sinful nature. As a result, they can live on spiritually, after their physical deaths, with God and his son.[15]

This belief in Christ's death and resurrection is, in large part, common to all Christian denominations.[16] What makes Catholicism unique is its belief that Christ's will is embodied in an earthly institutional structure, the Catholic Church, whose chief representative is the pope. The church's role is to interpret the will of God in the context of a shifting social reality.[17] During my research—which occurred under the papacy of Benedict XVI—some US nuns questioned the papacy's teachings on social issues such as abortion and same-sex marriage, but the sisters of Our Lady were extremely conservative in their adherence to the magisterium.[18] As one sister put it: "The Holy Father represents Jesus Christ. If we can't be faithful to Jesus's representative . . . then why are we doing what we are doing?"

Adherence to the papacy is reinforced by the sisters' views on the relationship between faith and works. As Father Stanley Brewer put it in our interview: "In the Catholic interpretation of salvation . . . humans are saved by grace through faith, but we are called to cooperate with that grace . . . by doing good works." Thus, in Catholicism, though faith is a precondition of salvation, works are valuable means of ensuring one's place in the spiritual realm of heaven and then afterward at the last judgment—when Christ will return to earth and cast his judgment on the materially resurrected dead.

The desire to do good works is the primary justification that the sisters I interviewed gave for the enormous sacrifices they make by entering religious life. As a sister I call Matilda explained:

> I've given my whole life because I believe this. I believe in the resurrection. I believe that one day our body and our souls will be reunited with the Lord, and we will go to heaven and be with the heavenly Father, the Trinity, all the saints, our relatives, our family members that have gone before us. . . . And I hope and pray that [Jesus] will say to me, "Well done, my good and faithful servant." Because that's what I long to hear, those words: "Well done, you have served me well. Come share my Father's joy."

Sister Matilda reaffirmed her belief that her works will give her a place in heaven. In this sense, she emphasized that she was not doing this work as an act of charity offered without hope of recompense. On the contrary, she worked for the recompense of resurrection, which can only be understood in terms of Catholic religious belief. This compensation justified the sister's sacrifice of her earthly life by entering the order. Indeed, though Matilda expressed her extreme joy at being a nun, she also emphasized that it had been a difficult decision for her because she had wanted to have a family. Such sacrifices were, in the sisters I interviewed, only comprehensible in the light of the resurrection.

It is by virtue of their understanding of compensation through resurrection that the sisters formulate a unique perspective on exactly *who* are the actors involved in end-of-life care. Through Sister Matilda's description of herself as "giving her own life," she drew an implicit parallel between her situation and that of Jesus, as well as God. As she noted later in our conversation, both God and Jesus had to make an enormous sacrifice—Jesus's very life—to save humanity. Through her own sacrifice of the life she could have enjoyed, Matilda is at once inspired by and representative of Jesus's sacrifice. In fact, Matilda referred to herself in the conversation as "on the cross" with Jesus. This identification with Jesus might seem narcissistic, but it is the very point that enables the sisters of Our Lady to empathize with their patients—people who represent the suffering of Jesus just as much as they do themselves.

Seeing Jesus

The sisters I spoke with were emphatic about their attempts to "see Jesus" in their patients. By seeing Jesus, the sisters treat each patient as if they were Jesus Christ—not the resurrected Christ, but Christ as he is dying. By seeing Jesus, the sisters attempt to provide patients with the care that they would give to Christ himself. Learning how to see Jesus is the key part of the sisters' religious training, which forms the basis for their medical education.

In end-of-life care, Christianity is perhaps uniquely qualified to foster such identification because it is a religion centered around a dying man and his grieving family. The nuns identify Christ with terminally ill patients, while understanding the patients' families through other key biblical figures, such as the Virgin Mary, Mary Magdalene, and St. Joseph. At times, this identification can be extremely literal, and it is facilitated by the iconographic representations of the crucifixion that are present in each of the home's rooms. One sister remarked to me that as dying cancer patients become increasingly thin, "their cheeks hollow out, and they look just like Jesus on the cross." But such a literal interpretation of seeing Jesus was rare among the sisters I spoke with; instead, Christ's iconographic body opened a gateway to a world of shared resemblances that undercut physical appearance.

As Father Brewer described, the identification between Jesus and dying patients would not, in a "mature" formulation, be based on physical resemblance but rather on a shared suffering that underlies surface appearances and contemporary medical categories. He explained the relationship of his practice of seeing Jesus in patients to his looking at the cross: "When I look at the cross of Christ, I think of [the patients] going through their cross. Or me going through my cross." Here, the physical suffering of Jesus on the cross is shown to have a broader meaning than its literal resemblance to the suffering of dying patients. It includes Brewer's own suffering, which is a universal aspect of the human condition even as it is grounded in his own particular life experience. Thus, the dying Jesus is present not only in the literal bodies of dying patients, but also in *all* bodies, including those of Our Lady's religious staff.

The universality of Jesus's suffering—its presence in our very embodiment—reconfigures the relationship between patient and provider at Our Lady. Rather than a binary opposition between the healthy and the sick, the patient and provider are both seen as sick and, in a sense, dying. As one sister commented: "So we see Christ in the patients and their families, and we hope they see Christ in us. And so it's just like a continuous thing of going from Christ to Christ to Christ." As the sister explained, at Our Lady there is no one outside of Christ. The practice of seeing Jesus breaks down the typical barriers structuring the delivery of medical care, revealing a common substance underlying both patient and provider.

Thus, though the sisters only accept patients who belong to the medical category of "terminal illness," their religious understanding of end-of-life care is a powerful rejection of this category. The home's sisters are, in this sense, every bit as "dying" as the human-God they worship and the patients they treat. And yet, though the sisters believe that all humans are, like Christ, bound toward death, the Christ narrative also assures them that death is not the end point of life.

The Resurrected Body

The sisters I spoke with highlighted the importance of mass in their daily activities. The sisters attend mass every morning at 6:30 a.m. and every afternoon at 4:00 p.m. At mass they relive the story of the death and resurrection of Jesus Christ. The service concludes with their receiving the communion wine and wafer. As Sister Matilda explained: "The mass is our food, our nourishment for the soul. Without that, I could go anywhere and be a nurse, do oncology work, do hospice." The mass, then—and specifically the Eucharist—gives care at Our Lady both its underlying meaning and its motivational force.

The mystical power of the communion wine and wafer is grounded in a Catholic understanding of the Eucharist. Father Brewer explained: "The resurrected Christ truly becomes present and alive to us . . . in the Eucharist. . . . We claim even though the elements appear still to be bread and wine, that it actually is Christ there. So when we receive it, Christ comes into our hearts and as such his power dwells in our hearts. To inspire us and to strengthen us to go out and to live the Catholic faith. To do the Christian work." As Brewer explained, the Eucharist is, for the sisters, the literal resurrected body of Christ. Taking communion every morning, then, not only affirms their faith in Christ's resurrection, but also allows them to take part in it. Though they suffer as Christ, they are also saved through him.

But to be saved through Christ is not enough. Such salvation contains within it the desire to spread it to others. But unlike missionary Christian denominations, Our Lady's sisters do not spread salvation through the holy word. Rather, they spread it through the holy body. The vehicle of this resurrected body is not the literal Eucharist. It is the medical care that they provide to dying patients and their families. Sister Matilda explained:

> We receive [Christ] into our soul through communion. And it's that that gives us strength, knowing that the Lord died on that cross. . . . We take in that divinity of Christ within us, and we have to be Christ bearers. . . . What would we do if we received him and did not take him to others? That's not what he wants us to do. What we do is, we take him out to the patients, the families, [the] visitors. In other words, that love of Christ has to dwell within us. It has to be something that nourishes us so that we can also nourish others, nourish them through the love of Christ.

Matilda noted that through communion the sisters become the bearers of the resurrected body of Christ. This resurrected body is the substance of the medical care they provide. Thus, Our Lady is not, in a strict sense, a medical institution. It is a religious institution oriented toward spreading Christ's resurrection. And yet, it spreads this resurrection not by proselytization, but rather through its high level of holistic end-of-life care.

This care is the vehicle that promotes freedom at the end of life. The promotion of freedom at the end of life at Our Lady is made possible by the home's Catholic foundation. This observation overturns the way we normally in the United States think about the relationship between religion and freedom in healthcare settings.

Balancing Freedoms at the End of Life

At Atlanta's Our Lady of Perpetual Help Home, Catholic nuns provide dying people with the same level of care as if they were Jesus Christ. As a result of this care, Our Lady's patients are freer than they were prior to their enrollment in the home. They have more and better options available to them. The constraints that would have affected them at home or in a nursing home are diminished. Thus, Our Lady's care gives its patients more freedom because of its religious foundation.

But we generally would not see it that way. Scholarship on religious healthcare institutions and freedom has focused on the question of so-called religious exemptions, which allow religious institutions to not offer services that violate the principles of their religion. These exemptions have been criticized for impinging on the freedom of patients who might want those services.[19] Thus, religious foundations are in general presumed by scholars to make healthcare facilities *less* free.

But this scholarship ignores that religious foundations are not solely prohibitive. They can be generative. Our Lady's religious foundation could lead it, in theory, to prohibit services that would be available in a secular hospice. But the same religious foundation makes it possible to provide services that secular providers do not: for example, long-term, inpatient end-of-life care. If we just focus on the services the home is exempt from, we miss those that it provides. This omission is significant for the question of freedom at the end of life.

Consider the following thought experiment. Were the right to die legal in Georgia, Our Lady would have petitioned to be exempt from providing it. Physician-assisted suicide would violate the home's religious commitment to the sanctity of life. Amberview Hospice, in contrast, as a secular facility might have chosen to provide PAS. As a result, it might seem that Amberview was *freer* than Our Lady.

But this analysis would ignore the services that Our Lady provides that Amberview does not. Amberview Hospice does not provide long-term, inpatient end-of-life care oriented toward the social inclusion of dying patients. By not doing so, it limits the freedom of dying patients without familial support. Our Lady, in contrast, gives these patients a freedom that Amberview does not allow them. As a result, it is arguably a freer institution.

Take Simon as an example. In this thought experiment, had Simon remained with his previous hospice, he might have been able to commit physician-assisted suicide. But this freedom to die would not have challenged the constraints that robbed him of his freedom in the first place. Our Lady, in contrast, largely removed them. Thus, his situation at Our Lady was freer than it would have been *even if* his original hospice offered the right to die. Simon's ability to move had been destroyed, his sustenance curtailed, his interactions with others eliminated. He lived in a virtual prison. Giving him PAS in that context would have allowed him a way out of this constraining environment. But you're not very free if your only choice is death.

At Our Lady, in contrast, Simon had a number of ways to be free. He could move without impediment, socialize with others, and live without significant pain or suffering. He might not have been able to choose to die "with dignity," but he could do many things that death with dignity would not permit him. With his previous hospice, he might have had the freedom to die, but he would not have been free in any other meaningful sense.

This does not mean that the freedom to die is negligible. It means that it must be understood in the broader context of the additional freedom available to patients at the end of life. Our Lady of Perpetual Help Home will likely never offer the right to die, but it is not inherently less free than its secular counterparts. Enjoying the home's freedom requires a trade-off. This trade-off is deeply relevant to Simon's case.

The Limits of Our Lady

Simon loved Our Lady. But this love did not keep him from, on occasion, feeling left behind. His family and friends were distant or busy. He was tired of life. He had beaten two fatal prognoses already. He did not put much value in the time that he had left. He was at Our Lady, and was extremely grateful for the time he had there. But this did not feel like his life anymore. "If I could," he said to me one day, "I'd just end it right now."

One could interpret this comment as a request on Simon's part for physician-assisted suicide. At the very least, it attests that even in cases of extremely competent care—like that which Simon received at Our Lady—terminally ill patients may wish to have control over their deaths. I have argued that such control should not be considered the only nor the primary way to expand freedom at the end of life. But that does not mean that it should not be considered at all.

One could argue that Our Lady's not offering PAS limited Simon's freedom. One could also argue against that point: claiming, for example, that it is impossible to freely choose death or that, even if such a choice increased freedom, it should still be limited due to the risks of a slippery slope. This is a reasonable argument to have, and it is, to a degree, the argument we have been having in the United States about the right to die.

But my view is that, whatever position one takes on PAS, it should not be the sole or even the primary way in which we debate freedom at the end of life. I am willing to concede the possibility that Simon's freedom was limited by his inability to die with dignity, but I challenge that this should be viewed as the primary limitation on his freedom.

Prior to his enrollment at Our Lady, Simon's freedom already was limited, irrespective of his right to die. Making the right to die available to him would have been a poor first option to realize his freedom. There were multiple ways to enhance his freedom that would not bring about his death, as his care at Our Lady showed. These should be considered prior to PAS, but in most discussions of

PAS, they are not considered at all. These discussions assume that dying patients are already free and that PAS merely extends their freedom. I have argued that this is not the case for patients with inadequate familial support.

Our primary goal should be to enhance the freedom of this patient population. One can debate whether PAS would do so. But this debate should be premised on the agreement that, regardless of PAS, we need to do more to provide care for dying people. Doing more is consistent with the goals of both supporters and opponents of physician-assisted suicide. If you support PAS, advocating for more and better services will strengthen your argument that the desire to die cannot be reduced to a lack of care. If you oppose PAS, providing more and better services will help give dying people the resources to make their lives more livable. Either way, instituting more nonlethal measures to promote freedom at the end of life furthers your goals regarding the right to die.

In fact, both sides of this debate, for the most part, share the same goal: improving freedom among dying people. They disagree on whether PAS does so and if it is worth the trade-offs. This is a reasonable disagreement, but it should not obscure the substantial common ground among supporters and opponents of the right to die. And it should not obscure the work that we need to do if we are to achieve our shared goal.

Achieving this goal can seem daunting, but it carries a lesser cost than attempting to ban or legalize PAS. Due to the decisions of the US Supreme Court, it is unlikely that there will ever be enough political momentum to either ban or legalize the right to die on a federal level.[20] The decision has been left up to the states, and given the demographic characteristics of various states, there is a ceiling on how many are likely to ban or legalize PAS.[21] To be sure, a state whose population in general considers physician-assisted suicide to be a violation of the sanctity of life can change its views. But the cost of such change is high, and its effects are limited to that state. That does not mean that it is not worth pursuing. It means that it should not be the *only* strategy to promote freedom at the end of life.

Attempting to promote freedom through nonlethal means is much more possible on a federal level. The Medicare Hospice Benefit is a federal piece of legislation that instantly established a reimbursement structure for hospice throughout the country. The benefit has had bipartisan support: it was passed under the Reagan administration and supported by liberals. In this book, I highlight its flaws, but it has nevertheless increased freedom for millions of dying Americans. It does so, however, to a considerably lesser extent for those Americans who lack adequate familial support. Right now, it is necessary to find a way to attend to the increasing numbers of this population group. The long-term, inpatient end-of-life care provided by Our Lady is one such way.

We should encourage the work of other charitable religious healthcare providers. Too often, the work of these providers is unacknowledged in discussions of healthcare justice.[22] But religious healthcare providers regularly provide services to patients who fall through the cracks of the US healthcare system. They do so because they operate according to a logic that differs from that of this system. Such differences are extremely valuable for the populations they serve. Religious healthcare providers also serve as valuable points to rethink—and, ideally, transform—the very nature of a US healthcare system that fundamentally needs to be rethought. In this sense, the work of Our Lady exemplifies the suggestion made by philosopher and bioethicist Jeffrey Bishop that "only theology can save medicine."[23]

But while generative, Our Lady's religious nature limits the home's ability to provide a solution to the crisis of US hospice care. In a religiously pluralistic country, the services provided by the charitable organizations of any one religious group will necessarily be patchwork. Our Lady of Perpetual Help Home has limited beds. It provides an invaluable service in the context of Atlanta's end-of-life care. But just as local hospices depend on the sisters to care for their patients, so too Our Lady's sisters depend on these hospices to accommodate the patients that they cannot. In this sense, Our Lady of Perpetual Help, though providing an alternative to US hospice care, itself depends on hospice.

There are other drawbacks to Our Lady's model. By its nature, the home removes patients from their familial environments. It is in a neighborhood in Atlanta that has limited resources and a high crime rate. At the same time, Our Lady has little direct interaction with its neighborhood, existing at times as an island apart. The result can be isolating. And no matter how excellent the care, it is being provided by people whom the patients did not previously know and in a building that is, to a degree, unfamiliar. Our Lady's sisters and staff do an incredible job of making the home accommodating, but even with the greatest skill and effort, there are limits.

Simon's loneliness in the last weeks of his life illustrates these limits. His loneliness was a product of him being housed in a home that, no matter how accommodating, was geographically distant from most of his family. But it was also a product of Simon's particular familial circumstances and, more broadly, the tensions of US society. Simon's family were scattered throughout the country. They were limited in the amount of time that they could spend with him, and they may have limited themselves due to previous disagreements. Thus, much of Simon's loneliness was due to circumstances out of the control of Our Lady or any end-of-life care facility.

Still, many things could have been done to improve Simon's life, even at the very end. Some actions would have been personal decisions by Simon and his family, but others were matters of public policy. Had Simon's brother been able to take a paid leave from his job as a trucker, he would have been able to spend more time with Simon. Had Simon's initial hospice care been better integrated with mental health services, perhaps his depression could have been lessened, if not completely ameliorated. Had Our Lady been situated in a neighborhood that was accessible and safe, he would have been able to interact more with his immediate community. Though perhaps not eliminated, Simon's loneliness could have been reduced.

Our Lady of Perpetual Help Home is not, in itself, an alternative to the crisis of freedom in US hospice care. But it does provide a starting point from which such an alternative can be formulated.

The Alternative to Come

For a time during my fieldwork, Our Lady's sisters began each morning mass with a prayer for an end to both abortion and euthanasia. They were "pro-life," and their commitment to the sanctity of human life shaped their voting priorities. It led them, in general, to support the Republican candidate, Mitt Romney, in the 2012 election.

On the surface, the politics of Our Lady could not have contrasted more with those of Amberview Hospice. Amberview's staff was generally liberal. When Barack Obama was reelected president, the home's chaplain began the staff meeting by saying, "Well, I assume everyone's happy, right?" Everyone nodded in agreement. In interviews with the staff, I found a diversity of opinions on assisted suicide: several members were in favor of it, and those who opposed it did so largely on procedural grounds—as opposed to an opposition based on the sanctity of life.

Yet, in spite of their divergent politics, the staffs of Amberview Hospice and Our Lady of Perpetual Help Home worked together. In part, this was because they needed each other. Our Lady could take in patients that Amberview couldn't, and vice versa. But the staffs of Amberview and Our Lady also worked together because they had a common goal: providing dying people with the best care possible. The manner in which they realized that goal differed, as did the reason they had it. But both the sisters at Our Lady and the staff at Amberview were frequently incensed at the treatment that dying people received in US society, and they were eager to do everything possible to make it better.

This partnership signals the alternative to the crisis of freedom in US hospice care: the political project of building a broad coalition of individuals dedicated to improving the way we care for dying people. Our Lady and Amberview Hospice are already doing this work in their collaboration. And in this, they are not alone. Across America, people are working together across political lines and ideological disagreements in order to provide better care for dying patients. Unfortunately, such local collaborations have not been reflected in the realm of national politics.

A significant reason that this is the case is because of our collective focus on physician-assisted suicide. Though Amberview's staff and that of Our Lady coordinated in many ways, they differed in general on this issue. Such a difference is emblematic. Assisted suicide is an issue that is polarizing and will remain so for the foreseeable future. Important issues are frequently polarizing, and perhaps they should be. But this polarization is negative because it obscures the agreement underpinning the provision of much of US end-of-life care.

In trying to find a consensus on a deeply divisive topic in bioethics, my argument builds on that of Charles Camosy's book *Beyond the Abortion Wars*.[24] Camosy's work is an attempt to find a consensus between "pro-life" and "pro-choice" positions on abortion. He argues that the widespread view that these two sides are irreconcilable is mistaken. Contrary to the perception of a "hopeless stalemate," the majority of Americans, Camosy writes, "actually agree about broad ideas with respect to abortion morality and law."[25] Camosy's book is directed to this (relatively silent) majority, proposing a public policy that coheres with their beliefs while also being backed by "the best ideas and arguments" on the topic. The result is to transform abortion into an issue that, far from stifling unified political action, can promote it in quite dynamic and radical ways.

I find Camosy's argument about abortion compelling. But I want to emphasize here that even if I did not, that does not mean that a consensus is impossible regarding freedom at the end of life. Rather, I encourage us to see the topic of freedom at the end of life, in general, and the right to die, in particular, as distinct from that of abortion. One can support abortion and be opposed to the right to die, or oppose abortion and support it. Either way, I argue that, though there is room for consensus on abortion, there is *more* room for consensus on the right to die and certainly on the broader topic of freedom at the end of life.

To see this consensus, it is necessary to disentangle the right to die from the context that has, to a significant degree, framed the way that the issue has been discussed in the US public sphere: the so-called culture wars.[26] The culture wars—a term originally attributed to conservative politician Patrick Buchanan—refers to the (largely) nonviolent conflict in the United States between liberals and conservatives. This conflict can be discussed in various terms, with race, economics, education, and geography all being central. But in his history of the culture wars, *A War for the Soul of America*, historian Andrew Hartman argues that in addition to—and intersecting with—these factors, a fundamental dividing line is religion and, more specifically, Christianity.[27]

The culture wars pit conservatives who identify in general as Christian or, at the very least, who are protective of what they refer to as "Christian values" against a coalition of groups identified with secular liberalism. Though Hartman, whose book was published in 2015, declared these wars to be over, he has since admitted that Donald Trump's rise to the presidency—fueled to a significant degree by evangelical support—has rendered that diagnosis premature.[28] These wars continue to shape our national conversation on a range of issues, from gun control to immigration, same-sex marriage to Homeland Security. Abortion is not only one of these issues. It is arguably the *central* issue, and it has shaped the culture wars as much, if not more, than it has been shaped by them.

The right to die has in general been viewed through the lens of the culture wars. As such, it pits secular liberals against religious conservatives. If you are a secular liberal who lives on the country's coasts, chances are that you are "pro-choice" and perhaps only know other people who support PAS. Alternatively, if you identify as a Christian and are from a less populated area in middle America, chances are that you identify as "pro-life" and are therefore against the right to die. Such identifications are largely tribal, a product of whom we identify as family, and they have been shown to be highly resistant to change.[29] So long as the right-to-die debate, then, remains locked in the culture wars framework, it will be difficult to build any effective political coalition.

But the right to die is a much more complex issue than the existing culture wars framework allows. For "pro-choice" advocates for PAS, the right to die raises the question of why this choice is *only* extended to dying people and whether doing so is an act of—and intensification of already existing—oppression. For "pro-life" opponents of PAS, the right to die is a conscious choice made by a consenting individual about their own body. It involves no additional person nor a fetus and as such is arguably coherent with a "small government" conservative philosophy based in religious liberty. Indeed, it was on the grounds of religious liberty that legal philosopher Ronald Dworkin made his argument for the right to die.[30]

There are thus compelling "liberal" reasons to oppose physician-assisted suicide and compelling "conservative" reasons to support it. This is true of abortion as well—as Camosy shows—but it is even truer of the right to die. In part, this seeming paradox stems from the analytical reasons I mentioned above. But it is also partly a result of contingent political factors related to how we form our identities in the United States. Abortion has been a highly politicized issue in this country for the past fifty years. It has not only been incorporated into our identities, but also defines them. Physician-assisted suicide, in contrast, is a much more recent issue, only rising to prominence in the 1990s.[31] It did not shape the culture wars. It was co-opted by them.

If we recognize this, we can perhaps use the right to die as an issue that might help us to escape the culture wars framework that has dominated US politics since the 1960s. But even if that is impossible, we can at least try to understand the issue on its own terms—terms that are, for both philosophical and political reasons, amenable to compromise. Such compromise does not involve abandoning our position in the culture wars. On the contrary, a coalition to reshape the US hospice system can further the goals of both the "pro-life" Right and the "pro-choice" Left. But recognizing such possibilities does require that we see the right to die as an issue that we can detach from this larger conflict. It is possible for us to work, at least in this context, across what remains an otherwise persistent national divide.

In this sense, the story of Pilar Martínez is not just an example of two end-of-life facilities coming together to provide outstanding care for a patient in need. Her story shows the kind of political networks that we need to form if we are to have an end-of-life system that works for dying people.

CHAPTER SIX

When the End of Life Begins

Julian's apartment opened before him: comfortable and small. He had lived there in the years since his divorce. The divorce had been painful, but also a relief. He had a new career as an addiction counselor. He loved helping people, and though not an addict himself, he could connect. When his treatment center shut down, it was a blow. But he had known worse. His dad had been a political prisoner in Kenya, tortured by the British. Julian had been an immigrant in America, arriving here without close contacts and washing dishes to pay his way through school. A black man in the South, he had managed to thrive. But then the door to his apartment closed.

It was a week before his cleaning lady discovered his unconscious body. Two weeks before he came to.

When he did, he was in hospice. This was surprising. Julian had no idea he was terminally ill. A doctor had examined him a few months prior for some discomfort in his abdomen, but he'd been sent away with a clean bill of health. Now he was dying. In truth, he was lucky to even be dying. The doctors who had first tended to his unconscious body had assumed that he was a goner. Before even starting to treat him, they were prepared to give up.

That's when his niece Angela had appeared. It had been years since they had spoken, even though they lived so close. But when she learned that her uncle was in the hospital, she had shown up, and it was good that she did. There was no one else for Julian. Even if someone else had shown up, he might well have died. But Angela was not just someone. She was a nurse. She knew that there were still procedures that could be done for her uncle, and she knew that the doctors tending to him were not doing their job. She let them know that if they didn't get to it, they would see her in court. They got to it. Julian survived.

He was sent to an inpatient hospice. Like practically all inpatient hospices, it was for short-term care. At first, this was fine, since Julian was expected to die almost immediately. But he kept living. He spent a few weeks sharing a room with a rotating coterie of the soon-to-be dead, which was difficult for him. He lost count of how many roommates died before his eyes. He had been disoriented already. Now he was on the brink of mental collapse. The resources of the inpatient unit were collapsing as well. They were losing money on him. But he couldn't return home to his apartment, and his niece had children and needed to work.

Julian was sent to Our Lady, where he thrived once again. His family visited him regularly. Friends he hadn't seen in years dropped by or, if they lived far away, sent him warm messages on Facebook. Volunteers—strangers—requested to sit with him. When I talked with him, our conversation was routinely interrupted by people waving as they walked or wheeled by.

Julian did not just receive care. He gave care. He was a counselor, a mental health professional. Beyond that, he was a good listener and a man who had lived a lot. He had interacted with a great many people through his life: poor and rich, white and black, gay and straight, Catholic and Baptist, Jewish and atheist. He contained multitudes: half Kikuyu, half Maasai, a Kenyan Catholic, and a child of the Mau Mau who had looked with sympathy on the white children expelled by Idi Amin. He knew how to belong to one group and many groups and how to create his own spaces in between.

Dying patients came to him to talk. Our Lady's staff came to him to talk. Volunteers came to him to talk. Even I came to him to talk. My mother had died a few months earlier. Her death provoked a series of familial conflicts whose end point would be the destruction of everything I had previously known as my life. My problems were tremendous but, compared to his, rather small. Still, he created a space where I could share them, and he listened to me and let me cry. He was loved by many. I loved him too.

Dying did not make Julian a better person than he already was. But he was well positioned to take advantage of the opportunities that it gave. This positioning was due in part to his arrival at Our Lady. It was due in part to Julian's family, who came together around their dying relative in a way that was rare. It was also due to Julian himself. Julian was not just ready to *die*. He was ready to *be dying*. In his dying, he adapted to the challenges before him with wit and wisdom, skill and grace and love. This does not mean that he was happy all the time. It means that he was able to recognize what was going on.

I have defined freedom at the end of life as the ability to control our dying. This ability is due in large part to the environment we live in. But it is also due to an ability to live in it—as exemplified by Julian—to be responsive to an environment that no matter how stable, how caring, is inherently one of dramatic transition. British psychoanalyst Donald Winnicott defined freedom as the ability to be psychologically flexible in response to change.[1] Such changes are inherent to dying.

Promoting freedom at the end of life requires that we be attuned to how to nurture such flexibility during transitions. This is not just an issue of the person's immediate environment. It is an issue of the environments that they have lived in their entire life and the character they have formed in relation to them. "The end of life does not begin at the end of life" was, as I noted in chapter 4, a common saying at Amberview Hospice. The same is true for freedom at the end of life. It is not just about the moment of death or any one moment. Freedom can only be understood within the totality of an individual's life. And it can only be promoted on a social level if we take such a life course approach.

It is in this spirit that I continue with Julian's story.

Julian's Story

Julian was born in Kenya in the early 1960s. He was the youngest son of a family of twelve. The British had just left the country. Though technically growing up in the postcolonial era, his childhood was marked in a particular way by colonial rule. Julian's father, Leopold, had been a political prisoner for a number of years because he had been a member of the Mau Mau, Kenya's primary anticolonial force.[2] The British treatment of colonial resisters had been brutal in Kenya—as throughout Africa—and Julian's father had suffered. Julian reported that Leopold had been tortured repeatedly during his time as a prisoner. Julian was the only child that he had sired following his release.

Julian's father was likely traumatized. Emotionally, he was not very involved in Julian's life. Julian described him as a quiet man, restrained, and physically diminutive. But as an ideal, he was gigantic. He was a real-life hero who transcended the tribal divisions that emerged in the wake of Britain's departure from the country. He was Maasai but had fought with the Mau Mau, who were predominantly Kikuyu. Along with his wife and children, Leopold lived in Kikuyu territory and was venerated there. He had been offered several political positions after his release but had turned them down out of a belief that such politics were tribal and corrupt. Julian looked at his father as a symbol of resilience in the face of impossible odds, of resistance to colonial power, and of cosmopolitanism amid tribal corruption. He may have been emotionally distant, but as an ideal, he was so powerful that Julian drew on him to confront the struggles that came later in his own life.

The ideal of his father was accompanied by the reality of his mother, who was his primary caregiver. She was a warm woman, as well as a strong one. She had raised eleven children by herself while her husband was a political prisoner. Other mothers routinely left their children with her. Thus, while Julian's biological siblings were significantly older than him, he grew up surrounded by an extensive network of nonbiological brothers and sisters. At the same time, he was cared for by the mothers of other village children. This informal kinship network, anchored in his mother, reinforced the same ideals of resilience and cosmopolitanism that he saw in his father, but gave them a fleshiness that his father was unable to provide.

This cosmopolitan resilience served Julian when he went to Catholic boarding school in a distant town. His father wanted his son to be grounded in Kenya but open to the world. He trusted Catholics to teach him that. Leopold had known many Catholics and considered them to be both highly educated and ethically principled. He knew that they would give his son opportunities he had not had. Julian, because of his upbringing, was able to take advantage of those opportunities. He was an excellent student. After his somewhat chaotic home life, he enjoyed the structure of school and of Catholicism itself. He fell in love with the rituals and converted while still a teenager.

Julian was accepted to Georgia Tech University in the United States. It was a long distance away, but he wanted the opportunity, and his family was supportive. He worked his way through college washing dishes and cooking as a line chef. He made friends with students at the university and people throughout Atlanta. He graduated and worked as an engineer until it became boring for him. He moved to Alabama, where he began a career as a small business owner, running a tie shop. Then he moved back to Atlanta and married his first wife, an African American woman from the area. They were together for more than ten years. He went to church with her—she was a Baptist—and integrated himself into her family. But with time they grew apart.

Out of the wreckage of his divorce, he decided to become an addiction counselor. Julian wanted to help people and had an intellectual bent. He liked sitting down with addicts and talking in order to understand what had driven them to use drugs. He liked giving them a structure and a relationship that could pull them into sobriety. He felt connected, grounded, good. Then, Georgia governor Nathan Deal rejected the Medicaid expansion that was part of President Obama's Affordable Care Act. Julian's facility lost its funding, and he lost his health insurance. Two months later, he collapsed unconscious.

He lived for almost a year following that moment. How he spent that year was shaped by relationships that had formed decades before.

From Early Life to the End of Life

As a result of his upbringing, Julian had a temperament that allowed him to flourish at Our Lady. He had a cosmopolitan outlook from his father and a great warmth from his mother. He also had a high degree of comfort around strangers and an ability to treat them like family. This openness was of significant help to him in navigating an end-of-life environment in which he was cared for by people whom he had not previously known. Early in his life, he had strong attachment figures in his parents, both of whom had been present throughout his childhood. As a result, Julian could form relationships with his caregivers at Our Lady, taking advantage of every opportunity the home offered.

Though Julian was attached to his caregivers at Our Lady, that did not mean he was deferential. His father had set a powerful example of the possibility and, indeed, the physical and moral necessity of resisting authority. Leopold's resistance against the British was the ultimate example of this. It motivated Julian in his occasional disagreements about his care with staff at Our Lady and other Atlanta medical institutions. Julian was able to be an effective advocate for himself as well as for other patients at Our Lady. He could communicate with a wide range of patients, and he spoke to the staff on their behalf.

Though Julian was willing to resist authority, he was also capable of obeying it when it suited him. His Catholicism allowed him to benefit from being present at Our Lady. He was able to take communion at the home, and he enjoyed attending mass. He had an institutional structure and system of authority that he believed in, and this ability to accept authority allowed him to survive without being in a state of constant rebellion. He also understood that the acceptance of authority is not unconditional. Authority is malleable. You can bend it to your own ends.

One example of this is the particular manner in which Julian related to Catholicism. As opposed to Our Lady's sisters, who, as I discussed in chapter 5, spoke regularly of Christ, Julian prayed directly to God. He identified with the Catholic Church but did not consider it to be a primary or necessary mediator of his relationship with the divine. Julian's direct relationship with God was a product of his continued identification as Maasai, who, he told me, pray to God. Even as he accepted Catholic authority, he transformed this authority so that it did not usurp his identity as Maasai.

Julian's personality was thus characterized by an enormous ability to adapt. This ability was a product of his upbringing and his attachment to his mother and father. These relationships gave him stability throughout his life. But his parents had also urged him to develop and change, modeling adaptability through their own behavior: his father as a resister to both British colonialism and the corrupt tribal order, and his mother as a dutiful caregiver to twelve children and as a central figure for the families of their village. Julian knew how to transition but also how to remain grounded. Most important, he knew how to do both at the same time.

These characteristics allowed Julian to adapt to being terminally ill. Julian was able to maintain his fundamental personality *while* dying. He was able to do so because to be dying was, though a distinct period in his life, also one in a lifelong series of transitions. Through each of these transitions, Julian had been able to remain attached to key figures and, indeed, to build on his early attachment relationships. This transition was different, however. Early in his life, he had transitioned from dependence to independence. In dying, he was transitioning from independence to dependence on those around him. But he was able to make this into a point not of rupture, but of development—one more movement, just at the end of his life.

Julian's early life history made it possible for him to enjoy a high degree of freedom at his life's end. He was able to control his dying process because his parents had given him tools he had used his entire life. His early life development enabled him to form strong attachments with his family, with Our Lady's staff, and with the numerous visitors who came to see him. It also allowed him to adjust to his changing body, to create a place for dying in a life that until then had been characterized by an unbelievable vitality. He experienced dying as a melancholy transition in his life, not a traumatic break from it.

While Julian's early life experience was fundamental to his freedom at the end of life, it was not in itself enough. His freedom required a certain institutional context and a family determined to make that institution into his home.

A Member of the Family, a Guest

Julian was able to die freely, but he was not able to do so on his own. He needed the help of others—and not just those who had raised him so long ago. He needed the help of people *now* to visit him, clean him, give him medicine, and make sure he was well fed. Without such support, no amount of psychic freedom would have been enough. And it is terrifying how close he had been to dying alone. He had no insurance, no immediate family, and a terminal disease. Even the best early life experience in the world would not have done him much good if he had awakened in a nursing home or, more likely, died in a hospital ward.

The first person who got him through it was Angela. Her advocacy ensured that he returned to consciousness after the doctors had given up on him. She came to visit him at Our Lady several times a week. These visits were to keep him company, but they were also to continue checking to make sure he was getting appropriate care. Angela did not have to do this. She and Julian had not been close for a while. But when her uncle was dying, she fought for him.

Cicely Saunders wrote about cancer as a "bringing together" illness, one that would heal previously broken families because of the proximity of death.[3] Maybe that is true for some. But evidence suggests that mostly it is not. Studies have shown that the outbreak of terminal illness can be an enormously disruptive and traumatic event for families.[4] At Amberview Hospice and Our Lady, terminal disease often seemed an excuse for already broken families to remain so. At other times, it took families that had a tenuous peace and ripped them apart. It is rare that massively traumatic events unify groups.[5] More often, they lead to further fragmentation. But that is not what happened with Angela and Julian. His terminal disease really did bring them together.

Why that happened is a complicated question, and I do not fully know the answer. It is easy to attribute their reunion to an amorphous "culture," and certainly culture did play a part. Angela, like Julian, identified as Maasai, and familial caregiving plays an important role in Maasai kinship structures.[6] Their family had stuck together through a lot. But she was also a strong and loyal person in her own right, and there were particularities to her relationship with her uncle, loyalties that had gestated over the course of their interactions in previous decades. Regardless of why she was there, her being there saved Julian's life, and her ongoing presence gave him a degree of control and pleasure throughout his dying that would have been inconceivable otherwise.

Angela's ability to help, however, would have been dramatically reduced had Julian been in a standard nursing home. Indeed, recall the case of Mary, whom I discussed in chapter 4. Mary had a dutiful caregiver in her son, but no matter how much her son tried to help, things kept going wrong: pain medicine undelivered, traumatizing falls, uncertainty on the part of Mary's son about what care his mother was getting or if she was getting care at all. Being there is not enough. There needs to be a place where a familial caregiver is welcome.

Our Lady provided Angela with such a place. She became a beloved presence in the home, much like Julian himself. She was on a first-name basis with his nurses and stopped by to visit with other patients from time to time. Occasionally, she brought food and small presents to the staff. Whereas at the nursing home, Mary's son was constantly having to reintroduce himself, at Our Lady Angela was a welcome fixture. The facility's embrace of her presence made it possible for her to better keep her uncle company and to monitor his care.

Without Our Lady, Julian would have been long dead. He knew this and was grateful for the home. Had he been left in his apartment, even with hospice care, his situation would have been grim. He would have no outlet for his warmth, no one to talk to, and no one to ensure that he took his medicine on time. At a nursing home, he likely would have been similarly constrained, lost in a sea of patients amid staff members who fluttered in and out. But at Our Lady he was able to have the kinds of bonds he needed, to be the kind of person that he was. There was a dynamic relationship among Julian, Angela, and Our Lady's staff. The end result of this relationship was the promotion of Julian's freedom.

Early in his time at Our Lady, Julian got in a fight with a staff member regarding the proper care for one of his wounds. The disagreement became so heated that the staff member threatened to have Julian thrown out of the home. Sister Matilda, the director, intervened in the dispute. She listened to Julian, decided that he was correct, and opted for his view of the situation over that of the staff member. Afterward, she confided to Julian that she would have sooner thrown the staff member out of the home than him. "You," she clarified, "are our guest."

This interaction shows the complex dynamic that existed between Our Lady's environment and Julian's self-advocacy. Because of his life experience, Julian felt comfortable fighting with a staff member who was giving him treatment that he believed (correctly) to be improper. At another institution, he might have been restrained from doing so, but at Our Lady, he was encouraged and given greater priority than the staff member.

At Our Lady, an ethic of hospitality privileges the wishes of patients over, at times, the directives of its staff. This is a radical form of empowering patient choice—promoting freedom even against what would seem to be the interests of the institution itself. Julian could take advantage of it because he had the temperament to do so. But had he been somewhere else, perhaps no amount of character would have been enough.

Julian's story is an ideal model of freedom at the end of life, in which the patient has the psychological, interpersonal, and institutional means to control their life until the very end. But this model is inaccessible to too many dying people. Making it a reality will require action on many fronts.

Integrated Long-Term and End-of-Life Care

The first step in repairing the crisis of freedom in US hospice care is to integrate long-term and end-of-life care. Fortunately, there are many people who have been thinking about how to do so for a long time. The Hawthorne Dominicans are but one example of this synthesis. Throughout the United States, there are innovative medical professionals who are finding new ways to combine these treatment modalities.[7] For their local communities, these professionals are providing an invaluable service. But their work suffers from size limitations that are similar to those of Our Lady, and we all suffer as a result.

It is necessary to institutionalize the integration of long-term and end-of-life care in the US health system. This integration must take place in both outpatient and inpatient care. In the outpatient context, this would require that hospices provide dying patients and their families with more extensive home health care. In the inpatient context, it would require finding ways to implement more effective end-of-life care delivery in long-term care facilities. In the short term, we should look for ways to better incentivize such integrated care within existing institutional structures: for example, by eliminating the competition between hospices and skilled nursing facilities for Medicare Part A funding. But in the long term, coordinating two distinct treatment modalities is likely to be difficult, costly, and ineffective.

A better solution is to add a more substantial long-term care component to hospice itself. This would streamline the process of integration, eliminating existing conflicts between long-term and end-of-life care providers and creating a shared incentive structure. At the same time, if long-term and end-of-life care providers worked together, they would become more knowledgeable about each other's treatments. This would lead to more effective collaboration and, ultimately, innovation. An integrated long-term care component within hospice will pay dividends well into the future.

The best vehicle for this integration is the Medicare Hospice Benefit. The benefit should be enhanced to include a more robust home health service, so that patients can remain longer in outpatient care. At the same time, it is necessary to increase the inpatient capacities of US hospices. Doing so means changing the requirement that, on average, 80 percent of a particular hospice's care be outpatient. This 80 percent requirement asks too much of dying patients and their families. It also asks too much of hospices. The benefit's regulations have made inpatient hospices financially unsustainable. Moving to a more flexible 50:50 ratio between inpatient and outpatient care—as hospice leaders suggested back in the early 1980s—would improve the situation for hospices, families, and dying patients.

There is also a need to address the problems of US long-term care. For decades, disability advocates have criticized our long-term care system's reliance on nursing homes. This reliance on nursing homes is one of the primary causes of the crisis of freedom in US hospice care. Disability rights advocates have long argued that nursing homes nullify the freedom of their disabled inhabitants;

they are quasi-segregated facilities whose regimented schedules and depersonalized services strip disabled people of any substantive control over their lives.[8] If this critique is true for people with disabilities, then it is also true for those who are dying. Nursing homes are—at least arguably—designed for disabled people. But their terminally ill residents find themselves trapped in a facility that is not designed for them—and is often mediocre even for its intended inhabitants. The result is the destruction of freedom for both groups of people.

Preventing this destruction means shifting toward independent living centers as the dominant way of coordinating long-term care. Such centers make it possible for disabled people to live safely and to integrate themselves into society.[9] They accomplish this by providing them with assistive technologies and by helping them receive personal care attendant services, generally funded through Medicaid. And yet, in spite of the proven benefits of the independent living model, nursing homes continue to be the dominant institution for organizing US long-term care. Increasing the federal funding for independent living centers will allow terminally ill people to stay longer in their own houses and be integrated into their communities. This will dramatically increase their freedom.

The same funding increase will also facilitate the delivery of hospice care by eliminating the conflict between hospices and nursing homes. Terminal illness is often preceded by an extended period of disability. But people with disabilities have been consistently, and understandably, fearful of institutionalization in a nursing home. More independent living centers would allow them to receive care earlier in an environment that they find safer. This more effective delivery of care will make it easier to provide dying people with hospice services and will allow them to stay at home, receiving hospice, much longer.

Independent living centers are not generally seen as serving dying people, but they should be. Giving them more power in the coordination of long-term care and end-of-life care will do a lot to increase the freedom of dying patients. Accomplishing this requires changing the funding of long-term care in the United States.

As I have discussed, long-term care in America is generally funded by Medicaid. Medicaid allows people, in theory, to choose between receiving personal care services (PCS) at home or going to a nursing home. In reality, the program has a strong bias toward nursing homes, even in cases where remaining at home could be possible if more help were given.[10] Having efficient coordination of hospice and nursing home care requires first overcoming this nursing home bias in general.

This bias is particularly strong at the end of life. In almost all US states, people receiving the Medicare Hospice Benefit are not eligible for Medicaid-funded PCS.[11] This creates situations where dying people are forced into nursing homes, even in cases where PCS access could enable them to stay at home. In order to have success in the coordination of hospice and independent living, we must first challenge this nursing home bias in the funding of US long-term care at the end of life. Fortunately, there is one hopeful example.

In 2016, the state of North Carolina changed its hospice policy for individuals who are eligible for both Medicaid and Medicare. In this change, individuals receiving Medicare-funded hospice care can also receive PCS funded by Medicaid.[12] This change may save these "dual eligibles" from the fragmentation that is inherent to the delivery of hospice care in the nursing home. It significantly enhances their freedom—and provides a model for the country as a whole.

The example of North Carolina should be emulated on a state-by-state basis. Doing so will be labor intensive due to the fragmented nature of the US health system. But in each state where it happens, it will create a significant improvement in the lives of dying people. It is notable that this improvement has already happened in a state whose legislature has been very hostile to social welfare programs.[13] The success of this policy in North Carolina illustrates how broadly it might be implemented. As the number of states that enact similar policies inches toward fifty, we will witness a categorical change in the freedom of dying people in America.

A Culture of Familial Care

I have chronicled the mismatch between the requirements of caregiving and the abilities of US families. This mismatch is in part a product of US hospice care, but it is also due to the current state of US families. Alleviating the crisis of freedom in US hospice care means looking for ways to support and nurture familial caregiving.

This will require a shift in cultural values. Over the course of the twentieth century, familial caretaking came to be denigrated. This rejection was a reasonable response to the gendered assumptions underpinning such caregiving: it would be carried out by women and should be women's primary role. The feminist rejection of women's consignment to the home is reasonable and good. But it has, to a degree, transferred to a denigration of caretaking itself, specifically a denigration of familial caregiving compared to the respect afforded to the paid labor of career advancement.[14]

The disparagement of caregiving has been assimilated by family members, including dying people. It underpins the fear among dying individuals that they will be a "burden." This is in part a product of a society that considers familial caregiving to be burden*some*. To the extent that this view predominates, it undermines both the willingness of family members to care for their dying relatives and that of relatives to receive this care.

Changing this perspective requires cultivating a culture that values familial caregiving. Such a culture would consider caregiving to be a fundamental part of being human. This was the case for Raúl Acosta's daughter, Marta, and for Julian's niece, Angela. Both understood caregiving not just as a duty, but also as a desire: something that they wanted to do, for they saw it as an affirmation of who they are. These desires, however, are often not valorized in a US popular culture that represents caregiving as a distraction from career advancement.

The movie *Still Alice* illustrates an exception.[15] Alice Howland, a linguistics professor, contracts early-onset Alzheimer's disease and becomes dependent on her family to care for her. For the most part, her family members refuse to help because of their commitment to their work. The exception is her daughter, Lydia, who sets aside her growing career as an actress to care for her mother. By doing so, she epitomizes the culture of care that needs to be supported on a larger scale.

She also illustrates why this culture is so difficult to cultivate. Lydia is able to abandon her career because her family has the material resources to support her. She does not need a job for financial reasons. As a result, she has the material ability to care for her mother, which most Americans lack. Marta had this ability as well, due to her husband's job and her father's benefits. If we are to support familial caretaking, we must make it materially possible.

To do so, we need to promote paid family leave.[16] Such leave is often touted as necessary at the beginning of life, but it needs to also be available for periods of terminal illness. We must make it materially possible for familial caregivers to tend to their dying relatives. In itself, this material advancement will help create a culture of care.

But paid familial leave is not enough. Even with such leave, familial caregivers will often need to obtain professional assistance provided by paid caregivers. Seeking out such assistance does not mean that families cease to be caregivers. On the contrary, Mary's son and Angela were both familial caregivers, even though they did not provide primary care themselves. Rather, seeking assistance means that the care required exceeds the abilities of the family member.

In such circumstances, familial caregivers need to have access to professional help that is both affordable and competent. But such help is in short supply. Long-term care is extremely expensive, and even if a family can afford it, it is often insufficient. Indeed, Mary's son was an extremely dedicated caregiver, but he was unable to protect his mother from the horrors of the Sunny Day Nursing Home. Fostering familial caregiving should thus not be seen as being in opposition to the need to improve the coordination of long-term and end-of-life care. Rather, the two are complementary.

Making paid caregiving better will be difficult unless we value it more. At present, paid caregivers make extremely little money.[17] These poor wages result in a high degree of turnover.[18] Furthermore, this work is disproportionately carried out by women, with a particularly high rate of participation by African Americans and Latinas. Because these women disproportionately care for others, they may be not be available to provide their own families with care.[19] Raising wages for home health workers would help to ameliorate this racial caregiving gap and, by diminishing turnover, would help those who give this care and those who receive it.

Familial caregiving is not just a cultural issue. It is also a labor issue. Without support for familial caregivers—both paid and unpaid—it will be extremely difficult to create a culture of care in US families. It will also be difficult to create such a culture if we do not change our framework for thinking about the economics of care. Philosopher Jennifer Parks has described our current approach: "Instead of seeing ourselves as a moral community with certain obligations to care for one another, we see ourselves as an economic entity with prior economic obligations that limit how much we are willing to spend on care."[20] The result is, for Parks, a reversal of our moral priorities. Though her argument focuses on home health care, its implications are relevant to the argument about end-of-life care that I am making in this book. Indeed, as psychiatrist and medical anthropologist Arthur Kleinman has argued, the denigration of caregiving is characteristic of our health system as a whole. For Kleinman, caregiving has no place in a healthcare system that takes as its starting point economic models "based on the narrowest calculations of what a 'rational' person would choose as most cost-effective."[21] Such models cannot accommodate caregiving, an activity that does not conform to strict measures of economic rationality. The subsequent exclusion of caregiving from our thinking about health care has "diminished professionals, patients, and family caregivers alike."[22]

In light of this problem, Kleinman calls for a "serious discussion" of the role of caregiving in medical practice, education, and research—and in the organization of health care more broadly. Indeed, he even goes beyond this, arguing that "once we open the door to the democratic implications of caregiving as moral and political practices, so much of the rest of our world from leadership to governance and from domestic to foreign affairs becomes a matter not just of markets, regulations, and security concerns, but of how we can enact care as humankind's shared project."[23]

Kleinman is right about the need for a greater place for caregiving in our discussions of health care, economics, and domestic and foreign politics. Including it will create the foundation for the flourishing of a culture that values familial caregiving.

Extending the Biological Family

The decline of marriage in the twentieth century was empowering for people of diverse backgrounds. But it also weakened the bonds between married people and between married couples and children. At the end of life, the diminishment of these bonds can leave dying individuals without sufficient support. It is not coincidental that three of the four dying individuals I have profiled in this book were divorced. Their not being married contributed to their not being able to maintain hospice care. Divorce may have also impacted the involvement of their children, since children of divorce may feel less commitment to either or both of their parents.[24]

Though the effects of divorce are real, terminal illness places strain even on still-married couples.[25] The physical and mental decline that accompanies terminal illness can be traumatizing even—perhaps especially—if the person witnessing it is a longtime spouse. In the best of circumstances, our resolve will be tested. But few US families, even intact ones, are living in the best of circumstances: poverty, unstable living conditions, concerns about employment and crime and incarceration, not to mention the stresses of family life, all have an impact. It is tough enough, but dying makes it so much harder.

Helping families to cope with these stresses requires greater social support. The problem in part is that discussions of such support in family policy have typically focused on the beginning of life, not the end.[26] This needs to change. We must explore ways to use social support to better care for familial caregivers. This support is not an *alternative* to a culture of caregiving. Without it, there will be no family to provide this culture.

An informal but extremely valuable source of support can be found in networks of extended kin. Such kinship networks need not be biological. They can be families of choice, in which two or more people who are not biologically related claim kinship with one another. These networks are valuable, first, as a substitute for the nuclear family, when such a family is not there. They are also valuable because even in cases where the nuclear family is intact, kinship networks provide support that is often necessary at the end of life.

In a classic ethnography, anthropologist Carol Stack observed one such kinship network in an African American community in an unidentified midwestern city.[27] These more flexible kinship networks are crucial in creating support systems to combat racism. They are also ideal for the end of life. They are capable of providing support to immediate family members, who may not always be able to provide enough care, and they are geographically localized in the dying individual's neighborhood. The African American community studied in Stack's book can serve as an example of extended kinship networks, but there are many others.

Hospice providers themselves epitomize such networks. This is true of the staff of Amberview Hospice, who often refer to caring for patients like "their families." And it was true of the grassroots hospices that emerged after the advent of the AIDS crisis in the 1980s.[28] Such hospices were designed to care for gay men who had been abandoned by their biological families. The kinship networks that formed successfully provided end-of-life care for a generation that was experiencing both social discrimination and biological destruction.

It is also possible to understand Our Lady of Perpetual Help Home in these terms. Part of seeing Jesus involves, for the sisters, putting themselves in the role of Christ's mother, the Virgin Mary, one of the witnesses of Jesus's death. The result is a rewriting of familial relations, in which the nuns claim kinship with the dying patients under their care. They create around these patients an extensive familial network that otherwise would not exist.

A kinship network should ideally include the broader community in which the dying person lives. The problem is that such communities are rarely equipped to recognize the needs of dying people, much less tend to them. Making them better equipped for this work requires the development of a comprehensive public health approach to end-of-life care. Such an approach would involve partnerships between public health agencies and local communities, with the goal of sustaining and, if necessary, creating the extended kinship structures that dying people need.

Sociologist Allan Kellehear has developed a compelling model for such partnerships, which he calls "compassionate communities."[29] This model redefines end-of-life care as the responsibility of not just the individual, the family, the healthcare system, and the state—but also the broader community. This diffusion of responsibility helps everyone, and the compassionate communities model has already been implemented with great success. Kellehear gives three examples: the partnership of St. Christopher's Hospice with area schools to pair local children with dying people; public efforts to recruit hospice volunteers in Shropshire,

England; and a national prize given out in Japan to the community that can demonstrate being the most dementia-friendly.[30]

These initiatives highlight the diverse forms that a public health approach to dying might take and are easily tailorable to the wide range of communal forms in America today.

Taking Familial Conflict Seriously

Even with sufficient material support, assistance from kinship networks, and conducive cultural norms, familial caregiving is more complex than it might appear. Marta did attribute her caregiving in part to "Hispanic culture," but she also saw it as a form of reimbursement. Her father had cared for her when she was a child. Now, she was caring for him. Thus, familial caregiving, though influenced by her culture, was part of the relationship between Marta and Raúl, a form of reciprocity for the care he provided.

Such reciprocity does not guarantee good care. Remember the woman, mentioned in chapter 4, who kept forgetting to give her husband pain medication. Amberview's staff attributed it to a desire for payback, born from the memory of her husband's mistreatment of her. Though difficult to know, it is possible. Before dying people are dying, they are just people. And people sometimes treat their family members badly, and their family members sometimes treat them badly in return. The result is familial conflict.

Such conflicts create problems in a hospice system dependent on familial caregiving. If a family member dislikes or is ambivalent about the dying individual, they may not provide reliable care. Worse, they may consider "caregiving" an opportunity to settle scores. The result can be neglect and abuse.

Culture is not in itself a solution to such conflicts. Though there are cultures that seemingly place a higher value on familial caregiving, people in those cultures still have issues with their family members, and such conflicts can lead to the subversion of care. The same is true of marriage. Marriage, when successful, can nurture emotional bonds that are conducive to caregiving. But not all marriages are successful. The mere state of being married to someone is not an indication of the desire or ability to care.

Creating such a desire requires working through familial conflicts. There is a tool to do so: counseling. Mental health counseling has been proven to help individuals work through interpersonal conflicts and form lasting attachments.[31] Such attachments are beneficial throughout the life course, including the end of life.

In theory, counseling is provided regularly by hospice social workers. In practice, this is less often the case. Social workers provide psychosocial care in hospice, but the "social" aspects of this care often crowd out the "psychological" ones. At Amberview, for example, social workers were almost entirely occupied with case management: signing patients up for hospice and placing them in appropriate care sites. This privileging of social care is in part a product of economic incentives. Under the current reimbursement structures, if a social worker signs up a new patient for hospice, they are creating a source of income that is directly related to the material survival of the organization and its personnel. The benefits of counseling are, from a financial perspective, much more amorphous.

Addressing this predicament requires integrating a new role into the hospice interdisciplinary team: the counselor. This person's role would be solely to care for the psychological well-being of the patient and family. This role could be filled by counselors, psychologists, or social workers, but whoever filled it would be dedicated to working only as a mental health professional. The social worker role, in contrast, would just focus on the social aspects of the patients care. The result would clarify the division of labor in hospice teams in a manner more attuned to the complex and intersecting needs of patients and families.

But taking familial conflict seriously cannot just begin at the end of life. It must be integrated throughout the life course. This requires the increased financing of mental health care in the US health system and specifically psychological counseling. Such financing can help create a culture of therapy—which exists in a number of urban centers throughout the globe—that will help individuals to better negotiate the familial conflicts that appear throughout the lifespan.[32] This will make them better able to address familial conflicts when they emerge, in heightened form, at the end of life.

Dying patients will benefit both directly and indirectly. They will have caregivers who are more willing and prepared to tend to their needs, and they will be better prepared to address the conflicts that come with dying. Such conflicts come through their interactions with family members, with healthcare professionals, and with themselves. A culture of therapy will better prepare dying people to confront these conflicts, significantly enhancing their freedom in the face of death.

Julian saw all of this acutely. He credited his training as a mental health counselor for his survival in the inpatient hospice facility before he arrived at Our Lady. He had been given a good basis in early childhood, which encouraged him to explore and develop his psychic life. This paid dividends for him throughout his life and allowed him to thrive at life's end.

Creating a culture of mental health counseling is thus a necessary part of rectifying the crisis of freedom in US hospice care. But without greater attention to the conflicts and deficiencies of US society, no amount of therapy will be enough.

The Social Roots of Freedom

A particular problem of US public policy is the belief that the family can rectify social ills. To a degree, this is true. Strong familial bonds can have a generative effect on individuals as well as social groups. But the family itself exists in a social context, and the current context of US society is such that without significant changes, the family—however defined—will flounder. The problems of US hospice care are not just problems of US hospice care. They are the problems of US society, and without addressing their social roots, US hospice care will fail.

Hospice in the United States is a caregiving modality based in the home. But for tens of millions of Americans, the home has become a precarious place. The problem is not just the decline in home ownership. It is the declining value of homes that are still owned and the inability to find a stable rental property. It is the increasing speed at which families are evicted. In his book *Evicted*, sociologist Matthew Desmond argues that eviction has become a widespread social catastrophe in the United States.[33] It is also a catastrophe at the end of life. In part, this is a question of a family, but it is also a question of housing. Fixing this problem requires giving Americans a stable home environment.

Desmond proposes the creation of a universal housing voucher program. Such a program would expand our existing federally funded Housing Choice Voucher Program, which serves more than 2.1 million low-income households.[34] Desmond suggests expanding this program to all poor families. We have the money for such an expansion, and, as Desmond highlights, it could even be implemented without any additional spending "if we prevented overcharging and made the [existing] program more efficient."[35] Such programs have already been successfully implemented throughout the industrialized world. Doing so here will significantly increase American freedom in general and particularly at life's end.

The benefits of a stable home are limited, however, if it is impossible for someone to move within it or outside it. This raises the question of accessibility. Many American homes are not accessible to dying people. They are unsafe environments that leave them prone to falls and with limited mobility. Meanwhile, the arrangement of the built environment makes it difficult for dying people to leave their home. Urban sprawl, lack of public transportation, and lack of curb cuts, ramps, and even basic infrastructure collude to create an environment that is especially difficult to navigate. This lack of access compounds the lack of housing and touches even those who do have a stable home.

The lack of accessible housing disproportionately affects racial minorities, particularly African Americans. As I discussed in chapter 3, African Americans have disproportionately been victims of housing discrimination. Such discrimination presents a severe barrier to the delivery of end-of-life care. Areas that have been subjected to housing discrimination have higher crime, lower employment, and less access to food, transportation, and health care. These "neighborhood effects" all have a negative impact on the delivery of hospice care.[36] As a home-based system in a country created by housing discrimination, US hospice care is in its design systemically racist. Alleviating this systemic racism does not, however, require changing hospice (though that would be helpful). It requires taking measures to alleviate the effects of housing discrimination.[37] Desmond's housing voucher program would go a long way toward this goal, though measures more targeted at housing discrimination's victims may additionally be necessary. Though such measures would not themselves involve end-of-life care, they would significantly bolster freedom at the end of life.

Violent crime in areas that have suffered housing discrimination weakens the social fabric and threatens the familial bonds necessary to sustain end-of-life care. But so does the current response to this crime: mass incarceration. Effective policing deters crime. Overpolicing destroys the social fabric. African American communities have been *under*policed in ways that encourage crime, while they have also been *over*policed in ways that bolster unnecessary incarceration.[38] The result has been *both* crime and incarceration. This has devastated black families, breaking the kinship bonds that are central to end-of-life care.

Mass incarceration is an end-of-life issue, first and foremost, for prisoners themselves. Most prisoners in the United States do not have access to hospice.[39] The result is that prisoners die without basic care. This is the equivalent to an extrajudicial punishment: a painful death. But mass incarceration also punishes the families of prisoners, including dying people who are not in jail—terminally ill individuals who are left at home, often in precarious, high-crime neighborhoods, with no relatives to provide protection or care.

There is thus a broad range of social problems undermining freedom at the end of life. The breadth of the solutions to these problems may seem counterproductive. After all, it has been hard enough to expand *hospice* policy. What is the purpose of pointing out that hospice policy is dependent on disability access, housing, and mental health care? There is a risk that with so many problems identified, it will be impossible to make progress on any of them—or that the problems inherent to hospice care will fall through the cracks.

But there is also a risk in limiting our framework. The organization of US hospice care must be taken into account, but if we just focus on hospice, we misunderstand it. Hospice is dependent on the family and on US society. To simply propose better integrated long-term and end-of-life care as a solution to the problem of freedom at the end of life would be progress. But it would also work against progress since it would obscure that if you are a victim of untreated childhood trauma currently living in a redlined neighborhood, for example, your freedom at the end of life will likely be highly restricted, even if the US hospice system were dramatically improved.

This is not just an intellectual question. It is political as well. Right now, there are political movements mobilizing on all of the issues I have identified in this chapter: family leave, mental health care, disability access, antiracism, and, yes, better end-of-life care. But these movements do not in general understand themselves to be related. This fragments us, limiting our numbers, and hindering our ability to achieve our goals. By highlighting the relationships among these issues, I hope to contribute to the formation of a political coalition that will be able to make progress on all of them. Without such a broad coalition, it is difficult to see how progress can be made at all.

The Value of Religious Freedom

In the United States, religious freedom is often taken to be inherently valuable.[40] This is correct. But by focusing on the inherent value of such freedom, this approach misses that religious freedom has tremendous instrumental value as well. Its instrumental value should not be given primacy over its inherent value, but by acknowledging it, we can have a better understanding of how religious institutions function in society.

There are some common misconceptions about what religious institutions do. For example, in chapter 5 I argued that contrary to popular perception, religious institutions do not solely limit freedom. They also promote freedom in ways that comparable secular institutions do not. Their doing so is not to be taken as a justification of their existence, but it does provide a greater appreciation of their value: specifically, they are not less instrumentally valuable than their secular counterparts. They are, rather, *different*, which is itself valuable.

Take Our Lady, for example. Our Lady cares for patients who fall through the cracks of the US hospice system. This is not an accident. It is due to the institution's design as a religious charity. As a charity, the home is organized to care for those patients who cannot get help elsewhere. The group of people it cares for is specific: dying cancer patients with insufficient familial support. But that group is also extremely broad. Our Lady cares for individuals of different racial groups, different religious groups, different genders, different personality types, and different life experiences. What unites these diverse residents is that, in some way, their personal characteristics make them unable to receive hospice care.

State action is necessary to alleviate the crisis of freedom in US hospice care. But that does not mean that state action should replace the role of charity. No matter how well social policy is designed, there will be people who fall through the cracks. Religious charitable institutions are designed for such people. They care for the neediest of the needy. Even if every problem that I have described in this book were solved immediately, Our Lady and institutions like it would still have an invaluable role. The population they care for will never go away.

Its members, however, will change. For example, following the financial crisis of 2008, Our Lady's patient profile shifted. Previously, the home had cared for a large population of terminally ill individuals who were homeless and mentally ill. But following the economic collapse, a wider range of people needed help. The home began caring for formerly middle-class professionals who had lost their jobs, their money, and their homes. These patients needed Our Lady's care. But because Our Lady was caring for them, the facility had fewer beds available for dying people who were homeless and mentally ill.

Religious charities provide an alternative to public policy, but they do not provide a replacement for it. Further, their actions are influenced and even hampered by public policy in subtle ways. The banking deregulation that led to the financial crisis was not designed to hinder the mission of religious charities. But one of its effects was to make it more difficult for religious charities like Our Lady to accommodate those most in need.

Thus, public policy makers need to be invested in religious charities. And supporters and practitioners of religious charity must be invested in policy. The two spheres are interdependent. Good charity plugs the holes that exist in even the best-designed policies. Good policy allows charities to focus their attention on those who need help the most.

Ideally, this relationship should inform policy design. Religious institutions operate according to worldviews that differ fundamentally from those of secular institutions. These worldviews can be limiting, but they can also spark innovative ways of caring for patients. Our Lady of Perpetual Help Home's integration of long-term and end-of-life care is but one example of such innovation. Our Lady's Catholic foundation cannot directly inform policy design in a secular society. But the model of care that has emerged from this foundation can, to a degree, be adapted. In this way, religious charities can spur innovations in health care.

Religious charities are thus important to the functioning of the secular health system. They care for patients who fall through the cracks. They can also help us understand *who* these patients are and provide models of how to serve them better. The benefits of this care are not in themselves a reason to justify religious freedom. But they help explain why protecting religious freedom is of central importance to addressing the crisis of US hospice care—and the problems in our health system more generally.

Health policy makers have at times infringed on religious freedom in the name of promoting healthcare access.[41] Such infringements can be justified. But they should not lead us to overlook the value to policy makers of protecting the religious character of institutions. Recognizing this value will benefit our health system, and it is useful politically.

Traditionally, there has been a split in US politics between those who value religious freedom and those who see it as an obstacle to progress. Understanding how religious freedom spurs progress in end-of-life care—and in general—can help to ameliorate this split. Healing the division is essential to gaining the political capital necessary to implement the substantive changes I have described.

An alliance will require some compromises, but even more it will require seeing the substantial common ground underpinning our political disagreements. We must see the benefits of collaboration, both in general and for our own interests: religious freedom bolsters progressive social change, and vice versa. Nowhere are the benefits of collaboration more visible than on the issue of the right to die.

Putting the Right to Die in Its Place

I began this book with an argument that the right to die is a poor lens through which to view the much broader issue of freedom at the end of life. By solely focusing on this one aspect, we have missed the crisis of freedom in US hospice care. Rectifying this crisis does not require either banning or supporting physician-assisted suicide, but it does require speaking to the interests of partisans on either side of the PAS debate.

Advocates for PAS claim that the practice is a way of giving dying people further control over their lives. If this is true, then proponents should be sensitive to the total lack of control facing dying individuals who have insufficient familial support. Even if we assume that PAS would advance their freedom, it is not the only way to do so. The suggestions I made above would also increase the freedom of dying people, and they are consistent with the principles underlying the right to die.

The same is true of "pro-life" opponents of PAS. Physician-assisted suicide may impugn the sanctity of human life. But we cannot argue that life is "sacred" while still routinely abandoning dying people to horrific fates. Opposing the right to die is not in itself sufficient to build a culture that recognizes the sanctity of life. The suggestions I make in this book would help do so.

My argument in this book is thus consistent with the principles underlying both support for and opposition to the right to die. But it is not only philosophically consistent with these positions. My argument represents a political compromise that advances the goals of both sides of the debate: expanding patient choice while honoring the sanctity of human life.

One argument against PAS is that individuals choose it in response to insufficient end-of-life care. This is, in a sense, true. In Oregon, 40 percent of individuals who request physician-assisted suicide do so because of their fear of being a burden on their family, friends, and caregivers.[42] This fear is not irrational. Our hospice system places the burden of care on familial caregivers. If dying people feel that they are burdens, it is in part by our design. Reducing this sense of being a burden is in the interest of both advocates of PAS and its opponents. For advocates, it would strengthen their argument that terminally ill people who opt to die are doing so not because of social pressure, but rather because of their own desires. For opponents, it will make fewer people want to die.

Such a reduction can be accomplished by the measures I have suggested here: better integration of long-term and end-of-life care, better mental health care for individuals and families throughout the lifespan, and the creation of a society that is at a basic level hospitable to dying people and their families. If implemented, these measures would make dying people feel less burdensome on their families because they would be less burdensome in reality. The result would be fewer cases of PAS and a stronger argument for its legitimacy. This is a compromise that advances the interests of both sides of the PAS debate. Still, it may seem unpalatable to many. After all, why compromise when you can win?

But there will be no winning the debate about physician-assisted suicide in the United States. As I noted in chapter 5, the Supreme Court has left the decision on PAS to the states.[43] It is extremely unlikely that this will change in the coming decades. This means that legal change will only be possible on a state-by-state basis. In many states, even incremental change will likely be impossible.

States whose populations skew libertarian—such as Oregon, Washington, and Vermont—will support physician-assisted suicide.[44] States that are more traditionally liberal—such as New York—may eventually support it, but they also may not. States that are more conservative—the majority of the country outside the Northeast and West Coast—will not. These demographic characteristics are not likely to change. With increasing political polarization, they may well intensify.

Achieving whatever limited changes may be possible in this context will require enormous resources. These investments may pay off initially. Advocates for physician-assisted suicide will accomplish relatively rapid legalization in states with libertarian populations; opponents will encourage resistance in states whose populations are more split. With time, these dynamics will settle. There will be states that practice PAS and will do so for the foreseeable future. There will be states that do not and likely never will. Neither PAS advocates nor PAS opponents will be happy with this stalemate. But this is our reality. Pouring more resources—economic, interpersonal, political, emotional—into changing the situation will bring diminishing returns. It is worth considering another way.

The compromise I have proposed provides a way forward. My suggestion is that both sides in the PAS debate should recognize that PAS is not the only nor the most important issue relevant to freedom at the end of life. The most important issue is repairing the gap between the requirements of US hospice care and the capabilities of American families.

We must recognize that state support of dying people is itself a condition of their freedom. Such support promotes freedom while honoring the sanctity of life. We must compromise in order to enable truly radical change.

The Practicality of Radical Change

One might argue that the changes that I have proposed are impractical. To be sure, they are extensive: restructuring the US hospice system, instituting mental health care throughout the lifespan, ameliorating housing discrimination, and protecting religious freedom in a secularizing age. Any one of these changes would be difficult. Together, they seem absurd.

But these changes need not happen all at once. They can be implemented in a piecemeal fashion when politically possible: for example, through a bill to include higher reimbursement for inpatient hospice care or to increase funding for fall prevention. Such piecemeal changes may seem unsatisfactory, but they are far more practical than attempts to change people's minds on the right to die.

The scope of my suggestions is also broader. They could be implemented nationally. If, through enormous efforts, the right to die was either approved or rejected in the state of New York, that decision would affect approximately 20 million people. A more generous reimbursement structure for inpatient hospice care would affect more than 300 million. It would also require less political effort to enact and would be safer from repeal once enacted.

But the issue is not just practicality. Even if PAS were legalized everywhere tomorrow, there would still be millions of Americans dying in situations that destroy their freedom. The same would be true if PAS were banned. This is not to say that legalizing or banning PAS would be irrelevant to the issue of freedom at the end of life, but however one interprets its relevance, it is less than any of the individual reforms that I have suggested.

A piecemeal approach brings its own limitations, of course. Enacting change in the US system requires coalitional politics. The issues that I have described here, though diverse, are unified in their relevance to freedom at the end of life. Recognizing this unity makes it easier to form the broad political alliance necessary to enact change. A diverse coalition can be difficult to achieve, but it is the most reliable way to make change.

Indeed, my argument might be criticized for being too narrow. I have left out many issues relevant to freedom at the end of life: for example, health insurance access, rural poverty, labor protections, the surveillance state, and travel restrictions targeting Muslim families. But my goal is not to be exhaustive. My aim is to redirect a conversation that has long been counterproductive and to create a different kind of space: a space where people with diverse and even conflicting interests can come together, united in a common goal of advancing freedom at the end of life.

Ultimately, that space is our country: the United States of America. The crisis of hospice care that I have described is an American one. It is a product of not just our hospice system, but also the manner in which we have imagined a series of ideals: family, freedom, dying, and America itself. There is no solution to this crisis outside of the country in which we live. By rethinking America from the perspective of the end of life, we can also adopt a fresh perspective on a broader crisis currently unfolding about the meaning of American national identity.

Conclusion

Estelle Sechster was a very American character. She was Jewish, and her mother had migrated to the United States from somewhere in what would become the "former Soviet Union." Estelle was born in Manhattan in 1921. In 1944, she became pregnant and gave birth to her daughter Andrea.

About six months after Andrea was born, Estelle's uncle Ike noticed something. He had been playing with Andrea while she was in her crib. When he made sounds—knocking on the crib's wooden bars, clicking his tongue, or saying, even shouting, her name—Andrea went on playing as if nothing was happening. She did not look up.

"I don't know, Esther," Ike said to Estelle, using her Hebrew name. "I think your kid can't hear."

The doctor she sought help from was less reserved in his assessment. "Profoundly deaf" were the words he used to describe Estelle Sechster's daughter, words that Estelle would remember for the remainder of her life. Estelle never fully recovered from that pronouncement.

But her husband, Harold, had it the worst. His parents had both died years before, and he had found solace in Orthodox Judaism. Every morning he davened, wrapping his arm in the long black tefillin, tying the box to his head, bending, and whispering the Shema. In the wake of his parents' passing, such prayers had brought comfort. But now they only seemed to provoke a sense of futility, even rage. Estelle was never entirely sure why. Perhaps it was because of what the Bible said about deaf people. Perhaps it was because having a deaf daughter, after the deaths of both his parents, was just too much bad luck for Harold to continue to believe that God exists. Perhaps it was because other people in the Jewish community, including his family, abandoned Harold and his deaf daughter, turning down invitations to visit, whispering poisonous words to themselves when they did come over, sometimes saying them to his face.

It was not just the Jews who shunned them. Estelle had to fight with practically every person or group that came in contact with her daughter. Andrea was bullied by neighborhood kids. A police officer—believing that she was willfully ignoring his commands—threw her in jail. But the cops and the neighborhood losers in the end were minor characters in the story of Andrea and Estelle. Their main enemies—the supervillains, if you will—were the schools.

In the New York area, public education for the deaf was "oralist." Oralism was a philosophy of education in which deaf people were not taught sign language. They were taught to attempt to speak with their mouths and to "hear" via lip reading. Oralism was a spectacular failure for generations of deaf people,[1] and Andrea Sechster was among them. She never learned to lip read or vocalize at anything resembling a "normal" level. At the same time, she was denied the use of a language that would have worked for her and found herself in a kind of linguistic exile that structured, built on, and intensified the exile imposed on her by the outside world.

The failure of oralism, however, cannot by itself explain the inability of Andrea Sechster to succeed at school. Everyone at the school she attended was deaf, and in theory, they were being failed the same way and to the same degree. But among the deaf children, Andrea was unique. She bit. She pinched. She laughed unexpectedly and seemingly without cue, loud fits of laughter that interrupted the entire classroom; she could not be made to stop. She erupted at times into what the school's principal referred to as "disgusting nose sounds." Sometimes she seemed distant, impossible to reach. At other times, she was too present, too forceful, too *there*. Even when the other children attacked her, everyone knew that somehow it had to have been her fault.

The principal thought he had no choice in the matter. She would have to leave. But where would she go? It was not his business to decide or even really to know. Surely there must be places for Andrea Sechster.

Andrea might have been sent to a special school for intellectually disabled people, if one existed. But given her multiple disabilities, it is more likely that she would have been sent to an institution. These were places where people with disabilities, like Andrea, were placed when no one knew what to do with them. Their parents—who were often trying their best in extremely difficult situations—were told that they would be well taken care of. But in reality, they were simply swept from public view: segregated, neglected, and often abused. Willowbrook—a home for intellectually disabled people—would in the 1970s be exposed as a site of rampant abuse, including nonconsensual scientific experiments.[2] Given the home's proximity to New York City—less than twenty minutes by car—it is possible that Willowbrook is where Andrea might have ended up.

But Estelle Sechster did not send her daughter to an institution. Instead, she kept her at home and hired a tutor, Helen Kaufman. It was Kaufman who finally gave Andrea Sechster a language of her own, sign language, although Andrea was almost ten years old when she finally learned it. Learning this language did not work miracles: Andrea had endured cumulative traumas whose duration and intensity researchers are just beginning to understand.[3] No amount of sign language—learned so late—could erase those traumas' horrific effects.

Even at age ten, however, sign language opened doors for Andrea that everyone—including Estelle Sechster—had believed to be forever closed. And Estelle was there with her daughter, accompanying Andrea through those doors and watching her when she insisted on going through them alone. Estelle learned sign language and advocated for her daughter for the rest of her life. Andrea went on to graduate high school, to get married, and to have a child. Were all these things complicated? Sure. But had she gone to Willowbrook, her life would have been much, much harder.

With extremely rare exceptions, no one hopes for their child to be disabled. And very few people imagine that it will happen to them. We in America frequently think of our families as finished objects, imagining our children graduating from Harvard long before they're even conceived. It is easy to mock such grandiose fantasies. But it is important to see them, at least in part, as a product of the enormous opportunities that America opened up to immigrant families like those of Estelle and Harold. Had they remained in Europe, the options available to them as Jews would have been extremely limited, with a fair chance that they would have suffered and died during World War II. America gave them the chance to rise: to have careers, to raise a family, and to live as Jews, however *they* wanted to define Judaism, without fear of the Nazis or a pogrom.

Immigrants fantasized about intergenerational upward mobility, but alas, within this idealized climb, there was little room for a child with disabilities. Andrea was not just deaf (which was bad enough) but also "something else." To have a child like that was to see Horatio Alger pushed from the top of the Empire State Building, to witness one's own family romance—which, however unrealistic in retrospect, was held in earnest—transform into what could only have been a nightmare.

Estelle Sechster could have accepted such a "nightmare" as reality. She could have abandoned her daughter and retreated to the cozy nook of fantasy, rather than work with the hand that she had been dealt. But she didn't. Instead, she abandoned the romance she had been given and began to create a new one, a vision of the family that not only would include her daughter, but would come *from* her: a family that was as much Andrea's as it was Estelle's. To create this new family, she had to re-create herself: learning sign language, becoming her daughter's constant companion throughout childhood and adolescence, and then supporting her as she moved out to claim her independence as an adult.

She even supported her when Andrea announced that she was planning on marrying a man whom Estelle believed to be deeply unstable. His name was Douglas, and at least at first, he appeared to be deaf. He also appeared to be standoffish, extremely controlling, even violent. But he was Andrea's first serious boyfriend, and she was thirty-five. Why not leave well enough alone? That approach changed when Douglas told Estelle that in fact he was *not* deaf. He could hear. He just had decided not to speak. Why? He would not reveal. He had posed as deaf for the duration of his relationship with Andrea—and, it seemed, for many years prior. What did Andrea know?

Estelle felt that the situation was bad enough to hire a private investigator to track her future son-in-law. It was bad enough to talk via telephone to his mother in North Carolina, who had not seen him in more than a decade and had assumed that he was dead. Bad enough to consider calling off her daughter's wedding. A conversation with the owner of the wedding venue changed her mind. The man, like her, had a deaf child. "They have so little in life," he said. "Just let her have a day to be celebrated." Estelle allowed the wedding to go on. And when her daughter, less than one year later, told her that she was pregnant with a child sired by her "deaf" husband, Estelle wrapped her arms around Andrea and let her know that she had her support.

It was a difficult pregnancy and a difficult birth. But what came after seemed even more difficult. The baby boy would almost certainly have to be given up for adoption. The family was so sure about it that he was circumcised by a mohel on the third day—instead of the eighth, as ordered by Jewish law. They did not think that he would last eight days with them, and they wanted to be sure that—wherever he went—he would know that he was a Jew. But though it seemed impossible, Andrea wanted to try to raise him. And her husband, however terrible he was, did too. Estelle decided that she would do everything in her power to help.

Everything in her power—in anyone's power—was not, in the end, enough. The boy's father was an abuser: he bathed the baby in scalding water, allowed him to cry through the day and night, believed that to comfort him would breed weakness, rejected any hired help Estelle sent to assist them, and threatened with violence anyone who came near.

But the problem was not just the boy's father. Andrea, too, was ultimately unable to provide the necessary care. She had never been a warm person, at least not in a conventional sense, had never really known how to hug in a way that made the other person feel like she was there. As a mother, she was severely limited. She played Go Fish at the kitchen table with her deaf friends while the baby lay crying in the crib just a few feet away. The ability to feed him, to hold him, to change his diaper, to put him to bed—none of it was there. Did she love him? In her own way, yes, and over the decades to come, she showed him that. But however much she loved her child, Andrea could not do the work to care for him.

This was a personal tragedy of immense proportions. Andrea had always wanted to be a mother. She had imagined having a child throughout those long years when she had been exiled to her home, sitting in the window, watching as other kids—kids who could hear—joyfully went to school. Sometime in the 1960s, in her early twenties, she had made a timeline of her life as she imagined living it. In the timeline, at the age of thirty-six, she had written "baby boy." And then, finally, it seemed that she had been granted what she had dreamed of. When she was nearly forty years old, she had her son. It must have been amazing. Just fourteen months later, however, it was clear that she would not be able to raise him, that she would have to give him up.

Three decades earlier, Andrea's mother, Estelle, had been given two options: either place her daughter in an institution or teach her on her own. Andrea now found herself with a pair of options to consider, these somehow even sadder than those that her mother had dealt with before. She could either give her son up for adoption to a stranger, or he could be raised by Estelle, who had volunteered, at the age of sixty, to take him.

Andrea's husband, Douglas, knew which option he wanted: adoption. If he could not raise their son, he never wanted to see him again. He tried to convince Andrea. He "trained" her, alone in their apartment, to tell the social worker that she wanted the boy put up for adoption. He imitated the social worker: "Do you want your mother to have the baby?" Andrea was supposed to answer: "No, no, no." Despite this, when they were all in the room and the social worker asked the question, Andrea shrugged her shoulders and wrote "yes." From that moment forth, the child had two mothers: Estelle, who would raise him as her own, and his biological mother, Andrea, who could not do the work of caregiving, but loved him all the same.

That child is me. I am the son of two generations of American women, each of whom was faced with a similar choice: either lose their family or lose their family romance, the idealized image of what they believed family life should be. Both of them made the same choice—family—and I was their great beneficiary, growing up in an environment rich in associations, in relations, in creativity, and in love.

In this book, I have argued that we in the United States face a similar choice with regard to our system of hospice care. We can persist in the fantasy that the family by itself will be enough, or we can recognize that the family, as it is, is not enough. We can abandon the hospice family romance and combine our familial caregiving with assistance from the state. The result will be a family that is strange in a way not unlike my own: a family that crosses accepted boundaries, merging public and private in a way that, at least on the face of it, is disturbing, weird, perhaps even "un-American."

And yet, such families make up the majority of American family life. There is no typical American family, at least not in the way that phrase is often understood. The typical American family is not the much ballyhooed nuclear family, a relatively recent invention that was, as historian Stephanie Coontz has shown, never as widespread as is generally believed and certainly not uniform in its benefits.[4] The "typical American family" is the family that Americans have always created when their ideas of what the family should be were found to be in conflict with the realities they were dealt. Such families are chosen—though frequently not in the best of circumstances—in acts of creative survival by individuals recognizing that, to quote the poet W. H. Auden, they have to learn to "love one another or die."[5]

But sometimes we must both love one another *and* die.[6] This confluence of familial love and inevitable death places a particular strain both on existing families and on the meaning of "family" itself. Throughout our history—in American popular culture and American politics—the family has typically been oriented toward life's *beginning*.[7] The typical American family is the child-rearing family, the family whose primary—and perhaps only—role is the procreation and rearing of children. This family, defined by a singular function, has been represented as having a singular form: the nuclear family, defined as two parents living together with their children in a house that they (preferably) own.[8] The exact terms of this family have been the subject of some political debate, most recently regarding the topic of whether homosexual couples should be allowed to marry.[9] But these debates have been almost exclusively oriented around the child-rearing family.

Families do not just raise children, however. They also tend to each other throughout the lifespan, including when their members eventually get sick and die. The family at the *end* of life has been significantly less studied and has not received nearly the same bipartisan political support as the child-rearing family.[10]

This is unfortunate. The needs of families at the end of life are as great as—and arguably greater than—at the beginning of life. Child-rearing, though extremely difficult, is a culturally normative experience in US society today, and it is invested with a certain degree of pride. Though end-of-life care was once similarly common, over the course of the twentieth century it largely disappeared from public view. As a result, families are less prepared for dying, and dying itself has come to seem a private affair, suffused not with pride, but with shame. This shame has carried over to the topic with which I began this book: the reluctance of families at the end of life to demand state resources on behalf of their loved ones. But it goes beyond that, terrorizing dying people and their caregivers even in what otherwise might seem the "best" of circumstances.

Changing this situation requires placing the dying family—the family at the end of life—at the forefront of our discussions of familial policy. Indeed, I believe that the dying family may itself provide an ideal model for that policy because the "end of life" does *not* begin at the end of life. Therefore, thinking about—and creating policy for—the dying family necessarily requires thinking about and creating policy for families throughout the lifespan. It also requires thinking of the *form* of the family in a much more expansive way. There is no nuclear family at the end of life. The end of life is when the nuclear family, even if it once existed, begins to die. This dying is tragic, but it is not the absolute end of the family itself. On the contrary, it can—and, to an extent, must—be the spark for a more creative articulation of the family's meaning and a dynamic reshaping of its form.

The dying family is not a tightly bounded entity, contained in a private house. It is the family that comes together when the walls of the house fall off: a family that is wild, sprawling, and unexpected, "hillbilly" in the phrasing of memoirist J. D. Vance or, as philosopher Judith Butler puts it, "queer."[11] This expansive character of the dying family corresponds to the range of individuals who may be included in it: parents and children, cousins and uncles, grandparents and great-grandparents, and nonbiological family members as well, like neighbors and friends, life partners, co-workers, paid and unpaid professionals, and sometimes even perfect strangers who, impelled by the urgency of dying, volunteer to help. It also corresponds to the volatility of emotions at the end of life: love and longing, sadness and regret are the typical emotions we associate with dying, but we shouldn't forget the atypical ones, which we tend not to think of so much, like anger, indifference, and hate.

There are few better examples of the dying family's expansive emotional life than the song "My Orphan Year" by the California punk rock band NOFX.[12] In

"My Orphan Year," the band's lead singer, Michael Burkett (aka Fat Mike), writes of the deaths of his mother and father. In both cases, Burkett situates his response to their dying in the context of his longer relationship with them. In regard to his father, Burkett remembers that there were "months" when he would not see him. When he did see him, his father would be out with his friends "all night," leaving Burkett "alone at only nine." In the case of his mother, Burkett recognizes the work that she did in raising him alone after his father abandoned the family.

The different ways that his parents treated him led Burkett to treat them differently at the ends of their lives. His father, he recalls, lay in bed "for months" with dementia. He would occasionally call Burkett to ask him to visit. Burkett would tell him that he was coming but then would have "things to do." "And so," Burkett sings, his father "died without his son." In the case of his mother, in contrast, Burkett "nursed her and . . . held her when time was running out." The night before her death he "drank scotch all night / And thanked her for everything she'd done." Raising him alone, Burkett acknowledges, "wasn't much fun."

Burkett's song encompasses a range of emotions. Toward his father, he expresses outright anger and the passive aggression of indifference. His lack of presence during his father's death was, at once, an act of sympathy with his younger self—sitting at home alone, terrified—and an act of judgment on his father's abandonment of him. In the case of his mother, Burkett expresses love, kindness, and an empathetic acknowledgment of the difficulties he put her through. The song fuses emotions that are unruly when taken in isolation and seemingly contradictory when incorporated into a whole: love and hate, anger and remorse, a desire for revenge and for reparation. Such unruly contradictions are characteristic of the dying family's emotional life.

They are also characteristic of the emotional life of the family throughout the lifespan. Consider the family at the beginning of life. Parenting is frequently described in extremely limited emotional language: the language of joy, love, and care. To be sure, it can—and should—include all of those emotions. But this idealized image of parenting fails to account for the negative emotions that also can—and perhaps inevitably do—accompany it: mourning for the life one no longer has, regret for how one got there, frustration, exhaustion, hopelessness, even hate. The failure to recognize this emotional richness can have terrible consequences for the parent-child bond. Indeed, as psychoanalyst Donald Winnicott argued, a mother's "hate" of the child is a natural partner to her love.[13] By acknowledging this hate, a mother can address it and parent appropriately. It is when hate goes unacknowledged that the mother acts out, hurting her child because she cannot consciously recognize the complexity of her own feelings.

In this sense, the dying family is not just different from the procreative family. It is a superior alternative to it, which should replace the procreative family as our model for conceiving—and legislating—the family as a whole. The dying family encompasses the family's functions throughout the lifespan (including procreation), even as it accommodates and nurtures a much wider range of family forms and familial emotions. It is a family that contains multitudes.[14] As such, it is an ideal model for future thinking on American family life.

As a model of thinking about the family, it also provides a new model for familial politics. The American family should remain a largely private entity, and we should cultivate a private sphere that accommodates a broad range of familial forms. But for such families to flourish, we must entertain a broader notion of the *public* family, a family that has a political dimension not just at the beginning of life, but throughout the lifespan, including and especially at life's end. For the dying family, the personal is not entirely political.[15] But the personal does have a political dimension, and vice versa. Thinking about the family at the end of life thus requires that we engage familial policy in a much broader and comprehensive fashion than has generally been the case.

It also requires that we expand our notion of the family's purpose. The family does not just exist to breed and raise future generations. It also exists to care for and mourn the generations that are both passing and past. Such mourning is intrinsic to the family at the end of life, but it is not external to the family's role throughout the lifespan. As generations of psychoanalytic thinkers have argued, development is itself a process of mourning, one that includes not just growth, but also grief over the loss of previous developmental stages.[16] Thus, thinking about the family as saturated with grief is a perspective that, while particularly suited to the end of life, is worth considering throughout the lifespan. Family life is not just oriented toward the open-ended future of procreation. It is also infused with longing for a past that is no longer there. That this very grief can be a component of future growth is a paradox that must be incorporated into our broader understanding of what the family is.

This broader understanding should change how we think about the relationship between freedom and the family. As I argued in the introduction to this book, neoliberal theorists view the family as the necessary grounding of freedom. To an extent, I agree with them. But to ground freedom in the dying family, as I have defined it, requires redefining and challenging the neoliberal definition of freedom.

Mourning to Be Free

In the introduction, I argued, drawing on the work of Melinda Cooper, that neoliberal policy makers have based their conception of freedom—both economic and political—on a particular notion of the family.[17] This family is the procreative family, oriented toward the rearing of children. Through a "good" family structure—specifically, a nuclear family structure—such families raise adults capable of responsibly exercising freedom in the marketplace. Essential to such freedom is the denial of state support. Such support, neoliberals argue, atrophies familial bonds and, in the process, freedom itself. This conception of freedom thus understands the family as oriented toward the future, and freedom itself is characterized by the ability to choose our future among a (relatively) open range of possibilities.

There is at present a broad public and political consensus in the United States that this understanding of the relationship between freedom and the family is incorrect with regard to the beginning of life. As political scientist Patricia Strach has shown, both Republicans and Democrats have abandoned the idea that families at the beginning of life should be left on their own.[18] Both major parties accept the necessity of familial support, simply differing on the best vehicle for that support: tax credits, universal basic income, universal childcare, or some variant of paid parental leave. Such support is, presumably, necessary to maintain suitable familial relationships so that individuals can achieve the freedom of adulthood. Thus, the idea that families do not need governmental support has already been largely rejected.

But this rejection has been far too limited in scope. I have argued for the need to provide dying people and their familial caregivers with far more extensive state support at the end of life. We should debate the nature of such support, but the discussion must be understood as a debate not just about dying people and their families, but about freedom itself. State support is not external to the freedom of dying people. It is a fundamental condition—not the only condition, but an essential one.

Though support is necessary for freedom at the end of life, the freedom that it provides carries a distinctive tone. In the child-rearing family, the goal is to provide the child with a foundation for a future that in theory is relatively open. But the future that dying people have is closed. They cannot look forward to college and career, to boyfriends and girlfriends, to new children of their own. Now that they are at life's end, everything that they have experienced is in the process of becoming lost. They do not have "no future," as literary theorist Lee Edelman put it, but the future they have is harshly shadowed by its limitations.[19]

This changes the nature of what freedom is and how it is experienced, even in the best of circumstances.

The lack of a future makes the freedom of dying people one that is, by its nature, tragic. People may choose to die. But no one chooses *to be dying*. Therefore, any choices made freely in the space of life's end are choices made in the knowledge that one has no choice in reality—that the very concept of "free choice" is a kind of farce. If we were really free to choose, then we would choose to live, to heal, to go on, and on, and on. But that is not one of our options. The freedom we are left with is, in a paradox, a freedom that is conscious of its inability to ever be entirely free.

As a result of this consciousness, freedom at the end of life is based in mourning.[20] It comes not from the hope of limitless possibilities, but rather from the recognition—grim and in a way futile—that the life of possibility has come to an end. It is freedom drenched in grief. This grief is anticipatory in the sense that it looks toward the ultimate loss: death.[21] In another sense, it is a reasonable reaction to a series of losses that have already occurred. On a micro level, these are losses of functionality, of status, of our former role. On a macro level, these smaller losses are representative of the larger loss of the sense that we formerly were *not dying*, that we were living, and would continue living. To know that we are losing our life is already to have lost "life" as we knew it. The dying person dies a personal death, which precedes and shapes the physical death that is to come.

Thinking of freedom alongside loss seems deeply counterintuitive. In fact, it goes against the dominant ways of imagining freedom in Western political philosophy, where freedom is associated with mastery, with control.[22] But dying people at a fundamental level do not have control and cannot have control, because if they could, they would not be dying in the first place. In this sense, the very state of dying seems anathema to freedom as it has been traditionally understood. The freedom of the dying person, rather, is based in the cold recognition that the choices available to them are all ones that the dying person would rather not have. In a tradition that equates freedom with choice and possibility, the tragic freedom I am describing here is, in a sense, unthinkable.

This unthinkability is the foundation of our debates about freedom at the end of life. These debates are not, in fact, about freedom *at* the end of life. They are about freedom *from* the end of life. They are about giving individuals the freedom to *not* be dying. The means through which freedom from dying might be achieved are debated, but there is no debate about what it might mean to be free *while* dying. We might argue that this lack of debate is due to the presumption that our existing concept of freedom is adequate for dying people. But this is not the case, because these debates are about *expanding* freedom to include the act of being assisted in the voluntary ending of one's life. Thus, there is an acknowledgment implicit in this formulation that our existing conception of freedom is not enough. Yet there is no concomitant attempt to reformulate this understanding of freedom in a manner that might maximize the freedom of people *while* they are dying. The only freedom that we can imagine for dying people is the freedom to no longer be.

In this book, I have imagined freedom at the end of life differently—which is to say that I am imagining it at all. I want us to recognize that there can be freedom even amid extreme constraint, that there are ways in which we can maximize the control that dying people have even as that control seems negated in its entirety. I have given a number of suggestions toward that goal, and I hope that others give many more. But if all the resources in the world cannot save a dying person from dying, then what is the point of freedom? Isn't it better to just get it over with as soon as possible? Perhaps in some cases it is, but not in general. And those exceptional cases should not be the foundation of the way that our nation imagines freedom at the end of life.

Mourning provides a starting point that is better. By embracing tragedy, mourning dramatically expands the boundaries of individual control. It gives the individual a degree of control over that which is uncontrollable: the inevitability of death, the persistence of radical loss, the knowledge that we are, in a way, always already dying, even if much of our life is lived, perhaps necessarily, in denial of that fact. This is not a passive acceptance of loss. It is accepting loss while also accepting the violent and overwhelming emotions that accompany it, including the desire to reject the loss itself.

This is the experience that freedom at the end of life can open up for dying people. But it can only do so if they are surrounded by and ensconced in their families: if they are surrounded by people who will mourn the dying person's future absence, which dying people are themselves mourning. Death in the abstract means nothing. Death matters because it is personal, because it is the loss forever of people who matter to us. Without the family present, dying people are limited in their ability to feel the imminent loss of their own life, because what they are losing in part are the people who make them who they are. For this reason, the biggest affront to freedom at the end of life is not death itself, but rather the obstacles that come between us and the anticipatory mourning of our own death: those obstacles that make us unable to feel what we are losing and that prevent us from recognizing that our loss is much greater than the loss of our own "self."

Such freedom is routinely denied in the US hospice system as it currently exists. The system claims to support the dying family. In reality, it keeps the family so busy managing the dying person's needs that it denies both them and dying people the ability to collectively mourn. This denial of mourning is a denial of freedom, the ultimate restriction of what the dying person can do. This restriction was felt keenly by Steven with his pot pies, by Mary with her bruised arms, and by many of the dying people whose care I observed at Amberview. Simon and Julian did achieve a modicum of freedom, ironically because they were given an option out of the hospice system through the care provided at Our Lady. Raúl also got to experience some freedom, but only due to great sacrifice on Marta's part, which was aided by a significant degree of both material resources and luck.

My goal is to create the conditions in US hospice care in which dying people and their families can experience the freedom of mourning. The form this mourning takes can be distinct and chosen by patients and families. Indeed, whether they mourn at all is an issue of choice. But our hospice system must provide dying people and their families at least with the opportunity, and at present, it does not do so nearly enough.

This is a problem that goes beyond hospice. It cuts to the core of the very idea of America. America is a unique nation in the extent to which its political life has been based in the idea of freedom.[23] This book is a rethinking of that idea. As such, it is necessarily a rethinking of America itself, which might seem external to the goal of improving US hospice care. But this is not so. The US hospice system exists in its current state because hospice, as an idea, does not cohere neatly with the idea of American freedom and therefore of America itself. To create a country that is supportive of hospice, we must redefine who we are. This will be of great benefit to dying people and to us all.

Expanding the Frontier

America is a large nation, and like any nation it has its myths. The most prominent of these is the myth of the expanding frontier. Even prior to our nation's founding, as historian Richard Slotkin has written, the frontier was the central feature of American identity.[24] It represents in our national mythology the promise of America. So long as US territory continues to expand there will be land and work and hope for anyone bold enough—which is to say, "American" enough—to explore them.

Explorers are our national heroes: Lewis and Clark, Daniel Boone, Neil Armstrong, and even Clint Eastwood. These frontier heroes are symbols of America and, more specifically, they are symbols of the promise of American freedom:

freedom as a limitless future and as the complete control of our life. Through our identification with explorers, generations of Americans have come to see ourselves *as* American. But the manner in which this Americanness—and its concomitant freedom—has been defined is very particular and worthy of some reflection.

Historian Howard Kushner has argued that the frontier hero, though seemingly a flat character, has a complex, if largely unconscious, emotional life. The hero's journey westward does not occur in a vacuum. It is almost invariably a response to something that he would not have chosen: a death in his family.[25] This death occurs in a particular context, which is defined by the lack of appropriate rituals for mourning. The soon-to-be frontier hero experiences a death, but his community, for a variety of reasons, does not give him the means to process it. He does not know how to recognize the death he has suffered nor how to imagine it as a meaningful part of his life. Having not been offered an appropriate venue for mourning, the frontier hero denies his own desire to grieve altogether. The form that this denial takes is the journey west.

Westward expansion in this view is not an innocent foray. It is a flight not from death but from the frontier hero's terrifying emotions in response to it—an escape from a depth of loss that he was never given the tools to understand. This flight is mental, but it manifests physically in the frontier hero's self-induced exile from all connection with familiar others. He journeys into a realm that is bereft of the community to which he had been accustomed. Interpersonal relationships are terrifying to the frontier hero because he remains under the belief that they bring only senseless pain.

The frontier hero thus carries forever the suffering of loss unassimilated. Because he cannot mourn, he cannot live again. All he can do is run. The result is the expansion of the frontier, which drives the explorer on to new discoveries in service to his nation. But these discoveries do not bring fulfillment. Any moment of accomplishment brings with it a moment of repose, but such repose cannot be tolerated. The frontier hero must keep moving.

The frontier hero is not actually free. He is trapped by a loss that he cannot acknowledge and from which, therefore, he cannot heal. He believes himself to be experiencing the freedom of limitless expansion, but no matter how many miles he travels, he cannot in any meaningful way expand. His life is limited to the point of impoverishment. He has no loved ones, no family, no friends. He can only act in one way—by fleeing—and he repeats this action compulsively. Worst, he believes this compulsion marks the hard limit on what he can be. The frontier hero, then, does not represent freedom but its opposite. He is a prisoner of his own limited emotional life, and he mistakenly sees this self-created prison as proof that he is free. To be held hostage by our own need for reckless expansion—that is the American mythology, our idealized way of life.

This pseudo freedom takes a heavy toll on the frontier hero. But the toll is even greater on the people he encounters along his way. The lands the frontier hero moves through are not, in fact, uninhabited. The frontier is populated by people—most significantly by native populations who have long lived there or who have recently been exiled from the East, in addition to other explorers moving westward.

The frontier hero cannot bring himself to have mutually sustaining relationships with any of these people—and so he conquers them. In this sense, the frontier hero does not exactly "avoid" relationships. It would be more accurate to say that he can only conceive of relationships in one form: violence. Frontier freedom, American freedom, thus has come to be synonymous with colonial domination. This domination structures the frontier hero's relationship with the outside world, and it also colors his interactions with whatever family he eventually has. Some explorers do marry. But their relationship to their spouse replicates their relationship with the native people, with the land, and with themselves. It is a relationship based in the violent subjugation of the other.[26]

Eventually, even the frontier hero reaches his limit. Perhaps there are no new territories to conquer. Perhaps his physical and mental tools are no longer sufficient for the violent work. Regardless, the frontier hero finds himself stripped of the freedom that has, in his mind, defined him. In response to this dispossession, he sees only one option: self-destruction. The frontier hero turns his expansive gaze onto the one territory he can still conquer: himself.

The frontier hero's story ends in suicide.[27] Such self-destruction was the fate of one of the original frontier heroes—Meriwether Lewis—and the potential for it follows all explorers who are not killed along the way. That such endings rarely appear—that the frontier hero's story as represented in literature and film frequently cuts out before he reaches the end of his life—is an indicator of our collective unwillingness to acknowledge the violent and perhaps pointless underbelly of what is our most prominent national myth.

There is no hospice on the frontier. There is no place where a hero, bereft of his earlier abilities, might find acceptance for himself. There is no place where he might connect with others through the mourning of what he has lost. This lack of hospice—or, more basically, of hospitality—is not because the land is barren. It is rather because the frontier exists mostly in the head and heart of the explorer, and he cannot recognize the value of life without domination, cannot accept that the ability to have relationships *not* based in violence is the essence of what it means to be free. So long as the American myth remains tethered to the frontier hero, creating freedom at the end of life will remain impossible, and hospice will be marginalized in American public and private life.

The material impoverishment currently experienced by hospice providers in the United States—their lack of funding to do the jobs that dying people need and that hospice workers frequently would like to do—is a direct product of the lack of any conceptual space for hospice in our national mythology. The neoliberal individual, trading without limit in an ever-expanding market, is but the latest articulation of this frontier character—distinct in some ways but not in others.[28] Part of the success of neoliberalism in the United States is likely due to the coherence of that ideology with deeper and older American national myths.

The same can be said of the success of our most recent president, Donald Trump. Trump's repeated boastings of his lack of empathy for—and violent desires toward—racial and religious minorities mark his character.[29] He marries this character to the threat of imperialist violence. His concern was not our war with Iraq, but rather that we were too limited in our plunder.[30] In this sense, Trump does not mark a break from the American tradition. He represents the most recent overt manifestation of its violent character. So long as the frontier hero polices the border of our national self-imagination, this will not be a country that welcomes dying people or that provides them with a real sense of freedom at the end of their life.

Fortunately for the frontier hero and for all of us, there is a way out: mourning. This mourning is personal, but it must be facilitated, according to Kushner, by a collective environment that makes the acknowledgment of loss possible—and recognizes it as valuable for the aggrieved individual, for the broader community, and perhaps even in itself.[31] Collective sites of mourning make it unnecessary for the explorer to flee to the frontier. But in a deeper sense, they open the would-be frontier hero's own borders: reconnecting him with others in a way that allows him to grieve his private loss and to develop a more emotionally flexible and interpersonally rich sense of self. Mourning, then, is the real way to expand the American frontier.

Mourning also can provide a more expansive—and truer—sense of American freedom. Kushner discusses mourning in largely cultural terms, as a product of collective rituals.[32] Though such cultural resources are necessary, we must also acknowledge grieving's political dimension. A key reason for the lack of mourning that impels the frontier hero's journey is the incompatibility of mourning with our broader conception of American freedom. This lack of mourning—the loss of tragedy, the loss, in a way, of loss—condemns American freedom to being little more than the endless process of what Slotkin calls "regeneration through violence."[33]

By opening ourselves to grief, we can ground freedom in a range of emotions and potential actions that are denied in our current political mythology. Thus, the postulation of mourning as central to our *political* understanding of freedom is necessary for the cultural shift that Kushner recommends and also for the possibility of freedom both at the end of life and in general.

A New American Mythology

Writing in the 1990s, Slotkin lamented the demise of the frontier's power in American public life. Though Ronald Reagan had extensively referenced the frontier throughout his presidency, such myths did not have the power to unify a broad swath of the American population as they had throughout the previous centuries. Instead, the frontier had become a kind of a simulacrum, a myth that is referenced without being broadly shared.[34]

The demise of the frontier has continued in the twenty-first century. This death is not represented in a lack of frontier imagery in our politics and popular culture, however.[35] As I pointed out above, the two dominant trends in US politics of the last decades—neoliberalism and right-wing populism—are themselves rethinkings of the frontier. Rather, it is evident in the inability of either of these narratives to unify the nation in a coherent and widely shared myth.

Trump may reference the frontier, but rather than unifying the country through this myth, he further polarizes it. Indeed, such polarization is his goal. The slogan "Make America Great Again" is a call to return to the frontier. But that frontier does not include the majority of the country's population; Trump and his supporters rebel against the expanding diversity of the nation. This myth is not being used to unify, but rather to divide. The goal is not a great national project. It is the prolongation and intensification of Trump's own project: the impossible satiation of his narcissism.

The loss of the frontier is, for Slotkin, something to be lamented, albeit in a complicated way. More than anyone else, Slotkin has chronicled the manner in which the frontier myth has fueled our national proclivity toward violence. Nevertheless, though the frontier has throughout US history propelled tremendous violence, it has also provided a useful rhetoric that has been drawn on even by opponents of our worst national tendencies. For example, Slotkin chronicles how frontier rhetoric was used in the service of feminism, civil rights, and the expansion of social benefits.[36] He believes that these political changes were only possible because of the existence of the frontier as a unifying national myth. Thus, in a dialectical fashion, the frontier myth provided the grounds for legitimate alternatives to the violence that it had traditionally justified. The loss of this myth thus represents the loss of the degree of national unity necessary to engage in any collective political action at all.

It is in response to this loss of myth that hospice can—and, I believe, must—be of use. Redefining our national mythology is necessary if we are to have effective hospice care in this country. But hospice is necessary if we are to continue to have "America" itself. Without the articulation of a new and compelling national myth—one that builds on the idea of the frontier while subverting its violent content—the very existence of the United States as a political community is at risk. It is here that hospice can be of its greatest value to us, not just as a form of caring for dying people, but as a new and necessary way of reimagining the identity of America.

Hospice *is* a form of caring for dying people, but beyond this narrow definition, it is a political community defined by the entanglement of mourning and freedom. The nature of this entanglement, including its specifically political character, has been only imperfectly grasped by US hospice leaders, who have tended to depoliticize their work. Mourning has always been central to the hospice identity, present in a common sense of grief that unites patients and providers.[37] Such grief can, for example, be found in the practice of seeing Jesus as undertaken by the Dominican Sisters of Hawthorne. It also pervades secular hospice facilities, like Amberview, where providers mourn alongside patients and their family members, even as such present-day mourning awakens in them the memory of the family members that they have lost. Thus, hospice providers are living examples of the existence of communities based in mourning. They serve as models of what our nation might one day be.

To realize this potential—the potential of America itself—it is necessary to politicize US hospice care. The dying family, as I have defined it, is one example of such politicization. I understand familial caregiving—the oft-unrecognized foundation of hospice—to be an inherently political endeavor, even as it is also a personal one. These personal and political aspects of caregiving are not identical, but they shape each other. Recognizing this shaping can provide genuine insight, which can spur us to further action. This action will invariably be personal. But it must also be political. Indeed, such political action—making demands on the state—is, given the present circumstances, particularly urgent.

Hospice, conceived in political terms, is particularly well suited to be a foundation for a reconstructed American national identity. American identity, in such a perspective, will naturally be based in those who are open to grief. Its tone will be melancholic. Such melancholy is, as historian Enzo Traverso has commented, "a necessary premise of a mourning process."[38] Yet, by facilitating mourning, melancholy does not mire us in passive brooding; on the contrary, it helps us to become active. But not just active *again*: active in ways that are fundamentally different, more expansive, and indeed, freer than before.

There is no better representative of this melancholic American identity than dying people. Not all dying people grieve, and perhaps not all dying people should grieve. But dying people—because of their cumulative and ongoing losses and because they are at the end of their life—generally are more melancholic, more prone to grief than they were before.[39] They are also more likely to be grieved by those around them, as their family members prepare for and experience their loss. Thus, dying people are potentially powerful symbols of an American identity founded in the recognition of value in and amid loss.

This raises the question: What would it mean to make a dying person the center of our nation? Such a shift would be quite radical. American freedom has always been synonymous with a particular kind of health: physical strength, unlimited mobility, a kind of superpower. When Donald Trump titled his book *Crippled America*, he was not using the term as a neutral descriptor, much less a compliment, but rather as an indicator of a national disability that he would erase.[40] Our contemporary political discourse is thus conceptually underpinned by what bioethicist and disability studies scholar Rosemarie Garland-Thomson calls "eugenic logic," a philosophy whose goal is the elimination of disability.[41] Dying people are arguably the most disabled among us. By making them the bearers of American identity, we can create a nation that works differently, a nation where "crippled America" or even " dying America" are not seen as pejoratives, but as terms of national unity.

The basis of this unity cannot be "pride" in a simple sense. On the contrary, this simple sense of pride is the problem: it represents a rejection not just of weakness, but of the inherent nature of loss. There is no space in it for mourning, much less melancholy. It is not a happy emotion, but it seems to crowd out all emotions other than happiness. Any space that this pride gives to dying people or disabled people is restrictive.[42] On a national scale it gives us "unity" in the form of an emotional straitjacket.

Better than pride, then, is maturity. I mean maturity in a sense that is existential: as the ability to maintain a state of relative well-being in the face of death. This "existential maturity" has been studied by researchers Linda Emanuel, Neha Reddy, Joshua Hauser, and Sarah Sonnenfeld. They argue that if we experience dying in the presence of nurturing, "holding relationships," it can allow us not to wither, but rather "to explore fearsome possibilities, to fragment and come together, and to regress and regrow."[43] This maturity is not a denial of loss. On the contrary, it explores loss and by doing so finds opportunities for experiences that are not restrictive, but full.

If such maturity before death were to form the basis for our identity as a nation, that would be something of which we could be genuinely proud.

The American identity that I am proposing here cannot be based just in a dying person. The dying person must be accompanied by their family. However defined, the dying person's family is, much more than cells and bones, the foundation of their very life.[44] Because of this, family members are also the foundation of their very loss. Indeed, it is arguably the loss of our family that makes dying so terrible. I am recommending that the dying person be the center of American national identity, but this center should include those who orbit around this vibrant but withering core.

Like the frontier hero, this melancholic American identity will also have its myths. Its heroes are not those who, out of fear of loss, flee contact with others, defining their identity through their lust to conquer and their fear of themselves. Instead, these heroes embrace loss and allow it to change them—opening them to a world that they did not know existed, a world in which caring for dying people is a gateway to caring for all. The alternative to the frontier heroes, then, are the hospice providers: the professionals who currently work in the US hospice system and those founders who, by dedicating their lives to making America into a country more hospitable to dying people also made it into a country that was significantly more faithful to its own ideals.

From this perspective, there is no better example of American heroism than Rose Hawthorne Lathrop. Lathrop has long been acknowledged as a Catholic hero, and she is currently up for sainthood.[45] I have no means or authority to judge her Catholic sainthood, but I believe she should be accepted into the pantheon of American saints. Her decision to give her life to the care of the dying poor is the kind of activity that should be considered foundational to our nation.

Her decision was steeped in loss: the loss of her son, who died at the age of three; the loss of her marriage; the loss of her father and mother.[46] But rather than narrow her world, the immense losses that Lathrop suffered allowed her to expand it and to connect with others. This connection can largely be attributed to the framework provided by her Roman Catholicism. Through its rhetoric of mourning—oriented around Christ's death—Catholicism gave her the means to experience and process, ritualistically, the losses that she experienced throughout her life. Her care of dying people was a response to this healing and perhaps a vehicle of it. The result was a significant increase in her freedom and that of the people she cared for.

Lathrop's conversion to Catholicism is a particularly American story in a country defined by religious freedom and oriented in its best moments toward the care of those in need. Acknowledging Lathrop as an American hero in no way diminishes her Catholic beliefs. On the contrary, her somber religiosity is precisely that which our nation might embrace. In a country that will for the foreseeable future be predominantly Christian, Lathrop presents a figure of the kind of Christian faith that even the nonbelievers among us (the resolutely secular, conspicuously Jewish author of this book included) might embrace.

She also provides a model of a Christlike devotion that some American Christians might do well to remember exists. As historian Kevin Kruse has documented, American Christianity over the course of the twentieth century became conflated in the minds of many believers with the worst ravages of market capitalism.[47] As journalists Elizabeth Bruenig and Matthew Sitman have pointed out, this conflation is both theologically dubious and politically pernicious.[48] So long as it persists, our country will be hindered from cultivating the political will necessary to ensure the freedom of its dying citizens. We must find new sources for American Christianity, sources whose fidelity to Christ leads them to reject the violence of the market.

There are few better symbols of an authentic American Christianity than Rose Hawthorne Lathrop. She was a Christian, an American, and a friend of the poor. This friendship was, for her, inextricably linked to her commitment to dying people—especially people dying *in poverty*. It led her to be a passionate critic of a nation that declares itself to be "Christian" even as it abandons its neediest citizens to the gutter. In a time when many American Christians have thrown their support behind a president who represents this abandonment in perhaps its most gleefully dystopian form, Lathrop serves as a reminder that a different kind of American Christianity has previously existed and, with the support of more Christian Americans, can exist again.

The American Hospice Tradition

Rose Hawthorne Lathrop was not a "Christian" in some general sense, however. She was Catholic. And her Catholicism matters. American Christianity has generally been very harsh to Catholicism.[49] The present status of American Catholics as members of a relatively uniform Christian Right is a new one, and it does not represent the reality in which Lathrop lived. She was a member of a despised religious minority. Honoring Lathrop as an American hero requires honoring our country's commitment to religious minorities—a group that should include those of us who identify as secular. To be American is to adopt a pluralistic creed.

This pluralism forms the foundation for the American hospice tradition. Like its European predecessor, this tradition is grounded in the care of dying people. But unlike its European predecessor, the basis for this care is not Christianity.[50] It is America: a country dedicated to religious pluralism, indeed whose national religion is plurality. The American hospice tradition will always have a prominent place for Christian Americans who live out both their faith and their citizenship through the practice of end-of-life care. But their place exists alongside those of the many Buddhists and Muslims, atheists and Jews, Hindus and others who have dedicated their lives to people who are dying.

In this book, I have been critical of the leaders of the modern US hospice movement. But such criticisms should not detract from the greatness of what they have accomplished. Hospice leaders in the United States—Florence Wald, Edward Dobihal, Dennis Rezendes, and many others—created, at great personal sacrifice, a system of end-of-life care that, for all its flaws, is immeasurably better than what preceded it. They did so at the cost of their own resources and without any guarantee that their efforts would come to success (quite the contrary). In an inhospitable environment, they continued to labor, sacrificing their time, money, and a significant part of their lives. They gave us much more than they probably realized, including the resources hospice needs to endure and mature. They are the kind of heroes who epitomize our country's commitment to dying people.

Such heroes still live among us. I am referring not just to the members of Hospice Inc. who remain alive. I mean also the people who actually work in hospice today. Over the course of the research for this book, I interviewed thirty-one hospice professionals. I was struck by a commonality in almost all their stories. They had voluntarily turned away from jobs that were higher paying in order to care for dying people. They had done so because through a variety of circumstances, they had come into contact with dying people. And this contact transformed them—in a manner that they thought was for the better, even as it was grounded in the most painful loss. The result was not just a decision to make an economic sacrifice. It was also a decision to *not* sacrifice their lives for remuneration that would be solely economic. They chose to do the work that they loved for the people that they loved: dying people.

We should not romanticize this sacrifice. We should, in fact, pay them better. But in their willingness to sacrifice money for love—or, rather, their unwillingness to sacrifice love for money—they are worthy inheritors of the American hospice tradition. We, as Americans, must work to be worthy of them.

The hospice tradition is large enough to include both proponents and opponents of physician-assisted suicide. The PAS debate is about the proper means by which the American hospice tradition might be best realized. The problem is that this debate has occurred prior to the establishment of an enduring American hospice tradition. Grounding this debate in this tradition will allow us to approach it from a different perspective. But before we can do so, we must affirm the hospice tradition's centrality to our country.

This cannot be accomplished without the dying family. This family, as I have defined it, is composed of those of us who have been caregivers for dying people. We are a group that is larger than any faction in the PAS debate, one that transcends the debate itself and includes many Americans who have not been engaged in it. We too are members of the American hospice tradition because we too have engaged, as family members and as Americans, in the labor of end-of-life care. By claiming our role in this tradition, we can give hospice the role it deserves in our larger identity as a nation.

The American hospice tradition *is* a national tradition, although we have hidden it from ourselves. In the present historical moment especially, this tradition seems particularly foreign. But it is not. It is *here*, in who we are, in who we have been, and in who we must be if we are to fulfill our country's promise. This is the promise of a nation of people who, rather than turning to hate, open themselves up to those among us who are most cast out. The stories of such people must become our new myths, myths that reject the violence of the frontier while epitomizing—indeed, radicalizing—its expansive possibilities.

These new myths reject the idea of freedom that is dominant in America today. By doing so, they are perhaps most faithful to what historian Eric Foner calls the "story of American freedom."[51] Foner is not talking about fidelity to the understanding of freedom that existed at any particular moment in American history, much less the moment of our nation's founding. He is discussing the story of those groups that have been excluded from the old ways of understanding freedom and who have responded to this exclusion by redefining freedom in a manner that could include them. The story of American freedom is, then, a story of perpetual revolt.

But it is also a story of perpetual fidelity—and profound love of country. The groups whose story Foner tells all challenged American freedom and, by extension, America itself. They never abandoned America, however. On the contrary, their very act of challenging America was the means by which they became most authentically *American*. To be American, in this view, is not to passively acquiesce before the reality of our country nor to flee in the manner of the frontier hero. It is to stay, to fight, and, by doing so, to make America into a country that is not locked in self-contradiction: a country that can become the "land of liberty" that it has always claimed to be.

The American hospice tradition epitomizes Foner's story of American freedom. It is the story of Americans who have aggressively challenged the way that dying people have been excluded from a country that claims to have already given them liberty. It is a story about how dying people should be the center of our country and its understanding of what it means to be free: a freedom grounded not in dominance and mastery but rather in the mourning of the most profound loss. It is a story that spills far beyond the borders of these pages, a story in which we all can form a part.

It is not enough, however, to retell our national myths. We must also retell our own personal stories and, by doing so, find a new way of being American ourselves.

Our Stories, Our Selves

To be an American is about more than a line on our passport. It is about identifying with that line: about feeling ourselves to be a member of this country. This membership can be due to an accident of birth. But with time, this birth may begin to feel not accidental, but essential. One can be born an American; but whether by birth or not, an American is something that one can also choose to become.[52]

"Why," you might ask, "should I?" This country can be extremely hostile to its citizens. This hostility could be a reason to reject it as a whole: to renounce our Americanness, to deny that it exists. I would not judge anyone who made such a decision, but it is not the only choice. To be an American, I argue, does not involve passively accepting the "America" that we are given. It requires actively changing it. Part of this change must include making this country into one that is less hostile and more hospitable.

This is in keeping with—and epitomized by—the American hospice tradition as I have described it here. But this tradition cannot simply exist in the pages of a book. We must each make the tradition our own—and by doing so make our country into one that is more hospitable to *all*. We must retell our public story as a nation.

This public story also must be threaded through the private stories that we tell ourselves: the stories that are central to our self-understanding. By renarrating our own stories, we can connect to our larger identity as a nation and as citizens of that nation—as Americans. In this sense, the American hospice tradition can only serve as a model for a reborn American identity if we first come to see ourselves as members of the dying family. We must see our own experiences with dying as specifically *American* experiences in both their public and private dimensions.

This work of political formation and national identification must be carried out individually. It can happen only on the basis of a self-conscious identification by individuals with the American mythology I have proposed. Such identification will naturally include an element of redefinition. My vision for America is subjective, and it will be different in some ways from your vision or anyone else's. But the particularity of this identification does not negate its potential commonality. It provides the very vehicle through which a common national identity might further come to be.

In this sense, seeing my mother, Estelle Sechster, as a very American character involves viewing her as someone like Rose Hawthorne Lathrop. And indeed she was. Like Lathrop, my mother responded to the loss of her family—the family that she wanted—by expanding her notion of what a family could and should be. The same was true of her daughter, Andrea, my biological mother, who responded to the recognition that she could not raise me by discovering a new way to care and to be my mom. These three American women epitomize a national identity based in the creative freedom unleashed by loss.

I too am part of this nation. For this reason, I conclude by telling you about one of my own greatest losses: the death of my mother, Estelle. This story is by necessity incomplete because it is but part of the story of my life with Estelle and part of Estelle's own story. It is also incomplete because Estelle is but one of my two mothers, and I will not address further the complex relationship that both of us had to my other mother, Andrea Braswell.

Estelle was the first person I recognized as my mother, and she was until the day she died my best friend. I still think about her daily, and I'm still figuring out, almost a decade later, how to live in the wake of her loss. Perhaps telling her story here will give me some clues about how to do so—which would be a satisfying personal outcome.

But any personal outcome, however fulfilling, must be tied to my political goal of providing you with the tools to see your own personal stories of familial caregiving for dying people as part of the larger political story of our nation. We are constituted in part by each other, by our family members, and also by others who are members of the same nation-state.[53] I am "Harold Braswell," but seeing myself as such also involves recognizing that I am also my mother's son and an American. To see ourselves this way can seem insulting. No one likes recognizing someone else's work on—and hold over—ourself. But it is necessary if we are to become free individuals and members of a people.

Acknowledging our interdependence is also necessary if we are to care for our family members, particularly as they die. Recognizing the complicated overlap of our familial relationships with our national identity is necessary if we want our relationships to flourish to the maximum degree. It is also necessary if we are to help the weakest among us, those most frequently effaced from our national narrative.

It is in the hope of remedying such effacement—which I too have been complicit in and am in part formed by—that I end this book by telling you about how my mother died.

Afterword
How My Mother Died

Out of the darkness, the baby wipe glowed. My mother was holding it as she shuffled down the hallway, keeping it at a slight distance from herself. She was coming from her bedroom en route to the kitchen, where she turned the corner and continued right past. She nodded in my direction and with the weary fortitude of an office worker completing just one last task, she deposited the baby wipe in the kitchen trash. There it lay, on top of a multitude of crumpled papers, discarded foodstuffs, and other used sanitary products, soiled and buried underneath. Its white blossom unfolded, revealing a smudge that was watery brown. My mother turned away from it and gave me a polite, distant smile.

"Wait, Ma," I said, as she continued on her way. "Did you just wipe your ass with that?"

My mother turned back to me. Her color had faded, her skin taking on the same phlegmy hue as the nightgown that she now always seemed to be wearing. She looked at me with patient exhaustion.

"Yeah," she said. Her shoulders shrugged. There was a pause, and then she gave me a nod and another smile and walked away.

This is the story of how my mother died. But it is not just the story of my mother. It is also the story of my father and me and of the family that we three made.

What kind of family? The kind that has an enormous amount of love. A family in which there was a sixty-year gap separating parents and child. A family that ate early bird specials together, that laughed with George Burns and Jackie Mason, that watched *Matlock* and *Murder, She Wrote*, that only ate the "good" kind of ice cream: Häagen-Dazs.

We were old Jews essentially—and one very young one, though I never felt my age difference much. Whatever I did, my parents were with me, even if they thought my passions were silly (video games) or scary (mosh pits) or almost certain to end in ruin (writing). They always made me feel welcome, even though I was six decades their junior, even though I was essentially eliminating their "golden years."

My mother and I were best friends. You might have seen us at the local library together, reading at a table or, when they got them, in the big comfy chairs. If you didn't see us there, we'd probably be reading somewhere else: at home, most likely, or perhaps at Barnes and Noble.

"I'm like a fish in water," said my mother in the library. And it was true. In another era, in another life, she might have been a scholar or perhaps a shrink. As it was, her own mother had forbade her from going to college. My mother would not go until her forties, after her daughter Andrea had grown up.

My mother, Estelle, liked that I liked learning. And I liked it, in large part, because I liked her. We understood each other, had the same sense of humor, enjoyed similar TV shows and foods. We joked a lot about *Ellen* and *Drew Carey*. But our favorite show was, of course, *Seinfeld*.

We'd laugh about it every time we ordered black-and-white cookies—which we did with relative abandon. "Heal the world," my mother would chuckle (a misquote, also typical) as she gently tore the cookie in half. She'd take the chocolate side. I was always partial to vanilla.

The only problem our family seemed to have was how close my mother and I were—so close that it made my father jealous. Though paranoid in many respects—a trend that increased as he aged—he was, in his feeling that he was being excluded, not entirely wrong.

My father, Bud, was my mother's second husband, a fact that she pointed out —to him, to me, to herself, really to anyone—whenever the opportunity emerged. Harold Sechster had died almost a decade before I was born: a heart attack in his sleep on the first night of Passover. It was a sudden, traumatic death, and my mother coped by idealizing the man whom she had lost. "Harold Sechster," she would say, giving his first and last names as a unit, as if he were a figure from the history books who had, through some quirk of providence, ambled into her life.

She would tell a story about her honeymoon with him. They had been walking, and he saw a red dress in a store window. "Excuse me," he said to the saleswoman, "I must see that dress on my wife." It was an anecdote that in the abstract seems laced with chauvinism. But in her telling, it was a story about how well he understood her. Because it really was a very beautiful outfit. And yes, in those days, she looked *good*.

An intellectual! A conversationalist! Never worked too much! Not too tired to go out at night! And he was *tall*, a *tall Jew*, could you believe it? *That* was who Harold Sechster was, and being his wife was who she was—and what she wanted. Later, whatever Harold Sechster was, Bud was invariably the opposite.

This contrast was simplistic—and false in some respects. But it was not entirely wrong, and my mother was still very much a woman in recovery, a woman with many suspicions, which is appropriate of someone who loves another person deeply—and then gets suddenly, irreparably hurt. Despite this, she did love my father, and they did make it work. He learned bridge so they could play together (though they were never partners). When they went to restaurants together —which they did frequently—they split a main course and plotted (wordlessly) how to smuggle home spare "complimentary" pieces of bread. They had love and understanding 95 percent of the time.

But that other 5 percent: he was not Harold Sechster. This created a problem in their relationship, one that impacted us all.

Because while my father was *not* Harold Sechster, I might as well have been. We shared the same first name, and I, like him, was the one who really *got* her. We shared a special connection. But this connection existed, in my mother's mind, in opposition to her husband. Against my father, I became a cudgel that my mother—how I loved her—would on occasion wield.

I was, I believe, eight years old the first time. She took me to a diner, just the two of us. Very strange. There, she told me that she was thinking of getting a divorce.

"Should I leave him, Harold?" she implored me, blurred pools at the bottom of her eyes. I chewed my burger, fingers tensing into the sesame seed bun.

She did not wait for a reply. I would later learn she never needed one. She always stayed. Happy enough but never *quite.*

I stayed too, her watchdog, infused with her suspicions toward my dad, a distaste she deposited in me so thickly that I still do not know where "it" ends and "I" begin. The truth was that my mother and I *were* in many ways different than my father. For simplicity's sake, it might be easiest to describe us as two different American Jewish types.

My mother and I were "Jews." *Jews,* you hear me, the kind you may have seen on TV. Not the religious kind, of course. (We kept kosher, but in case of emergency, there was always a bag of shrimp stored in the back of the freezer.) We were the kind of Jews who are neurotic and witty, nervous and intellectual, charming yet also strange. The kind of Jews who might—at one time for better, now almost certainly for worse—be identifiable as "somewhat like Woody Allen."

My father—not so much. Oh, he was just as Jewish as my mom and me. Like her, Yiddish was his first language. Like me, his *schmeckle* was missing a small part. But if not for these two traits, you might have mistaken him for that most *goyische* of creatures: a normal American male. He joked constantly without ever being funny, was intelligent but unintellectual, disliked reading yet pretended it was because of his eyes. He had been a submarine man in World War II and identified strongly as a veteran for all of his life. In football, he played on the line.

A large man, very dependable, with a chin on which you could sharpen a knife. His given name was Irving Shterberg, but at a young age he changed it to Bud Stirber. This name captured much better the man he was to become.

Though he was different from me, I loved him greatly. He was the practical one, the one who, I knew, would always give me everything I might need. And he was unusually sensitive for a man of his generation. The granite of his chin had a gentle wobble. I have never been held in a more powerful hug, and he insisted, every night, on saying "I love you," each time with a kiss on the lips. In short, he was a very good man. Of this I am certain: I will never love a better man more deeply.

My father, you understand, became my mother's husband after their children from previous marriages were grown. He had been married to her for less than two years when I came through the door. My mother had reasons to welcome me: I was her daughter's child, her blood. But my father had no such relationship to me. We were bound by neither law nor blood. I came into his life unanticipated at what, for many, would have been the worst possible time. He was sixty-two and had raised five children already, always working very hard. If he had pushed me away, who could blame him?

But instead my father took me in.

"I just held you in my arms," he said to me decades later. He gave a smirk before clarifying, with a "who me?" shrug: "It just felt right."

And it *was* right, because he was the best dad I could ever ask for. He drove me everywhere, worked hard to understand me, and always made me feel like he had time. He never made me feel like a burden, even though I almost certainly was. In this book, I have been talking about opening ourselves to the other, about the American tradition of hospice, and there is no one who epitomizes that tradition more to me than my dad.

I wish I had done more to let him know that when he was alive. (Yes, he's also dead.) I think that in some ways I did. But I was on my mother's side in the battle between them, and this more than anything was what sent my father over the edge.

"I know what you two are doing in there!"

He blasted through my bedroom door. My mother was on my bed, reading to me, as she did every night. I was perhaps nine or ten.

"Buddy," my mother said to him, book in hand, "are you out of your mind?"

"You." My father pointed a trembling finger at her. "You are making fun of me."

"Okay, Buddy," my mother replied, rolling her eyes. "Now go to bed."

My father in fact went to bed every night at seven and then left for work at three or four in the morning. He did not have to keep this schedule but claimed that it was an unshakable relic from his years in the navy. My mother rightly resented this, and it seemed that this time her barb hit home.

My father looked around confusedly for a minute. For the first time, I remember, he seemed old. As soon as he had stomped out of there, my mother and I rolled our eyes.

I do not mean to exaggerate any negative dynamic. Ours was a happy family. Moments like this generally bubbled in the background, creating a kind of habitual white noise. But problems did boil over, and they reached a height when my mother came to the end of her life.

The heat in our family increased substantially at one point due to my father's financial situation. My mother and father had always kept separate bank accounts. At the time of their marriage, my mother had a lot more money than he did. This money was from her first husband's life insurance policy, and perhaps out of fealty to him, she was reluctant to simply fork it over.

She also had some suspicions that, given the context of her life, were not unreasonable. Immediately following her first husband's death she had, in a posttraumatic haze, gotten remarried. The marriage lasted one week, and according to my mother, the man had just been in it to steal her money. It was so insignificant that my mother did not even include him in her tally of grooms. Yet the experience was traumatic enough to lead her to be wary regarding finances.

Besides, both she and my father had families of their own: children who, though now adults, were entitled to inheritances. It just made sense to keep things separate, though I suppose the situation was an indicator of problems to come. For around twenty-eight years, however, those problems never materialized.

Then came the recession of 2008. My father took a big hit to his savings. His business was suffering too. He owned a Hallmark store in the mall and, aside from the crisis, a series of sociological changes (i.e., Target, e-cards, Amazon) had made his business model obsolete. The crisis hit some of his children pretty hard too, and my father was worried about what he would be leaving behind. He was feeling pinched.

He began to ask my mother for money. And that perhaps is when things began to go to hell. My mother sometimes did give him money: thousands of dollars in fact. But other times she did not and got very mad at him for asking. She felt he was using her. "What am I," she'd yell at him, "your piggy bank?"

This reaction, in turn, led my father to feel hurt and get mad at her: "Twenty-eight years, Estelle." Then she got mad at him: "Who paid for the house? You've been living here for free." He responded: "What about all the jewelry I bought you?" And her-him, him-her, vice and versa, to infinity.

Then they both got dementia. Or, rather, let me place scare quotes around that "both." The matter remains of some debate. Not for my mother. In her case, the dementia came swiftly, and we knew it immediately. But in the case of my father, it was so gradual as to be imperceptible. I am not even sure whether my father was demented at this point in his life. But if he was *not*, then I had misjudged the man's personality. Around this time, he began to act in a manner that, though not completely out of character, was more insensitive, narcissistic, and harmful than I had ever known him to be.

I'll never know for sure. But I am going to choose, at least at this point in my life, to believe that he had dementia. Doing so allows me to more easily forgive him for the actions that I am about to describe. After many years, I have determined that I am ready to forgive. But though he may have been demented, at the time I had no idea that he was. This made his actions extremely shocking to me—difficult to understand, much less accept. I felt like he was choosing to no longer be my dad.

My father's actions both influenced and were influenced by the familial dynamics that I have described here. Were these dynamics perfect? No. But they worked, sometimes beautifully, almost always well enough. Then my mother fell ill, which opened my family to a world that we had, up to that point, not really known.

When it happened, it came as quite a shock. True, my mother was old: eighty-seven. But for me, "old" was what she always had been. She was sixty when she took me in. This was a sacrifice on her part. But she and I had rationalized this sacrifice by telling ourselves that I was keeping her young. Her continued good health through her sixties, her seventies, and much of her eighties seemed to be proof: her aliveness, as an octogenarian, was a justification of my existence, an argument for the magical power of our love.

The refutation of this argument came when she fainted one night while out to dinner with my father. They went to the ER. The diagnosis came soon: non-Hodgkin's lymphoma.

A person in their late eighties does not in general have a good chance of "beating cancer." Chemotherapy is incredibly taxing. It is difficult for a person in their twenties. For someone in their late eighties, it is extremely destructive and almost certainly pointless, with little chance of anything resembling "success." As a doctoral student researching end-of-life care, I either knew this already or quite easily could have figured it out. But I didn't. At first, I was emotionally stunned and geographically distant. I let that distance become an excuse to let other factors and other people take control. Even when I did get more involved, it was not to stop my eighty-seven-year-old mother from doing chemotherapy. It was to, at best, be supportive of her and, at worst—I am sick now thinking about this—to urge her on.

There was a series of terrible ordeals. The first occurred while I was still in Atlanta. My mother went into a chemotherapy session, and after a few minutes, she had an awful reaction. By my mother's account, this experience was terrifying and terrible. And yet, they—we—decided to give it one more shot. In a week, she would go in for her second round. If it didn't work, there would be no others. If it didn't, we should understand, it meant certain death. I decided to fly up to be with my mother on this "final" try. Medicine had failed my mother. But perhaps love would make it work.

Love, however real, is limited in its medical efficacy. I drove my mother to the chemo lounge and sat across from her. The chair she was in looked comfortable. There was even a personal TV. When they first attached the bag to her, she looked calm, even indifferent. We were going to watch TV and chat for a couple of hours. This wasn't going to be so bad.

Then the hand I was holding began shaking. I watched the shakes jolt up and down her forearm, past her elbow, to her bicep and shoulder. Her eyes began to rattle in their sockets, the edges of her pupils seemed to strain. I pleaded: "Come on, Mom, you can do this." But soon I was pleading with the nurses to come and quickly take her off.

"I'm sorry we beat up your mother today," said the oncologist to me afterward. He assured me that we were done.

At home, things seemed calmer. I planted my mother in her usual green recliner. I turned on *Fox News*. It was late in the afternoon by then, and I called a friend with whom I had previously made plans. A few hours later, he came to pick me up, and we went to a bar. Before going, I asked my mother how she was feeling. She felt great, she told me, with a smile that seemed close enough to typical: "Have fun."

When I got home at nine, my father was asleep in bed. My mother had drifted off in the chair. Both these things were normal and therefore consoling. But when I bent over to kiss her forehead, it was hot. This was the first time that I had ever felt a fever in another person. Having no children of my own, I had always been the one to receive that cautious, caring kiss. The heat of her skull was unmistakable.

"Mom, Mom." I tried to wake her up. At first, she did not respond and then only groggily: "Huh?" Her head lolled from side to side, taking the rest of her with it. I tried to keep her upright, but her withered body possessed a power both slithering and immense. She kept falling through my hands.

"I have to pee," she mumbled, and I hauled her to the bathroom. I got her through the door, but then she slowly collapsed through my arms, landing on the hard tiles below. From under the edge of her nightie, the urine spilled.

Instead of breakfast on the kitchen table, there was a document. My father sat behind it, trying hard to imitate an accountant or perhaps a judge. On the other side of the table was my mother with a confused look.

The document was my mother's will, and my father wanted to discuss it. He had found the will by "chance." What he had seen had shocked him to the core. Just $15,000! *That* was what she had left him—after twenty-eight years of marriage. True, they had married in their sixties, and both had been clear that their own children were their priority. True, he was in his late eighties, thus having little use for her money himself. True, she had given him a life estate in the house—a house he had never paid a cent for—which would allow him to remain there as long as he wanted. But however true all these minor things were, the tru*est* thing was the jewelry.

"Think of the jewelry, Estelle!" he pleaded with moist eyes, as my mother tilted her head to the side.

The will had to be changed. It was from more than fifteen years ago. She had to update it. She had to! And I—her son, his son, their son—had to convince her that it was the right thing to do.

"Do something, Harold!" he urged.

"Harold," my mother whispered. "What's going on?"

Had my mother not been demented, she would have screamed at him, hungry as ever for a fight. I understood that perspective, but I also felt sorry for my father. I felt loyal to him because he had always given me his love. But whatever mixture of hatred, sorrow, and love I felt, it was beside the point. My mother was demented. Even if she wanted to, she could not legally change her will. The question was, in a sense, resolved. But this resolution was, from my father's perspective, deeply unsatisfactory. The anger it generated in him would, as much as any terminal illness, consume my mother's life.

Shortly after my mother's diagnosis, I had succeeded in getting her to take antidepressants. In many ways, this had been a lifelong journey. As far as anyone knew, my mother had always been depressed. "That's just who she is," a relative said to me.

Maybe so, but it wasn't who she wanted to be. She had begun seeing a psychiatrist for talk therapy years before. He had recommended that she consider antidepressants, and he made this recommendation more forcefully once she got sick. Apparently, there is research that they can increase a dying person's lifespan. My mother and I were initially suspicious, but with few side effects and some potential benefits, why not? I picked up the pills at the store and placed them in her pillbox myself.

But when I came back from Atlanta a few weeks later, my father informed me that she would be taking them no longer. It was not a decision made by a doctor. He, from now on, would be the one running the show. What this meant was that my mother would not receive her pills. My father did not believe in medicine, or rather, he believed that medicine would accelerate my mother's death. Instead, he would give her *alternative* medicine, specifically gigantic horse pills made of mushrooms. My mother did not want to take them, but he forced her to choke down six a day, withholding food until she did.

"Estelle," he chided her, pointing with a finger, "don't you want to get better?"

In denying my mother her antidepressant pills, I believe that my father was sincere. He really did believe that the medicine was part of some foul plot. This delusion was perhaps due to his dementia. But I also think that he took particular joy in denying her the antidepressants because he knew they were pills that *I* had gotten for her. He was mad at me because of the will, mad at me because he sensed that my mother loved me more than him, and mad at her for both of these reasons. When she had been healthy, she had resisted his control. Now, finally, he would have his way.

His was the way of unassisted walking. For the previous two years, my mother's physicians had counseled her to use a walker. She had frail bones and problems with balance, both exacerbated by her cancer. She had obtained a walker free through insurance. But there it stood, an abandoned sentinel in the hall. My father forbade my mother from using it. He considered it to be enfeebling both physically and spiritually. He seemed to relish placing her in the most perilous situations, believing perhaps that the higher the degree of danger, the greater was unassisted walking's ameliorative effects. He would drop my mother off in front of the local diner, winter winds blowing, as he went to park the car. If she woke up in the middle of the night to pee, there was no walker by her bedside that might prevent her from stumbling in the dark.

She fell backward once, smacking her head against the corner of her hard wooden nightstand. She fell a few other times too: when he dropped her off in front of the diner and the winter winds blew her over onto the concrete; and in the house, while walking down the hallway or trying to make her way up the stairs. But these falls were so minor that—he judged—no emergency room trip was needed. There may have been a few more times beyond that, but those were so slight that no one needed to be told. The bumps, bruises, perhaps concussions, and potential broken bones were a small price for the fortifying benefits of walking on your own.

Unable to stem the tide of falls, I got my mother a Life Alert bracelet in the hope that I might at least be able to get help to her sooner. Without telling me or anyone else, my father disconnected the system.

Sitting on the toilet, I heard my father's voice through the wall. "You know, Estelle," he said to my mother, who was with him in the other room, "I think it's time we got you back on the road."

"Oh yeah," she responded nonchalantly, as if she had been thinking the exact same thing.

The image of her squinting behind the wheel made me chuckle. Of course, were it to come to fruition, the results would be catastrophic. But I took comfort in my belief that at least this one absurdity would remain in the realm of ideas.

My mother always hated driving anyway. At the time, she had a Buick that was two years old, but she had never driven it. My father drove it much more than she did, greatly preferring it to his own car, which was older and not as nice. So great was his desire for her car that, a few weeks after this conversation, he got my mother, while demented, to sign over its title. "She said she wanted me to have it, Harold," he insisted over the phone.

It was the baby wipe that provoked my breakdown, or rather, my recognition that things had already broken down long before. Seeing the baby wipe atop the kitchen trash, something in me realized that this couldn't go on. I had to either get my mother out of that house or put someone into it who would be able to ensure that she received adequate care. My plan was to call social services. I did not know what might come of this. At a minimum, I was hoping that someone would scare the shit out of my father, maybe make him more amenable to listening to me. But before I called social services, I called a relative, who had another, better idea.

By the beginning of the next week, my parents had been moved to assisted living.

The assisted living facility was nice. Were my mother fifteen years younger and not demented and with cancer, it would have been perfect. The facility was a geriatric country club, made for that generation of Jews who had been too discriminated against to get into the real thing. Yiddish lessons in the morning, bridge in the afternoon, cheesecake and gefilte fish available à la carte. All would have been perfect. Except my father wouldn't help my mother go to Yiddish class, and he wouldn't let her eat cheesecake. He wouldn't let her eat *anything* until she choked down the mushroom pills. And he still wouldn't let her use the walker, though at least now she would be falling on carpet.

My mother was not on hospice. She was not receiving any palliative care, perhaps receiving no medical care at all. It was more of a lifestyle facility. At least at first, that seemed to be enough.

It was not until around a week before she died that my mother was placed on hospice. She was eighty-nine. For two years, she had non-Hodgkin's lymphoma, stage 4. We knew that the disease would kill her, but we neglected to enroll her in hospice. There was no dramatic resistance to hospice nor to acknowledging the fact that my mother was dying. But no one told us to look into hospice. Even though I was researching the topic, I did nothing. By the time we did get her on service, it was too late.

I came into my parents' apartment when the hospice nurse was visiting. The nurse seemed pleasant, if not particularly helpful. Her presence allowed me to understand that my mother was "dying." But there was no one to talk with me about what that meant. I never spoke with a social worker or chaplain, not even a doctor. Nothing noticeable changed about my mother's care. My father continued with his mushroom pills, the rest of us with our lives.

A few days after I met the nurse, the assisted living facility had an outbreak of a stomach virus. My mother did not get sick, but the facility imposed a quarantine. In a way, it did not matter. I was already heading out of town to visit my fiancée's family in Massachusetts. I said goodbye to my mother over the phone. I told her that I loved her. I'd be back in New York in a few days. She said that she loved me too. It was about as normal a conversation as we could have.

Two nights later, a relative called. My mother was in the hospital. She had collapsed and been admitted for treatment. I said that I was on my way back. But there was a blizzard on Long Island. All the roads were closed.

I spoke to a nurse at the hospital. She assured me that my mother wasn't in imminent danger of dying. She saw cases like this all the time.

"So, if I were to drive down first thing in the morning, I should be able to see her?"

"Of course," she said. So I chatted with my fiancée, and we went to sleep. At around four in the morning, I got the call.

Sometimes, I try to imagine what it must have been like for my mom as she was dying. I can't. I can imagine how she might have experienced it if she had not been demented. It would have been terrible. But she was demented. As a result, she seemed to be unaware of what was going on. I don't know how much she suffered on a daily basis. I do know that she was often confused. Such confusion could lead to pain—for example, when she fell—and be painful in itself. Perhaps she felt lonely, since she was often left alone. I can imagine that she would have hid that information from me. More than anything, she did not want to be a bother.

Though I don't know what my mother was feeling, I do know that what happened to her was wrong. It began with her oncologist, who suggested that she undergo a treatment that, to paraphrase my dissertation advisor, was a modern form of bloodletting. It continued with the battles with my father over the will, the house, her treatment, her body, and, eventually, her estate. I was a part of this too, subordinating her needs to my own insecurities in a manner that kept me from advocating on her behalf. The process ended with her paying thousands of dollars a month to be housed in a facility that was not for dying people, a facility that by necessity had to ship her out to a hospital when her condition became worse.

Transferred from one location to another without any awareness of what was going on, divested of any power over her life, her dying body exploited, arguably even looted by the family members and professionals charged with her "care," my mother, as she lay dying, was not free.

Everyone involved in her care shares the blame: my father, myself, the oncologist, the assisted living facility, the hospital, the nurse who told me she would live. My mother might have planned better, might have seen more clearly the changes happening to her, might have anticipated them years, even decades in advance. These are all failures. They are significant and pathetic. But the nature of these failures is personal. They are not the topic of this book.

I have written this book because of failures of a political kind. The existence of numerous personal failures during my mother's final years does not negate the political ones she experienced. Nor does the political nature of these failures absolve us of our personal responsibility. We all failed my mother in her hour of greatest need. By writing this book and highlighting some of the ways in which she was failed politically, I do not excuse myself. On the contrary, this book is an act of personal responsibility that I can carry out on my mother's behalf, although it is an act suffused with mourning since she is not here to benefit from it.

I have made an inventory of what went wrong, and I will do what I can to make sure that it does not go wrong again. One major thing that went wrong for my mother and for all of us was that we did not receive timely hospice care. My mother was not put on service until it was too late to be of any use. This late arrival is not happenstance. It is systemic: dying people not receiving hospice until it is too late is one of the most widely cited problems in US hospice care.[1]

This problem is a product of the dependence of the US hospice system on familial care. This dependence allowed hospice leaders to bill their form of care as a method of cost savings. This conception of cost savings led hospice to be integrated into Medicare in a form so reduced that a significant number of dying people never receive it. A hospice system and a healthcare system that were adequately funded could have recognized that my mother was dying much earlier and provided her with care that would have made her considerably freer during the final period of her life.

The late arrival of hospice shaped my interactions with my mother up until her death. During the years that my mother was dying, I was constantly managing her care. Little of this management occurred through direct interactions with her. On the contrary, it happened almost entirely through interactions with my father. By managing him, I tried to manage her. There seemed to be no other options for me at the time. If I did not manage him, he would destroy my mother. I would have preferred to spend the time caring for her directly. But the best thing I could do, the only thing I could do, and the thing I ultimately failed to do was control my father.

I should have done better. But it is also reasonable to wonder, given the circumstances, if there might have been an easier way. There are professionals who do possess, at least in theory, the training to assist dying people and their family members in negotiating such tricky situations: social workers. Had my mother been on hospice earlier, I might have been placed in contact with a social worker.

This hypothetical social worker, if competent, could have been extremely helpful to me in negotiating the conflict between myself and my father over my mother's care. Indeed, this social worker could have been of great assistance in helping me to know when the situation in my parents' house had become unsustainable.

As it was, I almost called social services. But I did not, in part because I was worried that such a call would have resulted in the forceful removal of my mother from my father's care, against her will. Such a removal might have been necessary, but it likely would not have been, had a competent social worker been working with our family. There was no social worker, however, because my mother was not on hospice.

I am not sure the extent it would have mattered if she had been. As I noted in chapter 6, social workers in contemporary US hospice care are, in some circumstances, used to increase the censuses of hospice, even though that is not technically their job. The opportunities that social workers have for genuine familial counseling can be constrained by the profit motives of their employers. Even had a social worker been available with enough time to help us, it is possible that contemporary social work education—based in behaviorism and macro-level policy—might not have trained them to be of assistance in guiding my family through our various psychological conflicts. And even if such assistance had been available, the structure of US hospice care would have placed a hard limit on the level of freedom my mother would have been able to enjoy.

A major aspect of that limit was location. Even had my family's conflicts been completely worked through, there would still likely have been no suitable location for my mother to die. The care she received, up until her death, still would have been inadequate. Home care was impossible for my father to provide. The assisted living center where they moved was not a facility for dying people. When she did begin to die actively, she had to be sent somewhere else: to a hospital, where she eventually died. Even had there not been a blizzard on the night of her death, the ability of our family to be with her during her final hours would have been extremely restricted. An alternative to this predicament might have been a nursing home. But, as I have argued, nursing homes are an inherently flawed solution to the problems of US hospice care.

Thus, the difficult circumstances of my mother's dying cannot be attributed solely to my family or even to the medical professionals who attended to us. They were products of the way our country's end-of-life care system is designed. This is even true, to a degree, of the oncologist who advised our family to pursue chemotherapy. As anthropologist Sharon Kaufman has shown, medical providers are incentivized to recommend heroic measures that will likely be harmful to patients, including dying people.[2] This incentivization is part and parcel of the structure of Medicare, which reimburses providers for medical services. The lack of long-term care in Medicare is the flip side of this model: the medical bias of the system leads to the undercutting of nonmedical components. While individual providers should be more sensitive, so long as we leave this system in place, dying people, like my mother, will continue to be hurt.

At its highest level, my mother's death was a product of the country in which it occurred: the United States of America. Her difficulties were a natural outcome in a country that has not yet made a place for dying people and continues to be ambivalent about whether they should have any place in the nation at all. In this sense, my mother's death was, like her life, very American. My mother's life represents an America that exists at the margin of our national discourse, an America of people who experience their freedom through the creation of new familial relationships in response to loss. My mother's death epitomizes our dominant national discourse, with its focus on the flight from loss through the courtship of violent death. If this is the limit of our national imaginary, then we should not be surprised when people spend their last months of life uncared-for before finally dying alone.

My mother's death is representative of this country as we currently are. Her life was the America that we must become. This can seem like a daunting journey. But as her life shows, there are many aspects of that America that are already here. This is true even of my mother's life at its end. Though in many ways she died stripped of her freedom, there were moments in which another America became possible. Such moments were fleeting, but they provide some guidance for the country that can, if we will it, still come to exist.

I was hanging around with my mother in the house, just a little while after the chemotherapy had failed. Our time together had usually been spent out of the house, exploring the world. Now, due to her condition, we were homebound. Worse, there appeared to be nothing good on TV. It was then that I first pressed a button on the remote control labeled "On Demand." Neither my mother nor I had any idea what this button meant. She was old, and I did not own a TV. It was with a throbbing sense of possibility that we scrolled through these previously hidden listings before finally coming to a name that I recognized, a show called *Mad Men*. About it, I knew nothing in particular, except that it was popular and supposed to be "smart." I looked over at my mom and raised my eyebrows. She shrugged.

There are thirteen episodes in the first season of *Mad Men*. Each episode is approximately forty-five minutes in length. That's nine hours and forty-five minutes of television. I don't understand how we watched it all in one day. Indeed, that day blends together in my mind. Did we do it in one sitting? When we began, it was morning, and by the time we were done, it was pitch black. My butt hurt. But those details are secondary. Instead, what I remember from that ten-hour period is the conversation, a long conversation, grounded in nearly three decades of friendship and love, to which the show, however well made, was only a provocation and a backdrop.

My mother did most of the talking. She talked about what it was like to be alive in the 1960s, the period during which the show's action takes place, two decades before I was born. Though I knew that my mother was alive—indeed, already in her forties—in that period, I had never really pictured her living then. Her tales of raising my biological mother were so all-consuming that they seemed to exist outside of normal historical time. "Was *that* true?" I asked her about every detail that seemed strange and incomprehensible to me, which for much of her life had been the norm. Did people really litter like that? What was it like to be a nonsmoker? Was everyone happy that everyone else seemed to always be having sex?

There is a view that the end of life is part of a dying person's development.[3] I believe that this can be true. But the development experienced by a dying person exists in a context defined in part by their family. Provoked by the shift in a dying person's life, family members can see aspects of them that had hitherto been invisible, seeing them not as less than they previously were, but as more. Watching *Mad Men* with my mother, I began to be with her in a way that otherwise I likely never would have. Could this heightened perception have been possible in other circumstances? Maybe. But it was the end of life that brought it about.

Around three months before she died, I went to see my mother in assisted living. I was in town to book the venue for my wedding. We had scheduled the ceremony for the following summer, hoping that she would still be around. When I arrived at the apartment, my father was in the front room doing something on the computer. I could hear my mother breathing in the back room. She was in bed, but she tried to stand to greet me. I sat next to her, taking her by the hands.

I began talking about the wedding, the plans we had, and how excited I was that she would be taking part. But as I talked to her, I began to see that she wasn't listening. She was trying to keep her eyes on me, trying to make me feel like she was there. But she was already leaving me then. And she knew. My mother knew. But she kept wanting me to believe that she was there.

I began crying. Something in my chest snapped, and I felt my body pull into her. "No, Ma, no, Ma." She tried to wrap her arms around me, but she was weak. So I encircled her. I was wheezing, screaming that I didn't want this, I didn't want her to die. She tried to comfort me, to say my name "Harold, Harold." But she was sobbing too.

When I emerged from the room, my father looked up from the computer and smiled, the corners of his eyes blurred with red.

The week before my mother died, it was her birthday. On our way to see her, my fiancée and I passed a deli. Gripped by inspiration, I bought a box of black-and-white cookies. It had been a while since my mother and I had a cookie together. Now or never, I thought to myself—and when better than her birthday? We met her in the assisted living facility's private lunchroom, which was used for family visits. My father was there. One last time together.

I opened the box. Immediately, my mother raised her head. We giggled together, and I sighed. I took one of the cookies and pushed down on its center, tearing it in half.

Introduction

1. Mount Eerie, "Death Is Real," *A Crow Looked at Me* (2017), CD.

2. J. Lynn et al., "Defining the Terminally Ill: Insights from Support," *Duquesne Law Review* 35, no. 11 (1996): 311–336.

3. Nicholas A. Christakis, *Death Foretold: Prophecy and Prognosis in Medical Care* (Chicago: University of Chicago Press, 2001).

4. Cited in the Committee on Approaching Death, *Dying in America: Improving Quality and Honoring Individual Preferences near the End of Life* (Washington, DC: National Academies Press, 2014), 28.

5. "Maya" is a pseudonym, as are the names of all the individuals I discuss from my research. I have changed some aspects of their identity—including possibly their gender—in order to further protect them. This research was conducted under the supervision of Emory University's Institutional Review Board.

6. In my decision to use the pronoun "we" throughout this book, I was encouraged by Mark Lilla, *The Once and Future Liberal: After Identity Politics* (Oxford: Oxford University Press, 2018).

7. National Hospice and Palliative Care Organization, *Facts and Figures: Hospice Care in America* (rev. April 2018), https://www.nhpco.org/sites/default/files/public/2016_Facts_Figures.pdf.

8. National Hospice and Palliative Care Organization, *Facts and Figures*.

9. Kelly Noe, Pamela C. Smith, and Mustafa Younis, "Calls for Reform to the US Hospice System," *Ageing International* 37, no. 2 (2012): 228–237; Kelly Noe and Pamela C. Smith, "Quality Measures for the US Hospice System," *Ageing International* 37, no. 2 (2012): 165–180.

10. I discuss one such exception in chapter 5 of this book.

11. Stephen H. Kaye, Charlene Harrington, and Mitchell P. LaPlante, "Long-Term Care: Who Gets It, Who Provides It, Who Pays, and How Much?," *Health Affairs* 29, no. 1 (2010): 11–21.

12. On familial caregiving in hospice, see William E. Haley et al., "Family Caregiving in Hospice: Effects on Psychological and Health Functioning among Spousal Caregivers of Hospice Patients with Lung Cancer or Dementia," *Hospice Journal* 15, no. 4 (2001); Woung-Ru Tang, "Hospice Family Caregivers' Quality of Life," *Journal of Clinical Nursing* 18, no. 18 (2009): 2563–2572.

13. Since end-of-life care and long-term care are inherently intertwined, they demand an enormous amount of work by caregivers. For a comprehensive overview of the centrality of familial caregiving to our country's health and social service system, see Joseph E.

222 Notes to Pages 5–11

Gaugler and Robert L. Kane, eds., Family Caregiving in the New Normal (London: Academic, 2015).

14. Carol Levine, "Home Sweet Hospital: The Nature and Limits of Private Responsibilities for Home Health Care," Journal of Aging and Health 11, no. 3 (1999): 341–359; Sandra R. Levitsky, Caring for Our Own: Why There Is No Political Demand for New American Social Welfare Rights (New York: Oxford University Press, 2014).

15. Bruce Jennings, "Solidarity, Mortality: The Tolling Bell of Civic Palliative Care," in Our Changing Journey to the End: Reshaping Death, Dying, and Grief in America, vol. 2, ed. Christina Staudt and J. Harold Ellens (Santa Barbara, CA: Praeger, 2013), 272.

16. Jennings, "Solidarity, Mortality," 272–273.

17. Levitsky, Caring for Our Own.

18. Levitsky, Caring for Our Own, 91–118.

19. Levitsky, Caring for Our Own, 50.

20. Lynn Hunt, The Family Romance of the French Revolution (Berkeley: University of California Press, 1992).

21. Sigmund Freud, "Family Romances," in Standard Edition of the Complete Psychological Works of Sigmund Freud, vol. 9, trans. James Strachey (London: Hogarth, 1959), cited in Hunt, Family Romance, xiii.

22. Hunt, Family Romance, xiv.

23. See James Frederick Barger, "Life, Death, and Medicare Fraud: The Corruption of Hospice and What the Private Public Partnership under the Federal False Claims Act Is Doing about It," American Criminal Law Review 53, no. 1 (2016), https://papers.ssrn.com /sol3/papers.cfm?abstract_id=2747543.

24. Sandol Stoddard, The Hospice Movement: A Better Way of Caring for the Dying (New York: Vintage, 1992).

25. Interview with Florence Wald by Monica Mills, Oral History Archive, Connecticut Women's Hall of Fame, June 10, 2003, http://cwhf.org/media/upload/files/Transcripts /Wald%20Interview%20Transcript.pdf.

26. The basic framework of this argument can be found in Michael Brown, "Between Neoliberalism and Cultural Conservatism: Spatial Divisions and Multiplications of Hospice Labor in the United States," Gender, Place and Culture 11, no. 1 (2004): 67–82.

27. See Sara Margaret Evans, Personal Politics: The Roots of Women's Liberation in the Civil Rights Movement and the New Left (New York: Vintage, 1979).

28. Brown, "Between Neoliberalism and Cultural Conservatism," 77.

29. For three excellent studies of the rise of medical authority and its impact on dying people, see Emily K. Abel, The Inevitable Hour: A History of Caring for Dying Patients in America (Baltimore, MD: Johns Hopkins University Press, 2013); Jeffrey P. Bishop, The Anticipatory Corpse: Medicine, Power, and the Care of the Dying (South Bend, IN: University of Notre Dame Press, 2011); Shai Lavi, The Modern Art of Dying: A History of Euthanasia in the United States (Princeton, NJ: Princeton University Press, 2005).

30. Lavi, Modern Art of Dying.

31. Eric Foner documents the relationship between 1960s liberation movements and state resources in The Story of American Freedom (New York: Norton, 1998), 275–306.

32. Gary Gerstle, Liberty and Coercion: The Paradox of American Government from

the Founding to the Present (Princeton, NJ: Princeton University Press, 2017); Karen M. Tani, *States of Dependency: Welfare, Rights, and American Governance, 1935–1972* (Cambridge: Cambridge University Press, 2016).

33. Corey Robin, "Reclaiming the Politics of Freedom," *Nation*, April 6, 2011, https://www.thenation.com/article/reclaiming-politics-freedom.

34. Gerstle, *Liberty and Coercion*, 1–16.

35. Gerstle, *Liberty and Coercion*; Foner, *Story of American Freedom*.

36. Foner, *Story of American Freedom*.

37. Foner, *Story of American Freedom*, 316.

38. Milton Friedman and Rose Friedman, *Free to Choose: A Personal Statement* (New York: Houghton Mifflin Harcourt, 1990).

39. David Harvey, *A Brief History of Neoliberalism* (New York: Oxford University Press, 2007); Manfred Steger and Ravi K. Roy, *Neoliberalism: A Very Short Introduction* (Oxford: Oxford University Press, 2010).

40. Melinda Cooper, *Family Values: Between Neoliberalism and the New Social Conservatism* (Cambridge, MA: MIT Press, 2017), 106–117.

41. Cooper, *Family Values*.

42. For a similar argument, see bioethicist and anthropologist Jarrett Zigon's work on the affinity between neoliberalism and addiction treatment programs run by the Russian Orthodox Church. Zigon, *"HIV Is God's Blessing": Rehabilitating Morality in Neoliberal Russia* (Berkeley: University of California Press, 2011), 16.

43. See, for example, Hans Theodorus Blokland, *Freedom and Culture in Western Society*, trans. Michael O'Loughlin (London: Routledge, 1997); Richard A. Epstein, *Principles for a Free Society: Reconciling Individual Liberty with the Common Good* (New York: Basic, 2009).

44. Robin, "Reclaiming the Politics of Freedom."

45. Foner, *Story of American Freedom*, xiii.

46. Foner, *Story of American Freedom*; Robin, "Reclaiming the Politics of Freedom."

47. Isaiah Berlin, "Two Concepts of Liberty," in *Liberty: Incorporating "Four Essays on Liberty,"* ed. Henry Hardy (Oxford: Oxford University Press, 2002), 166–217.

48. Berlin, "Two Concepts of Liberty." See also the discussion of Berlin's essay in Nigel Warburton, *Freedom: An Introduction with Readings* (London: Routledge, 2001), 1–24.

49. Berlin, "Two Concepts of Liberty."

50. Berlin makes this argument explicitly with regard to disability: "If I say that I am unable to jump more than ten feet in the air, or cannot read because I am blind, or cannot understand the darker pages of Hegel, it would be eccentric to say that I am to that degree enslaved or coerced. Coercion implies the deliberate interference of other human beings in the area in which I could otherwise act. You lack political liberty or freedom only if you are prevented from attaining a goal by human beings." Berlin, "Two Concepts of Liberty," 169. Note that he mistakenly equates the ability to read with sight. Blind people can, in fact, read if they have access to education and works in braille.

51. Joseph P. Shapiro, *No Pity: People with Disabilities Forging a New Civil Rights Movement* (New York: Broadway, 1994); Doris Zames Fleischer and Frieda Zames, *The*

Disability Rights Movement: From Charity to Confrontation (Philadelphia, PA: Temple University Press, 2012).

52. Stoddard, *Hospice Movement*.

53. James I. Charlton, *Nothing about Us without Us: Disability Oppression and Empowerment* (Berkeley: University of California Press, 1998).

54. Charlton, *Nothing about Us without Us*; Shapiro, *No Pity*.

55. Charlton, *Nothing about Us without Us*; Shapiro, *No Pity*; Andrew I. Batavia and Kay Schriner, "The Americans with Disabilities Act as Engine of Social Change: Models of Disability and the Potential of a Civil Rights Approach," *Policy Studies Journal* 29, no. 4 (1996): 690–702.

56. Batavia and Schriner, "Americans with Disabilities Act."

57. Batavia and Schriner, "Americans with Disabilities Act."

58. Samuel R. Bagenstos, *Law and the Contradictions of the Disability Rights Movement* (New Haven, CT: Yale University Press, 2014).

59. Harold Braswell, "From Disability Rights to the Rights of the Dying (and Back Again)," *Laws* 6, no. 4 (2017), http://www.mdpi.com/2075-471X/6/4/31.

60. Braswell, "From Disability Rights."

61. Bagenstos, *Law and the Contradictions*; Ruth Colker, *The Disability Pendulum: The First Decade of the Americans with Disabilities Act* (New York: New York University Press, 2006); Kay Schriner and Richard Scotch, "The ADA and the Meaning of Disability," in *Backlash against the ADA: Reinterpreting Disability Rights*, ed. L. H. Krieger (Ann Arbor: University of Michigan Press, 2010), 164–188.

62. Bagenstos, *Law and the Contradictions*; Colker, *Disability Pendulum*.

63. Bagenstos, *Law and the Contradictions*, 131–150.

64. For a fuller articulation of this argument, see Braswell, "From Disability Rights."

65. Jamila Michener, "People Who Get Medicaid Are Made to Feel Powerless: That Pushes Them Out of Politics and toward Fatalism," *Washington Post*, August 17, 2017, https://www.washingtonpost.com/news/monkey-cage/wp/2017/08/17/people-who-get -medicaid-are-made-to-feel-powerless-that-pushes-them-out-of-politics-and-toward -fatalism/?utm_term=.7ddaf16fcb11. A more extensive version of this argument can be found in Michener's *Fragmented Democracy: Medicaid, Federalism, and Unequal Politics* (Cambridge: Cambridge University Press, 2018). My thinking on this issue is indebted to Corey Robin's Twitter thread of August 17, 2017: https://twitter.com/CoreyRobin/status /898181703948283906.

66. Shant Mesrobian, "Freedom for the Many," *Jacobin*, October 11, 2017, https:// www.jacobinmag.com/2017/10/medicare-for-all-single-payer-freedom.

67. Bagenstos, *Law and the Contradictions*; Schriner and Scotch, "ADA and the Meaning of Disability."

68. See numerous examples of familial advocacy in Lennard Davis, *Enabling Acts: The Hidden Story of How the Americans with Disabilities Act Gave the Largest US Minority Its Rights* (Boston: Beacon, 2016).

69. Charlton, *Nothing about Us without Us*.

70. The Institute of Medicine reports that "enrollment in hospice often occupies just the last few days of life." Institute of Medicine, *Dying in America: Improving Quality and*

Honoring Individual Preferences near the End of Life (Washington, DC: National Academies Press, 2014), 33. See also Nicholas A. Christakis et al., "Extent and Determinants of Error in Doctors' Prognoses in Terminally Ill Patients: Prospective Cohort Study," *BMJ* 320, no. 7233 (2000): 469–473.

71. Judith Butler, "Violence, Mourning, Politics," *Studies in Gender and Sexuality* 4, no. 1 (2003): 9–37. For a more extensive elaboration of the argument, see Butler, *Precarious Life: The Powers of Mourning and Violence* (London: Verso, 2006).

72. Peter Singer, *The Expanding Circle: Ethics, Evolution, and Moral Progress* (Princeton, NJ: Princeton University Press, 2011).

73. Oregon Public Health Division, Oregon's Death with Dignity Act, 2014, https://public.health.oregon.gov/ProviderPartnerResources/EvaluationResearch/Deathwith DignityAct/Documents/year17.pdf; Ji Eun Lee et al., "Caregiver Burden, Patients' Self Perceived Burden, and Preference for Palliative Care among Cancer Patients and Caregivers," *Psycho-Oncology* 24, no. 11 (2015): 1545–1551.

74. Levitsky, *Caring for Our Own*; Institute of Medicine, *Dying in America*, 42–43; Tracey A. Revenson et al., "Gender and Caregiving: The Costs of Caregiving for Women," in *Caregiving in the Illness Context*, ed. Tracey Revenson et al. (London: Palgrave Macmillan, 2016), 48–63.

75. Keri Thomas, Ben Lobo, and Karen Detering, eds., *Advance Care Planning in End of Life Care* (Oxford: Oxford University Press, 2017).

Chapter 1. Beyond the Right to Die

1. Ann Neumann, *The Good Death: An Exploration of Dying in America* (Boston: Beacon, 2016), 1–5.

2. Neumann, *Good Death*, 78.

3. G. T. Couser, "When Life Writing Becomes Death Writing: Disability and the Ethics of Parental Euthanography," in *The Ethics of Life Writing*, ed. Paul John Eakin (Ithaca, NY: Cornell University Press, 2004), 195–215; Diane Rehm, *On My Own* (New York: Knopf, 2016).

4. Neumann, *Good Death*, 34.

5. David J. Rothman, *Strangers at the Bedside: A History of How Law and Bioethics Transformed Medical Decision Making* (New Brunswick, NJ: Aldine, 2008).

6. See, for example, the discussion of end-of-life decision making in Helga Kuhse and Peter Singer, eds., *Bioethics: An Anthology*, 2nd ed. (Oxford: Blackwell, 2006); and Tom L. Beauchamp et al., eds., *Contemporary Issues in Bioethics*, 8th ed. (Boston: Cengage Learning, 2013).

7. For a fuller treatment of Nietzsche's idea of eternal return, see Karl Lowith, *Nietzsche's Philosophy of the Eternal Recurrence of the Same*, trans. J. Harvey Lomax (Berkeley: University of California Press, 1997).

8. See Harold Braswell, "Putting the 'Right to Die' in Its Place: Disability Rights and Physician-Assisted Suicide in the Context of US End-of-Life Care," *Studies in Law, Politics, and Society* 76 (2018): 75–99. Two edited volumes discuss both Medicare and physician-assisted suicide, but not in relation to each other: Timothy W. Kirk and Bruce Jennings, *Hospice Ethics: Policy and Practice in Palliative Care* (Oxford: Oxford University

Press, 2014); Timothy E. Quill and Franklin G. Miller, *Palliative Care and Ethics* (New York: Oxford University Press, 2014).

9. Susan C. Miller et al., "The Growth of Hospice Care in US Nursing Homes," *Journal of the American Geriatrics Society* 58, no. 8 (2010): 1481–1488.

10. Ira Byock, *The Best Care Possible: A Physician's Quest to Transform Care through the End of Life* (New York: Avery, 2012), 274.

11. Byock, *Best Care Possible*, 273.

12. A. B. Satz, "The Case against Assisted Suicide Reexamined," *Michigan Law Review* 100, no. 6 (2002): 1380–1407; R. F. Weir, ed., *Physician-Assisted Suicide* (Bloomington: Indiana University Press, 1997).

13. Tom L. Beauchamp, "The Justification of Physician-Assisted Deaths," *Indiana Law Review* 29 (1996): 1173–1201.

14. James Werth, *Rational Suicide? Implications for Mental Health Professionals* (Washington, DC: Taylor and Francis, 1996).

15. Neumann, *Good Death*, 144.

16. Lydia Saad, "U.S. Support for Euthanasia Hinges on How It's Described," *Gallup*, May 29, 2013, http://www.gallup.com/poll/162815/supporteuthanasiahingesdescribed .aspx.

17. Ezekiel J. Emanuel, "Euthanasia and Physician-Assisted Suicide: A Review of the Empirical Data from the United States," *Archives of Internal Medicine* 162, no. 2 (2002): 142–152.

18. Emanuel, "Euthanasia and Physician-Assisted Suicide."

19. See, for example, Gerald Dworkin, R. G. Frey, and Sissela Bok, eds., *Euthanasia and Physician-Assisted Suicide* (Cambridge: Cambridge University Press, 1998); Margaret Pabst Battin, Rosamond Rhodes, and Anita Silvers, eds., *Physician-Assisted Suicide: Expanding the Debate* (New York: Routledge, 1998).

20. Neumann, *Good Death*, 244.

21. J. F. Drane, "Physician Assisted Suicide and Voluntary Active Euthanasia: Social Ethics and the Role of Hospice," *American Journal of Hospice and Palliative Medicine* 12, no. 6 (1995): 310.

22. L. O. Gostin, "Drawing a Line between Killing and Letting Die: The Law, and Law Reform, on Medically Assisted Dying," *Journal of Law, Medicine and Ethics* 21, no. 1 (1993): 94101.

23. James Rachels, "Active and Passive Euthanasia," in Kuhse and Singer, *Bioethics*, 288–291.

24. See, for example, Compassion and Choices president Barbara Coombs Lee, "Statement on Canada Euthanasia Bill," April 28, 2016, https://www.compassionand choices.org/compassion-choices-pres-barbara-coombs-lees-statement-on-canada-euthanasia-bill.

25. For example, both Neil M. Gorsuch and Paul K. Longmore acknowledge and condemn uses of WLST as a form of suicide, but neither recommends banning WLST. Gorsuch, *The Future of Assisted Suicide and Euthanasia* (Princeton, NJ: Princeton University Press, 2009); Longmore, "Policy, Prejudice, and Reality: Two Case Studies of Physician-Assisted Suicide," *Journal of Disability Policy Studies* 16, no. 1 (2005): 38–45.

26. Erwin Chemerinsky, *Constitutional Law: Principles and Policies* (New York: Aspen, 2006), 847–854.

27. The advocacy organization Death with Dignity works, in part, to build support for PAS in different states. Its website describes its project as follows: "We're a growing movement that works to ensure terminally ill Americans have the freedom to choose from a full range of end-of-life options, including how they die." https://www.deathwith dignity.org.

28. Ronald M. Green, "Brittany Maynard Was Courageous and Right," *CNN*, November 3, 2014, http://www.cnn.com/2014/11/03/opinion/green-assisted-suicide/index.html.

29. Howard Ball, *At Liberty to Die: The Battle for Death with Dignity in America* (New York: New York University Press, 2012), 6.

30. Rafia Zakaria, "Assisted Suicide Should Be Legal," *Al Jazeera America*, October 24, 2014, http://america.aljazeera.com/opinions/2014/10/assisted-suicidebrittanymaynard oregondeathwithdignity.html.

31. Ronald Dworkin, *Life's Dominion: An Argument about Abortion, Euthanasia, and Individual Freedom* (New York: Knopf, 1993); Derek Humphry and Mary Clement, *Freedom to Die: People, Politics, and the Right-to-Die Movement* (New York: St. Martin's, 1998).

32. John B. Mitchell, "My Father, John Locke, and Assisted Suicide: The Real Constitution Right," *Indiana Health Law Review* 45 (2006): 45–101; John P. Safranek, "Autonomy and Assisted Suicide," *Hastings Center Report* 28, no. 4 (1998): 3236.

33. Isaiah Berlin, *Four Essays on Liberty* (Oxford: Oxford University Press, 1969); Nils Holtug, "The Harm Principle," *Ethical Theory and Moral Practice* 5, no. 4 (2002): 357–389.

34. Thaddeus Mason Pope, "Balancing Public Health against Individual Liberty: The Ethics of Smoking Regulations," *University of Pittsburgh Law Review* 61, no. 2 (2000): 419–498.

35. Bonnie Kristian, "Legalize Heroin," *Week*, September 23, 2016, http://theweek.com/articles/650384/legalize-heroin; Simona Botti and Sheena S. Iyengar, "The Dark Side of Choice: When Choice Impairs Social Welfare," *Journal of Public Policy and Marketing* 25, no. 1 (2006): 24–38.

36. Eric Foner, *The Story of American Freedom* (New York: Norton, 1998).

37. Georges Minois, *History of Suicide: Voluntary Death in Western Culture* (Baltimore, MD: Johns Hopkins University Press, 1999).

38. Minois, *History of Suicide.*

39. Sampedro, *Cartas desde el infierno* (Barcelona, Spain: Planeta, 2004),148 (all translations are mine); Alejandro Amenábar, dir., *The Sea Inside* (Mar Adentro) (Fine Line Features, 2004).

40. Sampedro, *Cartas desde el infierno,* 148.

41. Oregon Public Health Division, "Oregon Death with Dignity Act: 2015 Data Summary," February 4, 2016, 4, https://www.oregon.gov/oha/ph/providerpartnerresources /evaluationresearch/deathwithdignityact/Documents/year18.pdf.

42. For example, C. A. Rodriguez-Osorio and G. Dominguez-Cherit, "Medical Decision Making: Paternalism versus Patient-Centered (Autonomous) Care," *Current Opinion*

in Critical Care 14, no. 6 (2008): 708–713; Gordon M. Stirrat and Robin Gill, "Autonomy in Medical Ethics after O'Neill," *Journal of Medical Ethics* 31, no. 3 (2005): 127–130.

43. Leon Kass, *Life, Liberty, and the Defense of Dignity: The Challenge for Bioethics* (San Francisco, CA: Encounter, 2002).

44. Margaret P. Battin et al., "Legal Physician-Assisted Dying in Oregon and the Netherlands: Evidence concerning the Impact on Patients in 'Vulnerable' Groups," *Journal of Medical Ethics* 33, no. 10 (2007): 591–597; Neil Francis, "Physician Use of Misinformation to Speculate 'Assisted Dying Suicide Contagion' in Oregon," *Journal of Assisted Dying* 1, no. 1 (2016): 1–6.

45. Diane Coleman, "Assisted Suicide Laws Create Discriminatory Double Standard for Who Gets Suicide Prevention and Who Gets Suicide Assistance: Not Dead Yet Responds to Autonomy, Inc.," *Disability and Health Journal* 3, no. 1 (2010): 39–50. Coleman is president of the advocacy group Not Dead Yet (http://notdeadyet.org). See also the work of Wesley J. Smith, which brings together many of the critiques that I discuss in this chapter and some that I omit. Smith, *Forced Exit: Euthanasia, Assisted Suicide, and the New Duty to Die* (New York: Encounter, 2006); Smith, *Culture of Death: The Age of "Do Harm" Medicine* (New York: Encounter, 2016).

46. Howard I. Kushner, "Suicide, Gender, and the Fear of Modernity in Nineteenth-Century Medical and Social Thought," *Journal of Social History* 26, no. 3 (1993): 461–490; Dorothy Roberts, *Fatal Invention: How Science, Politics, and Big Business Re-Create Race in the Twenty-First Century* (New York: New Press, 2011); Sheldon Rubenfeld and Holocaust Museum Houston, *Medicine after the Holocaust: From the Master Race to the Human Genome and Beyond* (New York: Palgrave Macmillan, 2010).

47. Carol Gill, "The False Autonomy of Forced Choice," in *Contemporary Perspectives on Rational Suicide, ed. J. L. Werth (Philadelphia, PA: Brunner/Mazel, 1991)*, 171–180; Longmore, "Policy, Prejudice, and Reality."

48. Felicia Ackerman, "Assisted Suicide, Terminal Illness, Severe Disability, and the Double Standard," in *Physician-Assisted Suicide: Expanding the Debate*, ed. Margaret Pabst Battin, Rosamond Rhodes, and Francis Silver (New York: Routledge, 1998), 149–163.

49. Ackerman, "Assisted Suicide."

50. Joseph P. Shapiro, *No Pity: People with Disabilities Forging a New Civil Rights Movement* (New York: Broadway, 1994).

51. Shapiro, *No Pity*.

52. Longmore, "Policy, Prejudice, and Reality."

53. Atul Gawande, *Being Mortal* (New York: Metropolitan, 2014), 73.

54. Gawande, *Being Mortal*, citing Erving Goffmann, *Asylums: Essays on the Situation of Mental Patients and Other Inmates* (New York: Anchor, 1961).

55. Harriet McBryde Johnson, "The Disability Gulag," *New York Times Magazine*, November 23, 2003, https://www.nytimes.com/2003/11/23/magazine/the-disability-gulag .html.

56. Gawande, *Being Mortal*, 75.

57. There are nursing homes that are exceptions to this characterization, which might serve as models for future long-term care reform. But their existence should not distract

us from the functioning of the nursing home system as a whole, and they do not negate the validity of the disability studies critique.

58. Fiona Kumari Campbell, *Contours of Ableism* (Basingstoke, England: Palgrave Macmillan, 2009); Campbell, "Exploring Internalized Ableism Using Critical Race Theory," *Disability and Society* 23, no. 2 (2008): 151–162; Nick Hodge and Katherine RunswickCole, "'They Never Pass Me the Ball': Exposing Ableism through the Leisure Experiences of Disabled Children, Young People and Their Families," *Children's Geographies* 11, no. 3 (2013): 311–325.

59. Harold Braswell and Howard I. Kushner, "Suicide, Social Integration, and Masculinity in the US Military," *Social Science and Medicine* 74, no. 4 (2012): 530–536; Faye Gary, Hossein N. Yarandi, and Floydette C. Scruggs, "Suicide among African Americans: Reflections and a Call to Action," *Issues in Mental Health Nursing* 24, no. 3 (2003): 353–375; Diana van Bergen et al., "Suicidal Behaviour of Young Immigrant Women in the Netherlands: Can We Use Durkheim's Concept of 'Fatalistic Suicide' to Explain Their High Incidence of Attempted Suicide?," *Ethnic and Racial Studies* 32, no. 2 (2009): 302–322.

60. Carol J. Gill, "Suicide Intervention for People with Disabilities: A Lesson in Inequality," *Issues in Law and Medicine* 8 (1992): 37–53; Margaret J. Giannini et al., "Understanding Suicide and Disability through Three Major Disabling Conditions: Intellectual Disability, Spinal Cord Injury, and Multiple Sclerosis," *Disability and Health Journal* 3, no. 2 (2010): 74–78.

61. Gill, "False Autonomy of Forced Choice."

62. Andrew Batavia, "Disability and Physician-Assisted Suicide," *New England Journal of Medicine* 336, no. 23 (1997): 1671–1673; Lennard Davis, *The End of Normal* (Ann Arbor: University of Michigan Press, 2013), 95–107; Scott Jaschik, "Rift in Disability Studies," *Inside Higher Ed*, October 5, 2005, http://www.insidehighered.com/news/2005/10/05/disability.

63. Davis, *End of Normal*.

64. Davis, *End of Normal*.

65. Batavia, "Disability and Physician-Assisted Suicide"; Davis, *End of Normal*.

66. Davis, *End of Normal*.

67. Batavia, "Disability and Physician-Assisted Suicide"; Davis, *End of Normal*; Samuel R. Bagenstos, *Law and the Contradictions of the Disability Rights Movement* (New Haven, CT: Yale University Press, 2014), 95–115.

68. For some examples of this argument, see Ira R. Byock, "Consciously Walking the Fine Line: Thoughts on a Hospice Response to Assisted Suicide and Euthanasia," *Journal of Palliative Care* 9, no. 3 (1993): 25–28; David Cundiff, *Euthanasia Is Not the Answer: A Hospice Physician's View* (New York: Humana, 1992); Kathleen Foley and Herbert Hendin, eds., *The Case against Assisted Suicide: For the Right to End-of-Life Care* (Baltimore, MD: Johns Hopkins University Press, 2002).

69. Timothy E. Quill, Christine K. Cassel, and Diane E. Meier, "Care of the Hopelessly Ill: Proposed Clinical Criteria for Physician-Assisted Suicide," in *Health Care Ethics: Critical Issues for the Twenty-First Century*, ed. John F. Monagle and David C. Thomasma

(Sudbury, MA: Jones and Bartlett, 2005), 295–301; Franklin G. Miller et al., "Regulating Physician-Assisted Death," *New England Journal of Medicine* 331, no. 2 (1994): 119–123; Constance E. Putnam, *Hospice or Hemlock? Searching for Heroic Compassion* (Westport, CT: Greenwood, 2002).

70. For one example of such a critical appreciation, see Byock, *Best Care Possible*.

71. For example, see Shapiro, *No Pity*.

72. Les Gallo-Silver, David Bimbi, and Michael Rembis, "Reclaiming the Sexual Rights of LGBTQ People with Attendant Care Dependent Mobility Impairments," in *Disabling Domesticity*, ed. Michael Rembis (New York: Palgrave Macmillan, 2017), 195–213; Stephen H. Kaye and Charlene Harrington, "Long-Term Services and Supports in the Community: Toward a Research Agenda," *Disability and Health Journal* 8, no. 1 (2015): 3–8.

73. Neumann, *Good Death*, 135–162. For a characteristically witty and intelligent cataloging of distortions that PAS advocates make of disability studies arguments, see Carol J. Gill, " 'No, We Don't Think Our Doctors Are Out to Get Us': Responding to the Straw Man Distortions of Disability Rights Arguments against Assisted Suicide," *Disability and Health Journal* 3, no. 1 (2010): 31–38.

74. Margrit Shildrick, "Deciding on Death: Conventions and Contestations in the Context of Disability," *Journal of Bioethical Inquiry* 5, nos. 2–3 (2008): 209–219.

Chapter 2. Depending on the Family

1. Shirley Du Boulay, *Cicely Saunders, Founder of the Modern Hospice Movement* (London: Hodder and Stoughton, 1984), 33–34; Cicely Saunders, "A Place to Die," in her *Selected Writings, 1958–2004*, ed. David Clark (Oxford: Oxford University Press, 2006), 124–128; Saunders, "Hospice: A Meeting Place for Religion and Science," in her *Selected Writings*, 223–228.

2. Saunders, "Hospice," 224.

3. Du Boulay, *Cicely Saunders*, 33.

4. Du Boulay, *Cicely Saunders*, 34.

5. Du Boulay, *Cicely Saunders*, 36.

6. On the origins of the modern hospice movement, and its differences from and similarities to its religious forebears, see David Clark, "Originating a Movement: Cicely Saunders and the Development of St. Christopher's Hospice, 1957–1967," *Mortality* 3, no. 1 (1998): 43–63; Clark, "Religion, Medicine, and Community in the Early Origins of St. Christopher's Hospice," *Journal of Palliative Medicine* 4, no. 3 (2001): 353–360. See also Cathy Siebold, *The Hospice Movement: Easing Death's Pains* (New York: Twayne, 1992); Grace Goldin, "A Protohospice at the Turn of the Century: St. Luke's House, London, from 1893 to 1921," *Journal of the History of Medicine and Allied Sciences* 6 (1981): 383–415; Claire Humphreys, " 'Waiting for the Last Summons': The Establishment of the First Hospices in England, 1878–1914," *Mortality* 6 (2001): 146–166; Michelle Winslow and David Clark, "St. Joseph's Hospice, Hackney: Documenting a Centenary History," *Progress in Palliative Care* 14 (2006): 68–74.

7. Joan Craven and Florence S. Wald, "Hospice Care for Dying Patients," *American Journal of Nursing* (1975): 1816–1822, box 3, folder 28, acc. no. 2001-M-047, Florence and

Henry Wald Papers, Sterling Memorial Library, Yale University (hereafter, Wald Papers); Peter Hudson, Sanchia Aranda, and Linda J. Kristjanson, "Meeting the Supportive Needs of Family Caregivers in Palliative Care: Challenges for Health Professionals," *Journal of Palliative Medicine* 7, no. 1 (2004): 19–25; Joan K. Parry and Michael J. Smith, "The Significance of the Patient/Family as a Unit of Care in Working with Terminally Ill Patients," *Hospice Journal* 1, no. 3 (1985): 37–49.

8. Craven and Wald, "Hospice Care for Dying Patients."

9. Du Boulay, *Cicely Saunders*, 33–34.

10. Commonwealth War Graves Commission, Annual Report 2014–2015, 38, https://issuu.com/wargravescommission/docs/ar_2014–2015?e=4065448/31764375.

11. See John Bowlby, Emanuel Miller, and Donald Winnicott, "Letter to the British Medical Journal" (1939), and Donald W. Winnicott, "Children in the War" (1940), both reprinted in *Deprivation and Delinquency*, ed. C. Winnicott, R. Shepherd, and M. Davis (New York: Brunner Routledge, 1984), 13–14 and 25–30, both cited in Lisa Farley, "'Operation Pied Piper': A Psychoanalytic Narrative of Authority in a Time of War," *Psychoanalysis and History* 14, no. 1 (2012): 29–52.

12. Marc Calvini-Lefebvre, "The Great War in the History of British Feminism: Debates and Controversies, 1914 to the Present," *Revue Française de Civilisation Britannique / French Journal of British Studies* 20, no. 1 (2015): 1–17; Margaret R. Higonnet, *Behind the Lines: Gender and the Two World Wars* (New Haven, CT: Yale University Press, 1987).

13. David Clark, "Cradled to the Grave? Terminal Care in the United Kingdom, 1948–67," *Mortality* 4, no. 3 (1999): 225–247.

14. Clark, "Cradled to the Grave?"

15. Du Boulay, *Cicely Saunders*, 56.

16. Clark, "Cradled to the Grave?"

17. Du Boulay, *Cicely Saunders*, 56.

18. David Clark, "'Total Pain,' Disciplinary Power and the Body in the Work of Cicely Saunders, 1958–1967," *Social Science and Medicine* 49, no. 6 (1999): 727–736.

19. Clark, "Total Pain."

20. Du Boulay, *Cicely Saunders*, 110.

21. Du Boulay, *Cicely Saunders*, 61.

22. Cicely Saunders, "A Death in the Family: A Professional View," *British Medical Journal* 1, no. 5844 (1973): 31.

23. Sylvia A. Lack and Robert W. Buckingham III, *First American Hospice: Three Years of Home Care* (New Haven, CT: Hospice Inc., 1978).

24. M. J. Friedrich, "Hospice Care in the United States: A Conversation with Florence S. Wald," *JAMA* 281, no. 18 (1999): 1683–1685.

25. Florence Wald, "Untitled [Protocol for Nurse's Study of the Dying Patient]," box 20, folder 21, Wald Papers.

26. "Certificate of Incorporation: Hospice Inc.," box 3, folder 32, acc. no. 2001-M-047, Wald Papers.

27. Edward F. Dobihal, "To Honor All Life: The Case for Support of Hospice Inc.," 1975, 3, box 3, folder 23, Wald Papers.

28. "A Hospice for New Haven," May 5, 1972, box 9, folder 109, Wald Papers.

29. "A Hospice for New Haven."

30. Guidelines for Patient Selection, Home Care Program, August 7, 1972, box 1, folder 10, Wald Papers.

31. Minutes of Meeting, "Interdisciplinary Study of the Dying Patient," research conference, October 29, 1970, revised January 5, 1971, box 7, folder 79, Wald Papers.

32. Letter from Arthur Mazer to Robert A. Devries, April 3, 1973, box 9, folder 111, Wald Papers.

33. Letter from Florence Wald, Morris Wessel, Edward Dobihal, and Ira Goldberg to Margaret Arnstein, Frederik Redlich, Collin Williams, and Charles Womer, February 18, 1971, box 4, folder 34, Wald Papers.

34. Memorandum, Patient Care Spaces, from M. Carney, C. Gray, S. Isenberg, C. Tiernan, and F. Wald to Lo-Yi Chan, March 5, 1973, box 1, folder 3, Wald Papers; Lawrence Kerns, "A Study of the Creation of a Community Setting: Hospice," box 3, folder 24, Wald Papers.

35. Wald, "Untitled [Protocol for Nurse's Study of the Dying Patient]."

36. Memorandum from Members of the Planning Staff to Board of Directors, July 2, 1973, box 1, folder 11, Wald Papers.

37. "Patients Offered a Helping Hand," *Waterbury Republican*, April 24, 1974, box 1, folder 6, Wald Papers.

38. "Needed: Ethic Imperative for Death and Dying," *Roche Report: Frontiers of Psychiatry*, January 15, 1975, box 10, folder 124, Wald Papers. See also "Patients Offered a Helping Hand," which described the goal of hospice as being to keep patients "at home as long as possible before they have to be admitted to the in-patient program."

39. See, for example, Henry Wald, "A Hospice for Terminally Ill Patients," May 21, 1971, box 21, folder 41–42, 26, Wald Papers.

40. Wald, "Untitled [Protocol for Nurse's Study of the Dying Patient]."

41. Morris Wessel, "To Comfort Always," *Yale Alumni Magazine*, June 1972, box 3, folder 25, Wald Papers.

42. Wald, "Untitled [Protocol for Nurse's Study of the Dying Patient]."

43. Wald, "Untitled [Protocol for Nurse's Study of the Dying Patient]."

44. Wald, "Untitled [Protocol for Nurse's Study of the Dying Patient]."

45. Wald, "Untitled [Protocol for Nurse's Study of the Dying Patient]."

46. Wessel, "To Comfort Always."

47. "Needed: Ethic Imperative for Death and Dying."

48. "Needed: Ethic Imperative for Death and Dying."

49. Wald, "Untitled [Protocol for Nurse's Study of the Dying Patient]."

50. Wald, "Untitled [Protocol for Nurse's Study of the Dying Patient]."

51. Patricia McCormack, "Hospice Movement Helps Terminally Ill and Their Families," United Press International, March 10, 1977, box 4, folder 46, Wald Papers.

52. Memorandum on Religious Spaces from E. Dobihal, G. Goldin, H. Klein, S. Montgomery, K. Tripp, and F. Wald to Lo-Yi Chan, March 5, 1973, box 1, folder 3, Wald Papers; memorandum, Patient Care Spaces.

53. Board of Directors Meeting, August 13, 1973, box 1, folder 11, Wald Papers.

54. Newsletter, "Hospice . . . a Vision," April 1973, box 7, folder 86, Wald Papers; memorandum, Patient Care Spaces.

55. Kerns, "Study of the Creation of a Community Setting."

56. Arthur Mazer, "Summary of Meeting with Connecticut Blue Cross," June 11, 1973, box 9, folder 111, Wald Papers; Board of Directors Meeting, August 13, 1973. A larger description of the struggle for licensure is in Kerns, "Study of the Creation of a Community Setting."

57. Benjamin C. Bloom, "Reimbursement under Medicare and Medicaid for Hospice Inc.," box 4, folder 78, Wald Papers; Board of Directors Meeting, January 12, 1977, box 2, folder 18, Wald Papers; Board of Directors Meeting, August 10, 1977, box 2, folder 19, Wald Papers.

58. Kerns, "Study of the Creation of a Community Setting."

59. Annual Report of Planning of Hospice Coordinated Inpatient–Home Care Facility, January 1, 1974–August 31, 1974, box 1, folder 3, Wald Papers; letter from Lo-Yi Chan to Florence Wald, November 22, 1974, box 3, folder 24, Wald Papers.

60. Kerns, "Study of the Creation of a Community Setting," 1; "Certificate of Incorporation," 26.

61. Lack and Buckingham, *First American Hospice*, 17.

62. Letter from Franklin M. Foote to Reed Nelson, September 13, 1973, box 9, folder 105, Wald Papers.

63. Kerns, "Study of the Creation of a Community Setting."

64. Regional Hospice Development Program, "Progress Report for 1972–3," January 29, 1973, box 1, folder 6, Edward F. Dobihal Papers, Sterling Memorial Library, Yale University (hereafter, Dobihal Papers).

65. Regional Hospice Development Program, "Progress Report"; letter from Florence Wald to Members of the Board, January 4, 1974, box 10, folder 120, Wald Papers.

66. Memorandum, Kraushaar to Murdock, Spoor, Dobihal, and Ward, March 27, 1975.

67. Finance Task Force Meeting Minutes, May 21, 1973, box 9, folder 110, Wald Papers.

68. Bureau of Labor Statistics, CPI Inflation Calculator, https://www.bls.gov/data /inflation_calculator.htm.

69. Letter from Edward Dobihal to Florence Wald, February 5, 1975, box 9, folder 107, Wald Papers.

70. Board of Directors Meeting, August 13, 1973, and March 5, 1973, box 1, folder 11, Wald Papers.

71. Annual Report of Planning of Hospice Coordinated Inpatient–Home Care Facility.

72. Memorandum regarding Work Flow of Planning Staff, 5/1/73–6/21/73, from Planning Staff to Board of Directors, May 2, 1973, box 1, folder 11, Wald Papers.

73. Ned Thomas, "Hospice Aims for '76 Opening: Site Not Disclosed," *New Haven Register*, April 24, 1974, box 1, folder 6, Wald Papers.

74. Letter from Dobihal to Wald, February 5, 1975.

75. Mazer, "Summary of Meeting with Connecticut Blue Cross"; newsletter, *Hospice*, January–March 1977, box 1, folder 4, Dobihal Papers.

76. Board of Directors Meeting, January 12, 1977; Board of Directors Meeting, August 10, 1977.

77. Board of Directors Meeting, August 10, 1977.

78. Paul Starr, *Remedy and Reaction: The Peculiar American Struggle over Health Care Reform* (New Haven, CT: Yale University Press, 2011).

79. "AMA Panel Urges Sweeping Reforms," *Parade Magazine*, December 4, 1977, box 3, folder 26, Wald Papers.

80. "AMA Panel Urges Sweeping Reforms."

81. Hospice Planning Group, Philosophy Statement, April 7, 1971, box 1, folder 5, Dobihal Papers.

82. Discussion Group on Religious Foundations, September 22, 1971, box 1, folder 14, Dobihal Papers.

83. Summary of Meeting between Sara E. Hartman, David Stockton, and Henry Wald, December 6, 1971, box 1, folder 9, Wald Papers.

84. Memorandum, Donald C. Kraushaar to John A. Murdock, Ralph Spoor, Edward F. Dobihal, and Ralph W. Ward, March 27, 1975, box 4, folder 34, Wald Papers.

85. Letter from Paul Sanazaro to Edward Dobihal, January 27, 1972, box 6, folder 63, Wald Papers.

86. Special Meeting of the Board of Directors, January 30, 1974, box 2, folder 12, Wald Papers.

87. Special Meeting of the Board of Directors, January 30, 1974.

88. Edward Dobihal and Dennis Rezendes, Working Draft of "Goals of Hospice" for Hospice Structure Committee, August 6, 1975, box 1, folder 9, Dobihal Papers.

89. David Rhinelander, "Hospice Center Finds State Site," *Hartford Courant*, May 11, 1974, box 3, folder 25, Wald Papers.

90. Henry J. Wald, "Rethinking Care for the Terminally Ill: Hospice: Reason, Responsibility, and Reaction," January 14, 1978, box 21, folder 46, Wald Papers.

91. Letter from Henry J. Wald to Patrick Crossman, March 28, 1977, box 10, folder 125, Wald Papers.

92. Guidelines for Patient Selection, Home Care Program, August 7, 1972, box 1, folder 10, Wald Papers.

93. Summary of Meeting between Sara E. Hartman, David Stockton, and Henry Wald, December 6, 1971, box 1, folder 9, Wald Papers.

94. Kerns, "Study of the Creation of a Community Setting"; Board of Directors Meeting, February 16, 1978, box 2, folder 21, Wald Papers.

95. See, for example, Wald, "Hospice for Terminally Ill Patients."

96. Trish Hall, "Hospice Defended before State Panel," *Journal Courier*, May 21, 1974, box 3, folder 25, Wald Papers.

97. State of Connecticut, "State Department of Health [Regulations] concerning Short-Term Hospitals, Special, Hospice," January 18, 1979, box 4, folder 48, Wald Papers.

98. Board of Directors Meeting, August 10, 1977.

99. Board of Directors Meeting, August 10, 1977.

100. On Beecher's views regarding the right to be left alone, see Gary S. Belkin, *Death before Dying* (Oxford: Oxford University Press, 2014), 51.

101. Maxine Baca Zinn, "Family, Feminism, and Race in America," *Gender and Society* 4, no. 1 (1990): 68–82; Patricia Hill Collins, "It's All in the Family: Intersections of Gender, Race, and Nation," *Hypatia* 13, no. 3 (1998): 62–82; Martha Fineman, *The Neutered Mother, the Sexual Family and Other Twentieth Century Tragedies* (London: Routledge, 1995); Dorothy Roberts, *Killing the Black Body: Race, Reproduction, and the Meaning of Liberty* (New York: Vintage, 1995).

102. Collins, "It's All in the Family"; Fineman, *Neutered Mother*; Roberts, *Killing the Black Body*.

103. Brown, "Between Neoliberalism and Cultural Conservatism."

104. Emily K. Abel, "The Hospice Movement: Institutionalizing Innovation," *International Journal of Health Services* 16, no. 1 (1986): 71–85.

105. Abel, "Hospice Movement," 84–85.

106. Cathy Siebold, *The Hospice Movement: Easing Death's Pains* (New York: Twayne, 1992); Sandol Stoddard, *Hospice Movement: A Better Way of Caring for the Dying* (New York: Vintage, 1992); Nicky James and David Field, "The Routinization of Hospice," *Social Science and Medicine* 34, no. 12 (1992): 1363–1375; Foley and Hendin, *Case against Assisted Suicide*.

107. Dennis Rezendes, letter to Hospice Board of Directors and Greater New Haven Capital Fund Driven Committee re: D. L. Ansley Letter, March 3, 1976, box 2, folder 16, Wald Papers.

108. Hospice Inc., "Statement on Euthanasia," 1976, box 2, folder 16, Wald Papers; also available in box 8, folder 95.

109. James Rachels, "Active and Passive Euthanasia," in *Bioethics: An Anthology*, 2nd ed., ed. Helga Kuhse and Peter Singer (Oxford: Blackwell, 2006), 288–291.

110. Rachels, "Active and Passive Euthanasia"; Peter Singer, "Voluntary Euthanasia: A Utilitarian Perspective," *Bioethics* 17, no. 5 (2003): 526–541.

111. Rachels, "Active and Passive Euthanasia"; Singer, "Voluntary Euthanasia."

112. Howard Ball, *At Liberty to Die: The Battle for Death with Dignity in America* (New York: New York University Press, 2012).

113. Belkin, *Death before Dying*, 51.

114. On the importance of individual liberty to the American euthanasia movement, see Ian Dowbiggin, *A Merciful End: The Euthanasia Movement in Modern America* (Oxford: Oxford University Press, 2003).

115. Doris Zames Fleischer and Frieda Zames, *The Disability Rights Movement: From Charity to Confrontation* (Philadelphia, PA: Temple University Press, 2012).

116. Fleischer and Zames, *Disability Rights Movement*; Shapiro, *No Pity*; Richard Scotch, *From Good Will to Civil Rights: Transforming Federal Disability Policy* (Philadelphia, PA: Temple University Press, 2001).

117. Edward F. Dobihal, "Progress Report: First Observations and Impressions of St. Christopher's Hospice," September 15, 1970, box 1, folder 14, Dobihal Papers.

118. Emily K. Abel, *The Inevitable Hour: A History of Caring for Dying Patients in America* (Baltimore, MD: Johns Hopkins University Press, 2013), 57–87.

119. Fleischer and Zames, *Disability Rights Movement*; Shapiro, *No Pity*; Harriet McBryde Johnson, "The Disability Gulag," *New York Times Magazine*, November 23, 2003, http://www.nytimes.com/2003/11/23/magazine/the-disability-gulag.html.

120. "A particular focal point [of hospice] is the terminally ill patient and the inappropriate care arrangements which now exist to meet patient and family needs in the typical pattern of acute, general hospital, nursing home, chronic disease institutions, and home care." Connecticut Regional Medical Program Review and Evaluation Committee Report to Executive Committee, April 10, 1972, box 1, folder 10, Wald Papers.

121. Kerns, "Study of the Creation of a Community Setting."

122. This conflation is seen in the frequent representation of disability as a memento mori, which has been used to justify the denial of resources to people with disabilities. See Lennard Davis, introduction to *The Disability Studies Reader* (New York: Routledge, 1997), 1–6.

123. On the centrality of employment to disability rights, see Bagenstos, *Law and the Contradictions*; Ruth Colker, *The Disability Pendulum: The First Decade of the Americans with Disabilities Act* (New York: New York University Press, 2006).

124. Bagenstos, *Law and the Contradictions*; Lennard Davis, *Enabling Acts: The Hidden Story of How the Americans with Disabilities Act Gave the Largest US Minority Its Rights* (Boston: Beacon, 2016).

125. Davis, *Enabling Acts*, 10.

126. Davis, *Enabling Acts*, 11.

127. Davis, *Enabling Acts*, 11.

128. Section 504, Rehabilitation Act of 1973 (29 USC § 701), https://www.dol.gov /oasam/regs/statutes/sec504.htm.

129. Davis, *Enabling Acts*, 11.

130. Davis, *Enabling Acts*.

131. Letter from Mark R. Kravitz to Vincent Prota, August 9, 1977, box 3, folder 32, Wald Papers. This document was attached to a memorandum from Dennis Rezendes to the Building Committee, Executive Committee, Joint Conference Committee, and Lo-Yi Chan, August 22, 1977.

132. Letter from Kravitz to Prota, August 9, 1977.

133. Larry Beresford and Stephen Connor, "History of the National Hospice Organization," *Hospice Journal* 14, nos. 3–4 (1999): 15–31.

134. "Administrator Testifies on Hospice Legislation," *Connecticut Hospice Newsletter* 8, no. 1 (Winter–Spring 1982): 2, box 1, folder 4, Dobihal Papers.

Chapter 3. Birth of a Crisis

1. Ira Byock, *The Best Care Possible: A Physician's Quest to Transform Care through the End of Life* (New York: Avery, 2012), 250, emphasis in original.

2. Emily K. Abel, *Living in Death's Shadow* (Baltimore, MD: Johns Hopkins University Press, 2017), 117.

3. National Hospice and Palliative Care Organization, "The Medicare Hospice Benefit," October 2015, http://www.nhpco.org/sites/default/files/public/communications /Outreach/The_Medicare_Hospice_Benefit.pdf; Herbert Lukashok, "Hospice Care under Medicare: An Early Look," *Preventive Medicine* 19, no. 6 (1990): 730–736; L. F. Paradis and S. B. Cummings, "The Evolution of Hospice in America toward Organizational Homogeneity," *Journal of Health and Social Behavior* 27, no. 4 (1986): 370–386; Medicare Regula-

tions for Hospice Care, including the Conditions of Participation for Hospice Care, 42 CFR 418, current as of July 29, 2011, https://oregonhospice.org/media/Medicare Regulations-for-Hospice-Care-with-COPs-for-Hospice-Care-CFR418.pdf; Cathy Siebold, *The Hospice Movement: Easing Death's Pains* (New York: Twayne, 1992); Joy Buck, "'From Rites to Rights of Passage: Ideals, Politics, and the Evolution of the American Hospice Movement," in *Hospice Ethics: Policy and Practice in Palliative Care,* ed. Timothy W. Kirk and Bruce Jennings (Oxford: Oxford University Press, 2014), 13–34; Thomas Hoyer, "A History of the Medicare Hospice Benefit," *Hospice Journal* 13 (1998): 61–70.

4. Paradis and Cummings, "Evolution of Hospice in America."

5. Buck, "From Rites to Rights of Passage," 25.

6. Florence Wald, Henry Wald, and Zelda Foster, "The Hospice Movement as a Health Care Reform," article submitted to the *New England Journal of Medicine,* November 21, 1978, box 21, folder 40, Florence and Henry Wald Papers, Sterling Memorial Library, Yale University (hereafter, Wald Papers); Joy Buck, "Policy and the Re-Formation of Hospice: Lessons from the Past for the Future of Palliative Care," *Journal of Hospice and Palliative Nursing* 13, no. 6 (2011): 5; Larry Beresford and Stephen R. Connor, "History of the National Hospice Organization," *Hospice Journal* 14, nos. 3–4 (1999): 15–31.

7. Buck, "From Rites to Rights of Passage," 25–27.

8. Board of Directors Meeting, February 9, 1977, box 2, folder 20, Wald Papers.

9. Buck, "From Rites to Rights of Passage," 26.

10. On deinstitutionalization and neoliberalism, see Terry Carney, "The Mental Health Service Crisis of Neoliberalism: An Antipodean Perspective," *International Journal of Law and Psychiatry* 31, no. 2 (2008): 101–115.

11. Beresford and Connor, "History of the National Hospice Organization," 21; Buck, "From Rites to Rights of Passage," 26.

12. Lukashok, "Hospice Care under Medicare"; Paradis and Cummings, "Evolution of Hospice in America"; Medicare Regulations for Hospice Care; Siebold, *Hospice Movement.*

13. Lukashok, "Hospice Care under Medicare," 732.

14. Ann Neumann, *The Good Death: An Exploration of Dying in America* (Boston: Beacon, 2016), 34; Judy L. Meyers and Louis N. Gray, "The Relationships between Family Primary Caregiver Characteristics and Satisfaction with Hospice Care, Quality of Life, and Burden," *Oncology Nursing Forum* 28, no. 1 (2001): 73–82; R. G. Steele and M. I. Fitch, "Needs of Family Caregivers of Patients Receiving Home Hospice Care for Cancer," *Oncology Nursing Forum* 23, no. 5 (1996): 823–828.

15. Conditions of Participation for Hospice Care, 42 CFR 418.76.

16. Conditions of Participation for Hospice Care, 42 CFR 418.78.

17. Joan M. Teno et al., "Change in End-of-Life Care for Medicare Beneficiaries: Site of Death, Place of Care, and Health Care Transitions in 2000, 2005, and 2009," *JAMA* 309, no. 5 (2013): 470–477; P. J. Miller and P. B. Mike, "The Medicare Hospice Benefit: Ten Years of Federal Policy for the Terminally Ill," *Death Studies* 19, no. 6 (1995): 531–542.

18. "Administrator Testifies on Hospice Legislation," *Connecticut Hospice Newsletter* 8, no. 1 (Winter–Spring 1982): 2, box 1, folder 4, Edward F. Dobihal Papers, Sterling Memorial Library, Yale University.

19. Vincent Mor, with the assistance of Susan Masterson-Allen, *Hospice Care Systems: Structure, Process, Costs, and Outcome* (New York: Springer, 1987).

20. Michael Preodor and Sally Owen-Still, "Care of the Terminally Ill," *New England Journal of Medicine* 310, no. 17 (1984): 1127–1128, cited in Mor, *Hospice Care Systems*, 13.

21. Donald E. Gibson, "Hospice and the New Devaluation of Human Life," *Mental Retardation* 22, no. 4 (1984): 157–169, cited in Mor, *Hospice Care Systems*, 13–14.

22. Abel, *Living in Death's Shadow*, 127.

23. Emily K. Abel, *The Inevitable Hour* (Baltimore, MD: Johns Hopkins University Press, 2013), 58–62.

24. Paul Starr, *The Social Transformation of American Medicine* (New York: Basic, 1982), 73; Emily K. Abel, *Hearts of Wisdom: American Women Caring for Kin, 1850–1940* (Cambridge, MA: Harvard University Press, 2000); Abel, *Inevitable Hour*, 81–85.

25. Steven Mintz and Susan Kellogg, *Domestic Revolutions: A Social History of American Family Life* (New York: Free Press, 1988); Andrew J. Cherlin, *Public and Private Families: An Introduction*, 6th ed. (New York: McGraw-Hill, 2010), 315.

26. Philip N. Cohen, *The Family: Diversity, Inequality, and Social Change* (New York: Norton, 2015), 48.

27. Eli Zaretsky, *Capitalism, the Family and Personal Life* (New York: Harper and Row, 1976).

28. Abel, *Inevitable Hour*; Sharon Kaufman, *And a Time to Die: How American Hospitals Shape the End of Life* (Chicago: University of Chicago Press, 2005).

29. Starr, *Social Transformation of American Medicine*.

30. Shai Joshua Lavi, *The Modern Art of Dying: A History of Euthanasia in the United States* (Princeton, NJ: Princeton University Press, 2005).

31. Cohen, *The Family*, 42; Orlando Patterson, *Slavery and Social Death: A Comparative Study* (Cambridge, MA: Harvard University Press, 1982); Evelyn Nakano Glenn, *Forced to Care: Coercion and Caregiving in America* (Cambridge, MA: Harvard University Press, 2010).

32. David Peterson del Mar, *The American Family: From Obligation to Freedom* (New York: Palgrave Macmillan, 2011), 23–35; Russell Thornton, *American Indian Holocaust and Survival: A Population History since 1492* (Norman: University of Oklahoma Press, 1987); Andrea Smith, *Conquest: Sexual Violence and American Indian Genocide* (Durham, NC: Duke University Press, 2015).

33. Wilma A. Dunaway, *The African-American Family in Slavery and Emancipation* (New York: Maison des Sciences de l'Homme / Cambridge University Press, 2003); Deborah J. Jones and Kristin M. Lindahl, *Coparenting in Extended Kinship Systems: African American, Hispanic, Asian Heritage, and Native American Families* (Washington, DC: American Psychological Association, 2011).

34. Glenn, *Forced to Care*.

35. Roxanne Dunbar-Ortiz, *An Indigenous Peoples' History of the United States* (Boston: Beacon, 2014).

36. Mintz and Kellogg, *Domestic Revolutions*, 83–106; Zaretsky, *Capitalism, the Family and Personal Life*, 40–58; Cohen, *The Family*, 43.

37. Cohen, *The Family*, 22.

38. Del Mar, *American Family*.

39. Raven Molloy, Christopher L. Smith, and Abigail Wozniak, "Internal Migration in the United States," *Journal of Economic Perspectives* 25, no. 3 (2011): 173–196.

40. Larry Long, "Residential Mobility Differences among Developed Countries," *International Regional Science Review* 14, no. 2 (1991): 133–147.

41. Cohen, *The Family*, 61, citing Jeremy Greenwood, Ananth Seshadri, and Mehmet Yorukoglu, "Engines of Liberation," *Review of Economic Studies* 72, no. 1 (2005): 109–133.

42. Linda Gordon, "Voluntary Motherhood: The Beginnings of Feminist Birth Control Ideas in the United States," *Feminist Studies* 1, nos. 3–4 (1973): 5–22; Elizabeth Bortolaia Silva, "The Transformation of Mothering," in *Good Enough Mothering*, ed. Elizabeth Bortolaia Silva (London: Routledge, 1996), 10–36.

43. Glenn, *Forced to Care*; Anne-Marie Slaughter, "Why Women Still Can't Have It All," *Atlantic*, July–August 2012, http://www.theatlantic.com/magazine/archive/2012/07/why-women-still-cant-have-it-all/309020.

44. Cohen, *The Family*, 351.

45. Cohen, *The Family*, 351, citing Robert Schoen and Vladimir Canudas-Romo, "Timing Effects on Divorce: Twentieth Century Experience in the United States," *Journal of Marriage and Family* 68, no. 3 (2006): 749–758.

46. Cohen, *The Family*, 353.

47. Cherlin, *Public and Private Families*, 333.

48. Madison Park, "US Fertility Rate Falls to Lowest on Record," August 11, 2016, *CNN*, http://www.cnn.com/2016/08/11/health/us-lowest-fertility-rate.

49. Cohen, *The Family*, 33, citing Joyce A. Martin et al., "Births: Final Data for 2010," *National Vital Statistics Reports* 61, no. 1 (2012): 1–72.

50. Tony Mander, "Longevity and Healthy Ageing: Will Healthcare Be Drowned by the Grey Tsunami or Sunk by the Demographic Iceberg?," *Post Reproductive Health* 20, no. 1 (2014): 8–10.

51. Anne A. Scitovsky, "The High Cost of Dying: What Do the Data Show?," *Milbank Memorial Fund Quarterly* 64, no. 4 (1984): 591–608.

52. Lavi, *Modern Art of Dying*.

53. Abel, *Hearts of Wisdom*.

54. Sidney D. Watson, "From Almshouses to Nursing Homes and Community Care: Lessons from Medicaid's History," *Georgia State University Law Review* 26 (2009): 937–969.

55. Cherlin, *Public and Private Families*, 307.

56. Brian Gratton, and Carole Haber, "In Search of 'Intimacy at a Distance': Family History from the Perspective of Elderly Women," *Journal of Aging Studies* 7, no. 2 (1993): 183–194.

57. John Silk, "Caring at a Distance," *Ethics, Place and Environment* 1, no. 2 (1998): 165–182.

58. Paul Starr, *Remedy and Reaction: The Peculiar American Struggle over Health Care Reform* (New Haven, CT: Yale University Press, 2011), 41–50.

59. Omar Ahmad, "Medicaid Eligibility Rules for the Elderly Long-Term Care Applicant: History and Developments, 1965–1998," *Journal of Legal Medicine* 20, no. 2 (1999): 251–280.

60. "Evaluating the Success of the Great Society," *Washington Post*, May 17, 2014, http://www.washingtonpost.com/wp-srv/special/national/great-society-at-50.

61. Daniel B. Rodriguez and Barry R. Weingast, "The Positive Political Theory of Legislative History: New Perspectives on the 1964 Civil Rights Act and Its Interpretation," *University of Pennsylvania Law Review* 151, no. 4 (2003): 1417–1542.

62. Arnold R. Hirsch, *Making the Second Ghetto: Race and Housing in Chicago, 1940–1960* (Cambridge: Cambridge University Press, 1983); David M. Oshinsky, *Worse than Slavery: Parchman Farm and the Ordeal of Jim Crow Justice* (New York: Free Press, 1996).

63. Ira Katznelson, *When Affirmative Action Was White: An Untold History of Racial Inequality in Twentieth-Century America* (New York: Norton, 2005).

64. David R. Williams and Chiquita Collins, "Racial Residential Segregation: A Fundamental Cause of Racial Disparities in Health," *Public Health Reports* 116, no. 5 (2001): 404–416.

65. Douglas S. Massey and Nancy A. Denton, *American Apartheid: Segregation and the Making of the Underclass* (Cambridge, MA: Harvard University Press, 1993).

66. Carol B. Stack, *All Our Kin: Strategies for Survival in a Black Community* (New York: Harper and Row, 1974).

67. Melvin N. Wilson, "The Black Extended Family: An Analytical Consideration," *Developmental Psychology* 22, no. 2 (1986): 246–258.

68. Evelyn Nakano Glenn, "From Servitude to Service Work: Historical Continuities in the Racial Division of Paid Reproductive Labor," *Signs* 18, no. 1 (1992): 1–43; Rose M. Brewer, "Theorizing Race, Class and Gender: The New Scholarship of Black Feminist Intellectuals and Black Women's Labor," *Race, Gender and Class* 6, no. 2 (1999): 29–47.

69. Cohen, *The Family*, 404, citing Harriet B. Presser, "Race-Ethnic and Gender Differences in Nonstandard Work Shifts," *Work and Occupations* 30, no. 4 (2003): 412–439.

70. Wendy Brown, *Undoing the Demos* (New York: Zone, 2015); Melinda Cooper, *Family Values: Between Neoliberalism and the New Social Conservatism* (Cambridge, MA: MIT Press, 2017).

71. Cooper, *Family Values*.

72. Cooper, *Family Values*.

73. Cooper, *Family Values*, 65.

74. Cooper, *Family Values*, citing Marisa Chappell, *The War on Welfare: Family, Poverty, and Politics in Modern America* (Philadelphia: University of Pennsylvania Press, 2012).

75. Cooper, *Family Values*, 101.

76. Gregory Albo, "Neoliberalism from Reagan to Clinton," *Monthly Review* 52, no. 11 (2001): 81–89; David Harvey, *A Brief History of Neoliberalism* (New York: Oxford University Press, 2007); Vicente Navarro, *The Politics of Health Policy: The US Reforms, 1980–1994* (Cambridge, MA: Blackwell, 1994).

77. Sandra R. Levitsky, *Caring for Our Own: Why There Is No Political Demand for New American Social Welfare Rights* (New York: Oxford University Press, 2014), 47.

78. Max Ehrenfreund, "How Welfare Reform Changed American Poverty, in 9 Charts," *Washington Post*, August 22, 2016, https://www.washingtonpost.com/news/wonk/wp/2016/08/22/the-enduring-legacy-of-welfare-reform-20-years-later/?utm_term=.eee69499ea67. See also Kathryn Edin and H. Shaefer, *$2 a Day* (New York: Houghton Mifflin Harcourt, 2015), 7.

79. Rebecca Vallas and Jeremy Slevin, "Everything You Wanted to Know about the 1996 Welfare Law but Were Afraid to Ask," *TalkPoverty*, August 22, 2016, https://talk poverty.org/2016/08/22/everything-wanted-know-1996-welfare-law-afraid-ask.

80. Mary Corcoran et al., "How Welfare Reform Is Affecting Women's Work," *Annual Review of Sociology* 26 (2000): 241–269.

81. H. Luke Shaefer and Kathryn Edin, "Rising Extreme Poverty in the United States and the Response of Federal Means-Tested Transfer Programs," *Social Service Review* 87, no. 2 (2013): 250–268.

82. Jordan Weissmann, "The Failure of Welfare Reform," *Slate*, June 1, 2016, http://www.slate.com/articles/news_and_politics/moneybox/2016/06/how_welfare_reform_failed.html.

83. Randy Albelda, "Welfare-to-Work, Farewell to Families? US Welfare Reform and Work/Family Debates," *Feminist Economics* 7, no. 1 (2001): 119–135.

84. Evelyn Nakano Glenn, "Creating a Caring Society," *Contemporary Sociology* 29, no. 1 (2000): 84–94.

85. Glenn, "Creating a Caring Society," 93. Though Glenn is writing about maternity care in particular, her point is applicable more broadly.

86. Judith Feder, Harriet L. Komisar, and Marlene Niefeld, "Long-Term Care in the United States: An Overview," *Health Affairs* 19, no. 3 (2000): 40–56, 45.

87. "Long-Term Care Costs Continue to Rise," Associated Press, May 10, 2016, http://www.modernhealthcare.com/article/20160510/NEWS/160519999.

88. "Real Median Household Income in the United States," *FRED Economic Data*, https://fred.stlouisfed.org/series/MEHOINUSA672N.

89. William Galston, "Live Long and Pay for It: America's Real Long-Term Cost Crisis," September 12, 2012, *Atlantic Monthly*, https://www.theatlantic.com/business/archive/2012/09/live-long-and-pay-for-it-americas-real-long-term-cost-crisis/262247.

90. Carroll L. Estes, "Privatization, the Welfare State, and Aging: The Reagan-Bush Legacy," in *The Nation's Health*, 5th ed., ed. Philip R. Lee and Carroll L. Estes (Sudbury, MA: Jones and Bartlett, 1997), 199–209.

91. Galston, "Live Long and Pay for It."

92. SCAN Foundation, "Who Pays for Long-Term Care in the U.S.?," January 2013, http://www.thescanfoundation.org/sites/default/files/who_pays_for_ltc_us_jan_2013_fs.pdf.

93. Larry Light, "How to Pay for Nursing Home Care," *Forbes*, September 3, 2016, http://www.forbes.com/sites/lawrencelight/2016/09/03/how-to-pay-for-nursing-home-care/2/#5182fa8d7a1a.

94. Galston, "Live Long and Pay for It."

95. Katherine Morton Robinson, "Family Caregiving: Who Provides the Care, and at What Cost?," *Nursing Economics* 15, no. 5 (1997): 243–248.

96. Robinson, "Family Caregiving"; Ann Bookman and Mona Harrington, "Family Caregivers: A Shadow Workforce in the Geriatric Health Care System?," *Journal of Health Politics, Policy and Law* 32, no. 6 (2007): 1005–1041.

97. DeNeen L. Brown, "The High Cost of Poverty: Why the Poor Pay More," *Washington Post*, May 18, 2009, http://www.washingtonpost.com/wp-dyn/content/article/2009/05/17/AR2009051702053.html.

98. Steven Cummins, "Food Deserts," in *The Wiley Blackwell Encyclopedia of Health, Illness, Behavior, and Society* (2014), 562–564, https://onlinelibrary.wiley.com/doi/abs /10.1002/9781118410868.wbehibs450.

99. Imran Cronk, "The Transportation Barrier," *Atlantic*, August 9, 2015, http://www .theatlantic.com/health/archive/2015/08/the-transportation-barrier/399728; Rosabeth Moss Kanter, *Move: How to Rebuild and Reinvent America's Infrastructure* (New York: Norton, 2016).

100. R. Turner Goins et al., "Perceived Barriers to Health Care Access among Rural Older Adults: A Qualitative Study," *Journal of Rural Health* 21, no. 3 (2005): 206–213; Asheley Cockrell Skinner and Rebecca T. Slifkin, "Rural/Urban Differences in Barriers to and Burden of Care for Children with Special Health Care Needs," *Journal of Rural Health* 23, no. 2 (2007): 150–157.

101. Sheldon Danziger, Koji Chavez, and Erin Cumberworth, "Poverty and the Great Recession," Russell Sage Foundation and the Stanford Center on Poverty and Inequality, October 2012, https://inequality.stanford.edu/sites/default/files/Poverty_fact_sheet.pdf.

102. Don Peck, "Can the Middle Class Be Saved?," *Atlantic*, September 2011, http:// www.theatlantic.com/magazine/archive/2011/09/can-the-middle-class-be-saved/308600.

103. Denise A. Hines et al., "The Great Recession and Its Impact on Families," 2010 Massachusetts Family Impact Seminar, Briefing Report, https://www.purdue.edu/hhs /hdfs/fii/wp-content/uploads/2015/07/s_mafiso1report.pdf; Aaron Reeves et al., "Increase in State Suicide Rates in the USA during Economic Recession," *Lancet* 380, no. 9856 (2012): 1813–1814; Judith Warner, "What the Great Recession Has Done to Family Life," *New York Times*, August 6, 2010, http://www.nytimes.com/2010/08/08/magazine /08FOB-wwln-t.html.

104. Emily Badger, "How the Housing Crisis Left Us More Racially Segregated," *Washington Post*, May 8, 2015, https://www.washingtonpost.com/news/wonk/wp /2015/05/08/how-the-housing-crisis-left-us-more-racially-segregated.

105. Laura Kusisto, "Many Who Lost Homes to Foreclosure in the Last Decade Won't Return: NAR," *Wall Street Journal*, April 20, 2015, http://www.wsj.com/articles/many -who-lost-homes-to-foreclosure-in-last-decade-wont-return-nar-1429548640.

106. Prashant Gopal, "Homeownership Rate in the U.S. Drops to Lowest since 1965," *Bloomberg News*, July 28, 2016, http://www.bloomberg.com/news/articles/2016-07-28 /homeownership-rate-in-the-u-s-tumbles-to-the-lowest-since-1965.

107. Josh Boak, "1 in 4 Renters Use Half Their Pay for Housing Costs," Associated Press, May 3, 2015, http://www.usatoday.com/story/money/personalfinance/2015/05/03 /rental-costs/26753859.

108. G. Thomas Kingsley, Robin Smith, and David Price, "The Impacts of Fore-closures on Families and Communities," Urban Institute, May 2009, http://www .urban.org/sites/default/files/alfresco/publication-pdfs/411909-The-Impacts-of-Fore closures-on-Families-and-Communities.PDF; Lauren M. Ross and Gregory D. Squires, "The Personal Costs of Subprime Lending and the Foreclosure Crisis: A Matter of Trust, Insecurity, and Institutional Deception," *Social Science Quarterly* 92, no. 1 (2011): 140–163; Joseph Gaugler and Robert L. Kane, *Familial Caregiving in the New Normal* (Waltham, MA: Academic, 2015).

109. Ta-Nehisi Coates, "The Case for Reparations," *Atlantic*, June 2014, http://www
.theatlantic.com/magazine/archive/2014/06/the-case-for-reparations/361631; Hirsch,
Making the Second Ghetto.

110. David Leonhardt, "Middle-Class Black Families in Low-Income Neighborhoods,"
New York Times, June 24, 2015, http://www.nytimes.com/2015/06/25/upshot/middle
-class-black-families-in-low-income-neighborhoods.html; Sean F. Reardon, Lindsay Fox,
and Joseph Townsend, "Neighborhood Income Composition by Household Race and
Income, 1990–2009," *Annals of the American Academy of Political and Social Science* 660,
no. 1 (2015): 78–97.

111. Reardon, Fox, and Townsend, "Neighborhood Income Composition"; Richard D.
Alba, John R. Logan, and Brian J. Stults, "How Segregated Are Middle-Class African
Americans?," *Social Problems* 47, no. 4 (2000): 543–558.

112. Mike Konczal and Bryce Covert, "This Is the Key to Recovering Black Wealth in
America," *Nation*, January 13, 2015, https://www.thenation.com/article/key-recovering
-black-wealth-america.

113. Massey and Denton, *American Apartheid*; Dalton Conley, *Being Black, Living in the Red:
Race, Wealth, and Social Policy in America* (Berkeley: University of California Press, 1999).

114. Renae Merle, "Minorities Hit Harder by Foreclosure Crisis," *Washington Post*,
June 19, 2010, http://www.washingtonpost.com/wp-dyn/content/article/2010/06/18
/AR2010061802885.html; Jorge Newbery, "Whites Recover from Housing Crisis: African
Americans and Latinos Left Behind," *Huffington Post*, June 12, 2014, http://www.huffing
tonpost.com/jorge-newbery/whites-recover-from-housi_b_5480437.html.

115. Renee E. Walker, Christopher R. Keane, and Jessica G. Burke, "Disparities and
Access to Healthy Food in the United States: A Review of Food Deserts Literature,"
Health and Place 16, no. 5 (2010): 876–884; Neil Bania, Claudia Coulton, and Laura Leete,
"Public Housing Assistance, Public Transportation, and the Welfare-to-Work Transition,"
Cityscape: A Journal of Policy Development and Research 6, no. 2 (2003): 7–44.

116. Robert J. Sampson, Stephen W. Raudenbush, and Felton Earls, "Neighborhoods
and Violent Crime: A Multilevel Study of Collective Efficacy," *Science* 277, no. 5328
(1997): 918–924.

117. Sampson, Raudenbush, and Earls, "Neighborhoods and Violent Crime"; Gary LaFree,
Kriss A. Drass, and Patrick O'Day, "Race and Crime in Postwar America: Determinants of
African-American and White Rates, 1957–1988," *Criminology* 30, no. 2 (1992): 157–188.

118. Susan M. Wachter and Isaac F. Megbolugbe, "Impacts of Housing and Mortgage
Market Discrimination [on] Racial and Ethnic Disparities in Homeownership," *Housing
Policy Debate* 3, no. 2 (1992): 332–370.

119. Sentencing Project, "Trends in US Corrections," June 2018, http://sentencing
project.org/wp-content/uploads/2016/01/Trends-in-US-Corrections.pdf; Michelle Alexan-
der, *The New Jim Crow* (New York: New Press, 2010); Marie Gottschalk, *The Prison and the
Gallows: The Politics of Mass Incarceration in America* (Cambridge: Cambridge University
Press, 2006); Todd R. Clear, *Imprisoning Communities: How Mass Incarceration Makes
Disadvantaged Neighborhoods Worse* (New York: Oxford University Press, 2009); Glenn C.
Loury, "Crime, Inequality and Social Justice," *Daedalus* 139, no. 3 (2010): 134–140.

120. Lawrence D. Bobo and Victor Thompson, "Unfair by Design: The War on Drugs,

Race, and the Legitimacy of the Criminal Justice System," *Social Research* 73, no. 2 (2006): 445–472.

121. John Pfaff, *Locked In: The True Causes of Mass Incarceration and How to Achieve Real Reform* (New York: Basic, 2017); James Forman Jr., *Locking Up Our Own: Crime and Punishment in Black America* (New York: Farrar, Straus and Giroux, 2017).

122. Sentencing Project, "Trends in US Corrections."

123. Bruce Western and Christopher Wildeman, "The Black Family and Mass Incarceration," *Annals of the American Academy of Political and Social Science* 621, no. 1 (2009): 221–242; Dorothy E. Roberts, "The Social and Moral Cost of Mass Incarceration in African American Communities," *Stanford Law Review* 56, no. 5 (2004): 1271–1305.

124. Estes, "Privatization, the Welfare State, and Aging," 199–210; D. King and S. Wood, "The Political Economy of Neoliberalism: Britain and the United States in the 1980s," in *Continuity and Change in Contemporary Capitalism*, ed. H. Kitschelt et al. (Cambridge: Cambridge University Press, 1999), 371–397.

125. Buck, "From Rites to Rights of Passage," 27.

126. D. S. Greer and V. Mor, "How Medicare Is Altering the Hospice Movement," *Hastings Center Report* 15, no. 5 (1985): 5–9.

127. Greer and Mor, "How Medicare Is Altering."

128. J. E. Perry and R. C. Stone, "In the Business of Dying: Questioning the Commercialization of Hospice," *Journal of Law, Medicine and Ethics* 39, no. 2 (2011): 224–234.

129. National Hospice and Palliative Care Organization, *Facts and Figures: Hospice Care in America* (rev. April 2018), https://www.nhpco.org/sites/default/files/public/2016_Facts_Figures.pdf.

130. MedPAC, "Report to the Congress: Medicare Payment Policy," March 2010, 141, http://medpac.gov/docs/default-source/reports/Mar10_EntireReport.pdf?sfvrsn=0; MedPAC, "Report to the Congress: Reforming the Delivery System," 216, June 2008, http://www.medpac.gov/docs/default-source/reports/Jun08_EntireReport.pdf. Both sources are cited in Perry and Stone, "In the Business of Dying," 227.

131. Perry and Stone, "In the Business of Dying," 225–226.

132. Perry and Stone, "In the Business of Dying," 228–229; S. Halabi, "Selling Hospice," *Journal of Law, Medicine and Ethics* 42, no. 4 (2014): 442–454.

133. David S. Greer, "Hospice: From Social Movement to Health Care Industry," *Transactions of the American Clinical and Climatological Association* 97 (1986): 82–87.

134. Melissa W. Wachterman et al., "Association of Hospice Agency Profit Status with Patient Diagnosis, Location of Care, and Length of Stay," *JAMA* 305, no. 5 (2011): 472–479; Brad Stuart, "The NHO Medical Guidelines for Non-Cancer Disease and Local Medical Review Policy: Hospice Access for Patients with Diseases Other than Cancer," *Hospice Journal* 14 (1999): 139–154.

135. Wachterman et al., "Association of Hospice Agency Profit Status," 465.

136. Karl A. Lorenz et al., "Cash and Compassion: Profit Status and the Delivery of Hospice Service," *Journal of Palliative Medicine* 5, no. 4 (2002): 507–514; Richard C. Lindrooth and Burton A. Weisbrod, "Do Religious Nonprofit and For-Profit Organizations Respond Differently to Financial Incentives? The Hospice Industry," *Journal of Health Economics* 26, no. 2 (2007): 342–357.

137. Perry and Stone, "In the Business of Dying," 229.

138. Stuart, "NHO Medical Guidelines," 140.

139. Carol Levine et al., "Bridging Troubled Waters: Family Caregivers, Transitions, and Long-Term Care," *Health Affairs* 29, no. 1 (2010): 116–124; Robyn Stone, Gail Lee Cafferata, and Judith Sangl, "Caregivers of the Frail Elderly: A National Profile," *Gerontologist* 27, no. 5 (1987): 616–626.

140. Cathleen M. Connell, Mary R. Janevic, and Mary P. Gallant, "The Costs of Caring: Impact of Dementia on Family Caregivers," *Journal of Geriatric Psychiatry and Neurology* 14, no. 4 (2001): 179–187; Peter P. Vitaliano, Jianping Zhang, and James M. Scanlan, "Is Caregiving Hazardous to One's Physical Health? A Meta-Analysis," *Psychological Bulletin* 129, no. 6 (2003): 946–972.

141. Nancy Folbre, "Measuring Care: Gender, Empowerment, and the Care Economy," *Journal of Human Development* 7, no. 2 (2006): 183–199; Paula England and Nancy Folbre, "The Cost of Caring," *Annals of the American Academy of Political and Social Science* 561, no. 1 (1999): 39–51.

142. Greer, "Hospice," 84; Buck, "Policy and the Re-Formation of Hospice"; Joy Buck, "Netting the Hospice Butterfly: Politics, Policy, and Translation of an Ideal," *Home Healthcare Now* 25, no. 9 (2007): 566–571.

143. Greg A. Sachs, Joseph W. Shega, and Deon Cox-Hayley, "Barriers to Excellent End-of-Life Care for Patients with Dementia," *Journal of General Internal Medicine* 19, no. 10 (2004): 1057–1063.

144. Peter Whoriskey and Dan Keating, "Dying and Profits: The Evolution of Hospice," *Washington Post*, December 26, 2014, https://www.washingtonpost.com/business/economy/2014/12/26/a7d90438–692f-11e4-b053-65cea7903f2e_story.html.

145. Fran Smith and Sheila Himmel, *Changing the Way We Die: Compassionate End-of-Life Care and the Hospice Movement* (Berkeley, CA: Viva, 2013).

146. Whoriskey and Keating, "Dying and Profits."

147. E. G. Ward and A. K. Gordon, "Looming Threats to the Intimate Bond," *Omega* 54, no. 1 (2006): 7–8; M. A. Sontag, "A Comparison of Hospice Programs Based on Medicare Certification Status," *American Journal of Hospice and Palliative Care* 13 (1996): 32–41.

148. Ward and Gordon, "Looming Threats," 9, citing M. A. Sontag, "Hospices as Providers of Total Care in One Western State," *Hospice Journal* 11 (1996): 71–94.

149. Virginia Sendor and Patrice O'Connor, *Hospice and Palliative Care in the U.S.* (Lanham, MD: Scarecrow, 1997), 97.

150. National Hospice and Palliative Care Organization, "NHPCO Facts and Figures on Hospice Care in America," March 2012, https://www.nhpco.org/sites/default/files/public/newsline/2012/NL_March_12.pdf.

151. Haiden A. Huskamp et al., "Providing Care at the End of Life: Do Medicare Rules Impede Good Care?," *Health Affairs* 20, no. 3 (2001): 204–211.

152. Huskamp et al., "Providing Care at the End of Life," 208.

153. Centers for Medicare and Medicaid Services, "Medicare Care Choices Model," September 19, 2018, https://innovation.cms.gov/initiatives/Medicare-Care-Choices.

154. MedPAC, "Report to the Congress: Medicare Payment Policy," June 2007, http://www.medpac.gov/docs/default-source/reports/Mar07_EntireReport.pdf; Kathy L. Cermi-

nara, "Hospice and Heath Care Reform: Improving Care at the End of Life," *Widener Law Review* 17 (2011): 443–473.

155. Centers for Medicare and Medicaid Services, "Hospice Payment System," October 2017, https://www.cms.gov/Outreach-and-Education/Medicare-Learning-Network-MLN /MLNProducts/downloads/hospice_pay_sys_fs.pdf.

156. Cerminara, "Hospice and Health Care Reform," 459.

157. James Fredrick Barger, "Life, Death, and Medicare Fraud: The Corruption of Hospice and What the Private Public Partnership under the Federal False Claims Act Is Doing about It," *American Criminal Law Review* 53, no. 1 (2016): 1–65; Smith and Himmel, *Changing the Way We Die.*

158. Judy Feder, "The Challenge of Financing Long-Term Care," *St. Louis University Journal of Health Law and Policy* 8 (2014): 47–60.

159. David G. Stevenson and Jeffrey S. Bramson, "Hospice Care in the Nursing Home Setting: A Review of the Literature," *Journal of Pain and Symptom Management* 38, no. 3 (2009): 440–451; Susan Lysaght and Mary Ersek, "Settings of Care within Hospice: New Options and Questions about Dying 'at Home,'" *Journal of Hospice and Palliative Nursing* 15, no. 3 (2013): 171–176; Muriel R. Gillick and James E. Sabin, "No Place like the Hospital," *Journal of Pain and Symptom Management* 42, no. 4 (2011): 643–648.

160. Gladys Catkins Keidel, "Burnout and Compassion Fatigue among Hospice Caregivers," *American Journal of Hospice and Palliative Medicine* 19, no. 3 (2002): 200–205; Janette S. Dill and John Cagle, "Caregiving in a Patient's Place of Residence: Turnover of Direct Care Workers in Home Care and Hospice Agencies," *Journal of Aging and Health* 22, no. 6 (2010): 713–730.

161. Melissa D. Aldridge Carlson et al., "Hospices' Enrollment Policies May Contribute to Underuse of Hospice Care in the United States," *Health Affairs* 31, no. 12 (2012): 2690–2698.

162. Peter Whoriskey and Dan Keating, "Terminal Neglect? How Some Hospices Decline to Treat the Dying," *Washington Post*, May 3, 2014, https://www.washingtonpost .com/business/economy/terminal-neglect-how-some-hospices-fail-the-dying/2014/05 /03/7d3ac8ce-b8ef-11e3-96ae-f2c36d2b1245_story.html.

163. Teno et al., "Change in End-of-Life Care."

164. Susan C. Miller et al., "The Growth of Hospice Care in US Nursing Homes," *Journal of the American Geriatrics Society* 58, no. 8 (2010): 1481–1488. See also Teno et al., "Change in End-of-Life Care," which notes a 7 percent increase between 2002 and 2009.

165. Dan McGrath, "There Aren't Enough Nursing Home Beds to Meet Demand," *CNBC*, December 7, 2015, https://www.cnbc.com/2015/12/07/there-arent-enough-nursing -home-beds-to-meet-demand.html; Levitsky, *Caring for Our Own,* 66–90.

166. Levitsky, *Caring for Our Own,* 66–90.

167. Thomas M. Gil et al., "Distressing Symptoms, Disability, and Hospice Services at the End of Life: Prospective Cohort Study," *Journal of the American Geriatrics Society* 66, no. 1 (2018): 41–47.

168. Sharon Kaufman, *Ordinary Medicine* (Durham, NC: Duke University Press, 2015).

169. Kathy L. Cerminara, "Pandora's Dismay: Eliminating Coverage-Related Barriers to Hospice Care," *Florida Coastal Law Review* 11 (2009): 107–154.

170. Whoriskey and Keating, "Terminal Neglect."

171. JoNel Aleccia and Melissa Bailey, " 'No One Is Coming': Hospice Patients Abandoned at Death's Door," *Kaiser Health News*, October 26, 2017, https://khn.org/news/no-one-is-coming-hospice-patients-abandoned-at-deaths-door; Joan Kenen, "Hospice in Crisis," *Politico*, September 27, 2017, https://www.politico.com/agenda/story/2017/09/27/how-hospice-works-000526. For the entirety of Whoriskey and Keatings's "Business of Dying" series, see http://www.washingtonpost.com/sf/business/collection/business-of-dying.

172. J. M. Teno et al., "Examining Variation in Hospice Visits by Professional Staff in the Last 2 Days of Life," *JAMA Internal Medicine* 176, no. 3 (2016): 364–370.

173. Aleccia and Bailey, "No One Is Coming."

174. Aleccia and Bailey, "No One Is Coming."

175. Teno quoted in Aleccia and Bailey, "No One Is Coming."

176. Institute of Medicine, *Dying in America: Improving Quality and Honoring Individual Preferences near the End of Life* (Washington, DC: National Academies Press, 2014), http://www.nationalacademies.org/hmd/Reports/2014/Dying-In-America-Improving-Quality-and-Honoring-Individual-Preferences-Near-the-End-of-Life.aspx.

177. Institute of Medicine, *Dying in America*, 266.

178. Institute of Medicine, *Dying in America*, 266–267.

179. " 'I see no evidence of any upturn in fertility, and deaths continue to grow,' says Kenneth Johnson, senior demographer at the University of New Hampshire's Carsey Institute," in Josh Sanburn, "More Americans Dying as Birth Rate Hits Record Lows," *Time*, March 27, 2014, http://time.com/39500/census-more-deaths-fewer-births-in-u-s.

180. "In short, long-term care faces perhaps its most serious crisis in a century." David Barton Smith and Zhanlian Feng, "The Accumulated Challenges of Long-Term Care," *Health Affairs*, 29, no. 1 (2010), https://www.healthaffairs.org/doi/full/10.1377/hlthaff.2009.0507. For a more recent perspective focused on the crisis in home-based long-term care, see E. Tammy Kim, "Americans Will Struggle to Grow Old at Home," *Bloomberg Businessweek*, February 9, 2018, https://www.bloomberg.com/news/features/2018–02–09/americans-will-struggle-to-grow-old-at-home.

181. Brown, *Undoing the Demos*.

Chapter 4. What Happens to Dying People

1. Sandra R. Levitsky, *Caring for Our Own: Why There Is No Political Demand for New American Social Welfare Rights* (New York: Oxford University Press, 2014), 42–43.

2. Lynn Feinberg and Rita Choula, "Understanding the Impact of Family Caregiving on Work," AARP Public Policy Institute, Fact Sheet 271, October 2012, https://www.aarp.org/content/dam/aarp/research/public_policy_institute/ltc/2012/understanding-impact-family-caregiving-work-AARP-ppi-ltc.pdf.

3. This novelty is due to the pervasive lack of research on familial caregivers in US hospice care. As the Institute of Medicine notes: "Information about the number and responsibilities of caregivers specifically for those nearing the end of life is not available." *Dying in America: Improving Quality and Honoring Individual Preferences near the End of Life* (Washington, DC: National Academies Press, 2014), 102. The lack of information on

familial caregivers at the end of life is another reason for privileging an ethnographic approach.

4. On the limitations of existing quantitative approaches to US end-of-life care, see Institute of Medicine, *Dying in America*, 99.

5. For some statistics on PAS over time, see Oregon Public Health Division, "Oregon Death with Dignity Act: 2015 Data Summary," February 4, 2016, https://www.oregon .gov/oha/ph/providerpartnerresources/evaluationresearch/deathwithdignityact/Docu ments/year18.pdf. For a defender of PAS citing its low rate of usage, see Arthur Caplan, "Brittany Maynard Did Nothing Unethical," *USA Today*, November 3, 2014, https:// www.usatoday.com/story/news/health/2014/11/03/brittany-maynard-death-assisted -suicide-cancer-kaplan/18415085.

6. For ethnographies that perform a similar function with respect to American debates about the end of life, see Sharon Kaufman, *And a Time to Die: How American Hospitals Shape the End of Life* (Chicago: University of Chicago Press, 2005); James W. Green, *Beyond the Good Death: The Anthropology of Modern Dying* (Philadelphia: University of Pennsylvania Press, 2012). Though not a strict ethnography, medical anthropologist Andrea Sankar's book also contains extremely illustrative vignettes. Sankar, *Dying at Home: A Family Guide for Caregiving* (Baltimore, MD: Johns Hopkins University Press, 1991).

7. Conditions of Participation for Hospice Care, 42 CFR 418.56.

8. Conditions of Participation for Hospice Care, 42 CFR 418.78.

9. National Hospice and Palliative Care Organization, *Facts and Figures: Hospice Care in America* (rev. April 2018), https://www.nhpco.org/sites/default/files/public /2016_Facts_Figures.pdf.

10. Robert Bullard, Glenn S. Johnson, and Angel O. Torres, *Sprawl City: Race, Politics, and Planning in Atlanta* (Washington, DC: Island Press, 2000).

11. Miriam Fiedler Konrad, *Transporting Atlanta: The Mode of Mobility under Construction* (Albany: State University of New York Press, 2009).

12. The circumstances of Steven's death were influenced by two contingencies that are worth clarifying: First, why did he call 911, rather than hospice? Second, why did receiving a blood transfusion lead his body donation program to reject his corpse? I do not have absolute certainty with regard to either issue, but I have two relatively compelling explanations.

With regard to Steven's 911 call, he probably panicked. This panic was likely due, in part, to the skittish nature of his personality; it was also almost certainly due to the sudden onset of extreme pain. He was in an overwhelming situation, which may have been made even more overwhelming by when he died: a weekend. On weekends—particularly Sundays—hospices frequently have less staff than during the week. This lack of staffing may lead to fewer nursing visits. Indeed, hospice researchers have found that patients who die on a Sunday are three times less likely to receive a skilled visit compared to patients who die on a Tuesday. Perhaps Steven attempted to get in contact with his hospice but did not receive a prompt response. In the meantime, he called 911, setting in motion the events that led to his transfusion. For more information relevant to this possibility, see JoNel Aleccia and Melissa Bailey, " 'No One Is Coming': Hospice Patients Abandoned at Death's Door," *Kaiser Health News*, October 26, 2017, https://khn.org/news/no-one-is

-coming-hospice-patients-abandoned-at-deaths-door; J. M. Teno et al., "Examining Variation in Hospice Visits by Professional Staff in the Last 2 Days of Life," *JAMA Internal Medicine* 176, no. 3 (2016): 364–370.

Regarding why Steven's blood transfusion led to his body being rejected: Given the severity of Steven's condition, the blood transfusion he received was likely large. This large blood transfusion immediately prior to his death may have made it impossible to conduct a valid serology test to determine if he was infected with HIV and/or hepatitis B and C. Some body donation services might have tried to get a pretransfusion sample of blood from the hospital's laboratory—but not all. Without suitable serology test results, Steven's body donation service would have had problems assigning his body to an end user, since a researcher would likely be unwilling to accept untested anatomical material. On these grounds, the decision of Steven's body donation service to reject his body was not particularly unique. I thank Angela McArthur, the director of the Anatomy Bequest Program at the University of Minnesota, for providing this possible rationale for the rejection of Steven's body.

13. João Guilherme Biehl, *Vita: Life in a Zone of Social Abandonment* (Berkeley: University of California Press, 2005), 130–137.

14. Biehl, *Vita*, 2.

15. Erving Goffman, *Asylums: Essays on the Situation of Mental Patients and Other Inmates* (New York: Anchor, 1961).

16. Timothy Quill, *Caring for Patients at the End of Life: Facing an Uncertain Future Together* (Oxford: Oxford University Press, 2001), 59.

17. Quill, *Caring for Patients*, 60.

18. James E. Allen, *Nursing Home Federal Requirements Guidelines to Surveyors and Survey Protocols, 2006: A User-Friendly Rendering of the Centers for Medicare and Medicaid's (CMS) Nursing Home Inspection and Requirement Forms* (New York: Springer, 2007).

19. Allen, *Nursing Home Federal Requirements Guidelines*, § 483.5.

20. Emily Mullin and Lisa Esposito, "How to Pay for Nursing Home Costs," *US News and World Report*, November 16, 2016, http://health.usnews.com/health-news/best-nursing-homes/articles/2013/02/26/how-to-pay-for-nursing-home-costs.

21. AARP, *Nursing Facilities, Staffing, Residents and Facility Deficiencies, 2001 through 2007, across the States: Profiles of Long-Term Care and Independent Living* (Washington, DC: AARP Public Policy Institute, 2009).

22. K. Aragon et al., "Use of the Medicare Posthospitalization Skilled Nursing Benefit in the Last 6 Months of Life," *Archives of Internal Medicine* 172, no. 20 (2012): 1573–1579.

23. Jane Banaszak-Holl and Marilyn A. Hines, "Factors Associated with Nursing Home Staff Turnover," *Gerontologist* 36, no. 4 (1996): 512–517; Nicholas G. Castle, John Engberg, and Aiju Men, "Nursing Home Staff Turnover: Impact on Nursing Home Compare Quality Measures," *Gerontologist* 47, no. 5 (2007): 650–661; Nicholas G. Castle and John Engberg, "Organizational Characteristics Associated with Staff Turnover in Nursing Homes," *Gerontologist* 46, no. 1 (2006): 62–73.

24. John F. Schnelle et al., "Accuracy of Nursing Home Medical Record Information about Care-Process Delivery: Implications for Staff Management and Improvement," *Journal of the American Geriatrics Society* 52, no. 8 (2004): 1378–1383.

25. Institute of Medicine, *Dying in America*, 297.

26. Stephen R. Connor et al., "Comparing Hospice and Nonhospice Patient Survival among Patients Who Die within a Three-Year Window," *Journal of Pain and Symptom Management* 33, no. 3 (2007): 238–246; Jennifer S. Temel et al., "Early Palliative Care for Patients with Metastatic Non-Small-Cell Lung Cancer," *New England Journal of Medicine* 363, no. 8 (2010): 733–742.

27. Institute of Medicine, *Dying in America*, 275.

28. Sharon Kaufman, *Ordinary Medicine* (Durham, NC: Duke University Press, 2015), 8.

29. Wendy Brown, *Undoing the Demos* (New York: Zone, 2015), 128.

30. Brown, *Undoing the Demos*, 128.

31. Milton Friedman and Rose Friedman, *Freedom to Choose: A Personal Statement* (New York: Houghton Mifflin Harcourt, 1990), 28.

Chapter 5. Caring across the American Political Divide

1. Ann Feather Davis, "Medicare Hospice Benefit: Early Program Experiences," *Health Care Financing Review* 9, no. 4 (1988): 99–111.

2. I am not using a pseudonym for either the Dominican Sisters of Hawthorne or Our Lady of Perpetual Help Home in accord with the agreement I made with the Hawthorne Dominicans regarding my research. I have, however, changed the names and identifying information of all individuals, including patients and both secular and religious professionals.

3. Nicholas G. Castle, John Engberg, and Aiju Men, "Nursing Home Staff Turnover: Impact on Nursing Home Compare Quality Measures," *Gerontologist* 47, no. 5 (2007): 650–661.

4. Raymond Benedict Flannery, "Psychological Trauma and Posttraumatic Stress Disorder: A Review," *International Journal of Emergency Mental Health* 1, no. 2 (1999): 135–140; Patricia K. Kerig et al., "Numbing of Positive, Negative, and General Emotions: Associations with Trauma Exposure, Posttraumatic Stress, and Depressive Symptoms among Justice-Involved Youth," *Journal of Traumatic Stress* 29, no. 2 (2016): 111–119.

5. Timothy E. Quill and M. Pabst Battin, eds., *Physician-Assisted Dying: The Case for Palliative Care and Patient Choice* (Baltimore, MD: Johns Hopkins University Press, 2004); Kathleen M. Foley and Herbert Hendin, eds., *The Case against Assisted Suicide: For the Right to End-of-Life Care* (Baltimore, MD: Johns Hopkins University Press, 2002).

6. Patricia D. Valenti, *To Myself a Stranger: A Biography of Rose Hawthorne Lathrop* (Baton Rouge: Louisiana State University Press, 1991), 100.

7. Valenti, *To Myself a Stranger*, 129.

8. Valenti, *To Myself a Stranger*, 137.

9. Valenti, *To Myself a Stranger*, 144.

10. Valenti, *To Myself a Stranger*, 152.

11. Valenti, *To Myself a Stranger*, 166.

12. United States Conference of Catholic Bishops, *United States Catholic Catechism for Adults* (Washington, DC: USCCB Communications, 2006).

13. United States Conference of Catholic Bishops, *United States Catholic Catechism*, 67–77.

14. Diarmaid MacCulloch, *Christianity: The First Three Thousand Years* (New York: Viking, 2009), 146–147.

15. United States Conference of Catholic Bishops, *United States Catholic Catechism*, 77–88.

16. MacCulloch, *Christianity*.

17. United States Conference of Catholic Bishops, *United States Catholic Catechism*, 32.

18. Stephanie Simon, "Vatican Crackdown on U.S. Nuns a Long Time Brewing," Reuters, April 20, 2012, http://www.reuters.com/article/2012/04/20/us-usa-vatican -nuns-idUSBRE83J1B720120420.

19. Samuel T. Grover, "Religious Exemptions to the PPACA's Health Insurance Man-date," *American Journal of Law and Medicine* 37, no. 4 (2011): 625–653; Rebecca Hall, "The Women's Health Amendment and Religious Freedom: Finding a Sufficient Compro-mise," *Journal of Health Care Law and Policy* 15 (2012): 401–424.

20. Erwin Chemerinsky, *Constitutional Law: Principles and Policies* (New York: Aspen, 2006); Neil M. Gorsuch, *The Future of Assisted Suicide and Euthanasia* (Princeton, NJ: Princeton University Press, 2009).

21. Twenty-first-century PAS legislation has generally succeeded in more libertar-ian states, failed in more conservative states, and had mixed success in states typically considered liberal. Catherine Glenn Foster, "Deciding Death," *US News and World Report*, October 2, 2017, https://www.usnews.com/opinion/civil-wars/articles/2017-10-02/state -courts-are-right-to-leave-physician-assisted-suicide-to-legislature.

22. See, for example, the discussions of charity in Rosamond Rhodes, M. Pabst Bat-tin, and Anita Silvers, *Medicine and Social Justice: Essays on the Distribution of Health Care*, 2nd ed. (New York: Oxford University Press, 2012).

23. Jeffrey Bishop, *The Anticipatory Corpse: Medicine, Power, and the Care of the Dying* (South Bend, IN: University of Notre Dame Press, 2011), 313.

24. Charles C. Camosy, *Beyond the Abortion Wars: A Way Forward for a New Generation* (Grand Rapids, MI: Eerdmans, 2015).

25. Camosy, *Beyond the Abortion Wars*, 4.

26. Andrew Hartman, *A War for the Soul of America: A History of the Culture Wars* (Chicago: University of Chicago Press, 2015).

27. Hartman, *War for the Soul of America*, 101.

28. Hartman, *War for the Soul of America*, 290. For Hartman's updated perspective on the end of the culture wars, listen to episode 69 of the podcast "Common Ground," https://www.stitcher.com/podcast/common-ground-2/e/52102998.

29. Danielle Kurtzleben, "Despite Constant Debate, Americans' Abortion Opinions Rarely Change," *NPR*, September 21, 2015, https://www.npr.org/sections/itsallpolitics /2015/09/21/441510600/despite-constant-debate-americans-abortion-opinions-rarely -change.

30. Ronald Dworkin, *Life's Dominion: An Argument about Abortion, Euthanasia, and Individual Freedom* (New York: Knopf, 1993).

31. Ian Dowbiggin, *A Merciful End: The Euthanasia Movement in Modern America* (Oxford: Oxford University Press, 2003).

Chapter 6. When the End of Life Begins

1. Donald Winnicott, "Freedom," in his *Home Is Where We Start From: Essays by a Psychoanalyst* (New York: Norton, 1986), 228–238.

2. Caroline Elkins, *Imperial Reckoning: The Untold Story of Britain's Gulag in Kenya* (New York: Holt, 2005); Wunyabari O. Maloba, *Mau Mau and Kenya: An Analysis of a Peasant Revolt* (Bloomington: Indiana University Press, 1993).

3. Cicely Saunders, "A Place to Die," in her *Selected Writings, 1958–2004*, ed. David Clark (Oxford: Oxford University Press, 2006), 124–128.

4. Susan Duke, "An Exploration of Anticipatory Grief: The Lived Experience of People during Their Spouses' Terminal Illness and in Bereavement," *Journal of Advanced Nursing* 28, no. 4 (1998): 829–839; Ibrahim Aref Kira, "Taxonomy of Trauma and Trauma Assessment," *Traumatology* 7, no. 2 (2001): 73–86.

5. Teresa Evans-Campbell, "Historical Trauma in American Indian/Native Alaska Communities: A Multilevel Framework for Exploring Impacts on Individuals, Families, and Communities," *Journal of Interpersonal Violence* 23, no. 3 (2008): 316–338; Susan L. Ray and Meredith Vanstone, "The Impact of PTSD on Veterans' Family Relationships: An Interpretive Phenomenological Inquiry," *International Journal of Nursing Studies* 46, no. 6 (2009): 838–847.

6. Carol Levine, "One Loss May Hide Another," *Hastings Center Report* 34, no. 6 (2004): 17–19; Elizabeth Edna Wangui, "Livelihood Strategies and Nutritional Status of Grandparent Caregivers of AIDS Orphans in Nyando District, Kenya," *Qualitative Health Research* 19, no. 12 (2009): 1702–1715.

7. See "Imagining a Care-Full Society," in Ira Byock, *The Best Care Possible: A Physician's Quest to Transform Care through the End of Life* (New York: Avery, 2012), 250–271.

8. Harriet McBryde Johnson, "The Disability Gulag," *New York Times Magazine*, November 23, 2003, http://www.nytimes.com/2003/11/23/magazine/the-disability-gulag .html; Joseph P. Shapiro, *No Pity: People with Disabilities Forging a New Civil Rights Movement* (New York: Broadway, 1994).

9. Gerben DeJong, "Independent Living: From Social Movement to Analytic Paradigm," *Archives of Physical Medicine and Rehabilitation* 60, no. 10 (1979): 435–446; James Elder-Woodward, "Independent Living: The Frontier of Communitarian Welfare?," *Disability and Society* 28, no. 2 (2013): 274–278.

10. See Samuel R. Bagenstos, *Law and the Contradictions of the Disability Rights Movement* (New Haven, CT: Yale University Press, 2014), 145–148.

11. The scale of this problem is not known, but I base my analysis here on correspondence and conversations with several hospice policy scholars and advocates.

12. "Concurrent Hospice and Personal Care Services for Adults," *North Carolina Medicaid Special Bulletin*, December 1, 2015, https://files.nc.gov/ncdma/documents /files/1215_SPECIAL_BULLETIN_Hospice.pdf.

13. Tyler Norris, "North Carolina: The New Model for Conservative Rule—and

Progressive Renewal," *NC Policy Watch*, August 30, 2017, http://www.ncpolicywatch.com/2017/08/30/north-carolina-new-model-conservative-rule-progressive-renewal.

14. Evelyn Nakano Glenn, *Forced to Care: Coercion and Caregiving in America* (Cambridge, MA: Harvard University Press, 2010); Anne-Marie Slaughter, "Why Women Still Can't Have It All," *Atlantic*, July–August 2012, http://www.theatlantic.com/magazine/archive/2012/07/why-women-still-cant-have-it-all/309020.

15. Richard Glatzer and Wash Westmoreland, dirs., *Still Alice* (Sony Pictures Classics, 2014).

16. Gillian Lester, "A Defense of Paid Family Leave," *Harvard Journal of Law and Gender* 28, no. 1 (2005): 3–83.

17. Howard Gleckman, "What the Battle over Home Health Care Worker Pay Is Really About," *Forbes*, March 18, 2015, http://www.forbes.com/sites/howardgleckman/2015/03/18/what-the-battle-over-home-health-care-worker-pay-is-really-about/#36bdb67d54fe.

18. Nicholas G. Castle et al., "Job Satisfaction of Nurse Aides in Nursing Homes: Intent to Leave and Turnover," *Gerontologist* 47, no. 2 (2007): 193–204.

19. Philip N. Cohen, *The Family: Diversity, Inequality, and Social Change* (New York: Norton, 2015), 404, citing Harriet B. Presser, "Race-Ethnic and Gender Differences in Nonstandard Work Shifts," *Work and Occupations* 30, no. 4 (2003): 412–439.

20. Jennifer A. Parks, *No Place like Home? Feminist Ethics and Home Health Care* (Bloomington: Indiana University Press, 2003), 121.

21. Arthur Kleinman, "Caregiving as Moral Experience," *Lancet* 380, no. 9853 (2012): P1550–1551.

22. Kleinman, "Caregiving as Moral Experience," P1551.

23. Kleinman, "Caregiving as Moral Experience," P1551.

24. Andrew J. Cherlin, *Public and Private Families: An Introduction*, 6th ed. (New York: McGraw-Hill, 2010), 333.

25. Duke, "Exploration of Anticipatory Grief."

26. For example, see the textbook by Karen Bogenschneider, *Family Policy Matters: How Policymaking Affects Families and What Professionals Can Do*, 3rd ed. (New York: Routledge, 2014).

27. Carol B. Stack, *All Our Kin: Strategies for Survival in a Black Community* (New York: Harper and Row, 1974).

28. Susan L. Waysdorf, "Families in the AIDS Crisis: Access, Equality, Empowerment, and the Role of Kinship Caregivers," *Texas Journal of Women and Law* 3 (1994): 145–220.

29. Allan Kellehear, "Compassionate Communities: End-of-Life Care as Everyone's Responsibility," *QJM: An International Journal of Medicine* 106, no. 12 (2013): 1071–1075.

30. Kellehear, "Compassionate Communities." For other examples, see Klaus Wegleitner, Katharina Heimerl, and Allan Kellehear, eds., *Compassionate Communities: Case Studies from Britain and Europe* (London: Routledge, 2015).

31. Jonathan Shedler, "The Efficacy of Psychodynamic Psychotherapy," in *Psychodynamic Psychotherapy Research*, ed. Raymond Levy, Stuart Ablon, and Horst Kächele (New York: Springer, 2012), 9–25; William J. Whelton, "Emotional Processes in Psychotherapy:

Evidence across Therapeutic Modalities," *Clinical Psychology and Psychotherapy* 11, no. 1 (2004): 58–71.

32. Nancy Caro Hollander, "Buenos Aires: Latin Mecca of Psychoanalysis," *Social Research* 57, no. 4 (1990): 889–919.

33. Matthew Desmond, *Evicted: Poverty and Profit in the American City* (New York: Crown, 2016).

34. Desmond, *Evicted*, 302.

35. Desmond, *Evicted*, 311.

36. Robert J. Sampson, Jeffrey D. Morenoff, and Thomas Gannon-Rowley, "Assessing Neighborhood Effects: Social Processes and New Directions in Research," *Annual Review of Sociology* 28 (2002): 443–478.

37. Ta-Nehisi Coates, "The Case for Reparations," *Atlantic*, June 2014, http://www.theatlantic.com/magazine/archive/2014/06/the-case-for-reparations/361631; William Darity, "Forty Acres and a Mule in the Twenty-First Century," *Social Science Quarterly* 89, no. 3 (2008): 656–664.

38. Khalil Gibran Muhammad, *The Condemnation of Blackness: Race, Crime, and the Making of Modern Urban America* (Cambridge, MA: Harvard University Press, 2010); Jill Leovy, *Ghettoside: A True Story of Murder in America* (New York: Spiegel and Grau, 2015).

39. Kevin N. Wright and Laura Bronstein, "An Organizational Analysis of Prison Hospice," *Prison Journal* 87, no. 4 (2007): 391–407.

40. See Vincent Muñoz, "Two Concepts of Religious Liberty: The Natural Rights and Moral Autonomy Approaches to the Free Exercise of Religion," *American Political Science Review* 110, no. 2 (2016): 369–381.

41. Katherine Lepard, "Standing Their Ground: Corporations' Fight for Religious Rights in Light of the Enactment of the Patient Protection and Affordable Care Act Contraceptive Coverage Mandate," *Texas Tech Law Review* 45 (2012): 1041–1070.

42. Oregon Public Health Division, Oregon's Death with Dignity Act, 2014, https://public.health.oregon.gov/ProviderPartnerResources/EvaluationResearch/DeathwithDignityAct/Documents/year17.pdf.

43. Lawrence O. Gostin, "Deciding Life and Death in the Courtroom: From Quinlan to Cruzan, Glucksberg, and Vacco: A Brief History and Analysis of Constitutional Protection of the 'Right to Die,'" *JAMA* 278, no. 18 (1997): 1523–1528.

44. Charles C. Camosy, "There's Nothing Progressive about Legalizing Assisted Suicide," *Dallas News*, October 2015, http://www.dallasnews.com/opinion/commentary/2015/10/15/charles-c.-camosy-theres-nothing-progressive-about-legalizing-assisted-suicide.

Conclusion

1. See Harlan Lane, *The Mask of Benevolence: Disabling the Deaf Community* (San Diego, CA: DawnSign, 1999); Thomas Hehir, "Eliminating Ableism in Education," *Harvard Educational Review* 72, no. 1 (2002): 1–33; Marek Meristo et al., "Language Access and Theory of Mind Reasoning: Evidence from Deaf Children in Bilingual and Oralist Environments," *Developmental Psychology* 43, no. 5 (2007): 1156–1169.

2. David J. Rothman and Sheila M. Rothman, *The Willowbrook Wars: Bringing the Mentally Disabled into the Community* (New Brunswick, NJ: Aldine Transaction, 2005).

3. Hall, Levin, and Anderson have coined the term "language deprivation syndrome" to refer to individuals deprived of language at an early age, and they discuss their hypothesis specifically in reference to deaf people. Wyatte C. Hall, Leonard L. Levin, and Melissa L. Anderson, "Language Deprivation Syndrome: A Possible Neurodevelopmental Disorder with Sociocultural Origins," *Social Psychiatry and Psychiatric Epidemiology* 52, no. 6 (2017): 761–776. See also Tom Humphries et al., "Language Acquisition for Deaf Children: Reducing the Harms of Zero Tolerance to the Use of Alternative Approaches," *Harm Reduction Journal* 9, no. 1 (2012): 16–25; Rachel I. Mayberry et al., "Age of Acquisition Effects on the Functional Organization of Language in the Adult Brain," *Brain and Language* 119, no. 1 (2011): 16–29. There are also two excellent videos on language deprivation: "Language Deprivation Syndrome Lecture" by Dr. Sanjay Gulati, April 1, 2014, https://www.youtube.com/watch?v=8yy_K6VtHJw&t=1s; and Nyle DiMarco Foundation, "What Is Language Deprivation?," December 20, 2016, https://www.you tube.com/watch?v=cUTymzn5FEc.

4. Stephanie Coontz, *The Way We Never Were: American Families and the Nostalgia Trap* (New York: Basic, 1992).

5. W. H. Auden, "September 1, 1939," https://www.poets.org/poetsorg/poem/septem ber-1-1939.

6. In this formulation, I draw on Auden's own revision of his poem. For context, see Maria Konnikova, "When Authors Disown Their Work, Should Readers Care?," *Atlantic*, August 28, 2012, https://www.theatlantic.com/entertainment/archive/2012/08/when -authors-disown-their-work-should-readers-care/261615.

7. Lauren Gail Berlant, *The Queen of America Goes to Washington City: Essays on Sex and Citizenship* (Durham, NC: Duke University Press, 1997); Lee Edelman, *No Future: Queer Theory and the Death Drive* (Durham, NC: Duke University Press, 2004).

8. Coontz, *The Way We Never Were*.

9. Andrew Sullivan, ed., *Same Sex Marriage, Pro and Con: A Reader* (New York: Vintage, 2004).

10. For example, Karen Bogenschneider's excellent textbook *Family Policy Matters: How Policymaking Affects Families and What Professionals Can Do*, 3rd ed. (New York: Routledge, 2014) does not discuss the end of life at all. Nor does Janet Zollinger Giele, *Family Policy and the American Social Safety Net* (London: Sage, 2012).

11. Judith Butler, *Antigone's Claim: Kinship between Life and Death* (New York: Columbia University Press, 2002); J. D. Vance, *Hillbilly Elegy* (New York: Harper, 2016), 243. Butler and Vance are ostensibly on opposite sides of the culture wars, but this perspective misrepresents their views. They share an appreciation for sprawling families. And neither suggests integrating such sprawling families into the institutions of government —in the manner that I am doing here. This may be due to their shared skepticism about government itself.

12. NOFX, "My Orphan Year," *Coaster* (Fat Wreck Chords, 2009), CD. I highly recommend the acoustic version of the song on NOFX, *Cokie the Clown* (Fat Wreck Chords, 2009), CD.

13. Donald W. Winnicott, "Hate in the Counter-Transference," *International Journal of Psychoanalysis* 30 (1949): 69–74.

14. Walt Whitman, "Song of Myself," http://www.english.illinois.edu/maps/poets /s_z/whitman/song.htm.

15. I am adapting the well-known feminist catchphrase.

16. See Sigmund Freud, *The Ego and the Id* (New York: Norton, 1961); Melanie Klein, "Mourning and Its Relation to Manic-Depressive States," *International Journal of Psychoanalysis* 21 (1940): 125–153; Hans W. Loewald, "Internalization, Separation, Mourning, and the Superego," *Psychoanalytic Quarterly* 31, no. 4 (1962): 483–504; John Bowlby, "Processes of Mourning," *International Journal of Psychoanalysis* 42 (1961): 317–340; André Green, "The Dead Mother," in his *On Private Madness* (London: Routledge, 2018), 142–174. Three more recent works are Jonathan Lear, "Mourning and Moral Psychology," *Psychoanalytic Psychology* 31, no. 4 (2014): 470–481; Susan Kavaler-Adler, *Anatomy of Regret: From Death Instinct to Reparation and Symbolization through Vivid Clinical Cases* (London: Routledge, 2013); Stephanie Brody, *Entering Night Country: Psychoanalytic Reflections on Loss and Resilience* (London: Routledge, 2015).

17. Melinda Cooper, *Family Values: Between Neoliberalism and the New Social Conservatism* (Cambridge, MA: MIT Press, 2017).

18. Patricia Strach, *All in the Family: The Private Roots of American Public Policy* (Stanford, CA: Stanford University Press, 2007).

19. Edelman, *No Future.*

20. Though my phrasing and perhaps some of my theoretical moves are different, the notion of freedom that I develop here is, I believe, compatible with what religious studies scholar David Kyuman Kim has called "melancholic freedom." See Kim, *Melancholic Freedom: Agency and the Spirit of Politics* (Oxford: Oxford University Press, 2007).

21. Irwin Gerber et al., "Anticipatory Grief and Aged Widows and Widowers," *Journal of Gerontology* 30, no. 2 (1975): 225–229.

22. Hans Theodorus Blokland, *Freedom and Culture in Western Society*, trans. Michael O'Loughlin (London: Routledge, 1997).

23. Eric Foner, *The Story of American Freedom* (New York: Norton, 1999).

24. Richard Slotkin, *Frontier Nation: The Myth of the Frontier in Twentieth Century America* (Norman: University of Oklahoma Press, 1998).

25. Howard I. Kushner, "The Persistence of the 'Frontier Thesis' in America: Gender, Myth, and Self-Destruction," *Canadian Review of American Studies* 22, no. 1, suppl. (1992): 53–82.

26. Kushner, "Persistence of the 'Frontier Thesis.'"

27. Kushner, "Persistence of the 'Frontier Thesis.'" See also Howard I. Kushner, *Self-Destruction in the Promised Land: A Psychocultural Biology of American Suicide* (New Brunswick, NJ: Rutgers University Press, 1989). To clarify: the frontier hero's suicide is not an analogue for PAS. It is an analogue for our national self-destruction. The relationship of this self-destruction to attempts to either ban or legalize PAS is an interesting and important question, but it is not my topic here.

28. See, for example, Slotkin's discussion of the Reagan presidency in *Frontier Nation*, 624–662.

29. See Leigh Cuen and Politifact, "Donald Trump Lies about Race and Communities of Color," *Teen Vogue*, August 23, 2017, https://www.teenvogue.com/story/donald-trump -lies-about-race-and-communities-of-color.

30. Michael T. Klare, "Trump Wants to Steal Middle East Oil, and He's Not Alone," *Foreign Policy*, October 13, 2016, http://foreignpolicy.com/2016/10/13/trump-wants-to-steal-middle-east-oil-and-hes-not-alone-iraq-war-elections.

31. Kushner, "Persistence of the 'Frontier Thesis.'"

32. Kushner, "Persistence of the 'Frontier Thesis.'"

33. Richard Slotkin, *Regeneration through Violence: The Mythology of the American Frontier, 1600–1860* (Middletown, CT: Wesleyan University Press, 1973).

34. Slotkin, *Frontier Nation*, 624–662.

35. On the persistence of frontier imagery, see Carl Boggs, *The Hollywood War Machine: US Militarism and Popular Culture* (London: Routledge, 2017).

36. Slotkin, *Frontier Nation*, 624–662.

37. See David Clark, "Originating a Movement: Cicely Saunders and the Development of St. Christopher's Hospice, 1957–1967," *Mortality* 3, no. 1 (1998): 43–63. For a more contemporary treatment, see Katherine Froggatt, "Rites of Passage and the Hospice Culture," *Mortality* 2, no. 2 (1997): 123–136.

38. Enzo Traverso, *Left-Wing Melancholia: Marxism, History, and Memory* (New York: Columbia University Press), 45.

39. Eric W. Widera and Susan D. Block, "Managing Grief and Depression at the End of Life," *American Family Physician* 86, no. 3 (2012): 259–264; Joanna Oi-Yue Cheng et al., "A Pilot Study on the Effectiveness of Anticipatory Grief Therapy for Elderly Facing the End of Life," *Journal of Palliative Care* 26, no. 4 (2010): 261–269.

40. Donald Trump, *Crippled America: How to Make America Great Again* (New York: Threshold, 2015).

41. Rosemarie Garland-Thomson, "The Case for Conserving Disability," *Journal of Bioethical Inquiry* 9, no. 3 (2012): 339–355.

42. There has been an increasing recognition in disability studies of the need to accommodate mourning alongside disability pride. See Alison Kafer, *Feminist, Queer, Crip* (Bloomington: Indiana University Press, 2013), 6.

43. Linda L. Emanuel et al., "'And Yet It Was a Blessing': The Case for Existential Maturity," *Journal of Palliative Medicine* 20, no. 4 (2017): 318–327, 323.

44. See Judith Butler, *Frames of War: When Is Life Grievable?* (London: Verso, 2010), 1–33.

45. Ron LaJoie, "Rose Hawthorne's Cause for Sainthood Moves to Rome," *Catholic New York*, April 17, 2013, http://cny.org/stories/Rose-Hawthornes-Cause-For-Sainthood-Moves-to-Rome,9204.

46. Valenti, *To Myself a Stranger*.

47. Kevin Kruse, *One Nation under God: How Corporate America Invented Christianity* (New York: Basic, 2015).

48. Elizabeth Stoker Bruenig, "Why the Left Needs Religion," *Dissent* (Fall 2015), https://www.dissentmagazine.org/article/why-left-needs-religion; Matthew Sitman, "Against Moral Austerity: On the Need for a Christian Left," *Dissent* (Summer 2017), https://www.dissentmagazine.org/article/moral-austerity-need-christian-left.

49. Josh Zeitz, "When America Hated Catholics," *Politico*, September 23, 2015, https://www.politico.com/magazine/story/2015/09/when-america-hated-catholics-213177.

50. David Clark has written compellingly on how St. Christopher's Hospice adopted a more pragmatic orientation toward Christianity in order to further the advancement of hospice in England. See Clark, "Religion, Medicine, and Community in the Early Origins of St. Christopher's Hospice," *Journal of Palliative Medicine*, 4, no. 3 (2001): 353–360. But there is no question that Cicely Saunders was deeply Christian in a country whose denomination of Christianity mirrored her own. This differentiates her from Rose Hawthorne Lathrop and from the founders of the modern US hospice movement, who were a religiously diverse group of Christians, atheists, and Jews. The need to be more pluralistic—compared to St. Christopher's—figured prominently in the early discussions of the modern US hospice movement's leaders. See Minutes of Meeting, "Interdisciplinary Study of the Dying Patient," October 29, 1970, revised January 5, 1971, box 7, folder 79, Florence and Henry Wald Papers, Sterling Memorial Library, Yale University.

51. Foner, *Story of American Freedom.*

52. My phrasing here is influenced by Simone de Beauvoir's famous formulation: "One is not born, but rather becomes, a woman." Beauvoir, *The Second Sex*, trans. Constance Borde and Sheila Mavalony-Chevallier (New York: Vintage, 2011), 283.

53. Butler, *Frames of War*, 1–33.

Afterword

1. Institute of Medicine, *Dying in America: Improving Quality and Honoring Individual Preferences near the End of Life* (Washington, DC: National Academies Press, 2014), 33.

2. Sharon Kaufman, *Ordinary Medicine* (Durham, NC: Duke University Press, 2015).

3. See, for example, Elisabeth Kübler-Ross, *Death: The Final Stage of Growth* (New York: Scribner, 1997).

INDEX